ASSESSMENT FOR INTERVENTION

The Guilford School Practitioner Series

EDITORS

STEPHEN N. ELLIOTT, PhD
Vanderbilt University

JOSEPH C. WITT, PhD
Louisiana State University, Baton Rouge

Recent Volumes

Assessment for Intervention: A Problem-Solving Approach
RACHEL BROWN-CHIDSEY, Editor

Individualized Supports for Students with Problem Behaviors:
Designing Positive Behavior Plans
LINDA M. BAMBARA and LEE KERN

Think First: Addressing Aggressive Behavior in Secondary Schools
JIM LARSON

Academic Skills Problems Workbook, Revised Edition
EDWARD S. SHAPIRO

Academic Skills Problems: Direct Assessment and Intervention,
Third Edition
EDWARD S. SHAPIRO

ADHD in the Schools, Second Edition:
Assessment and Intervention Strategies
GEORGE J. DuPAUL and GARY STONER

Helping Schoolchildren Cope with Anger:
A Cognitive-Behavioral Intervention
JIM LARSON and JOHN E. LOCHMAN

Child Abuse and Neglect: The School's Response
CONNIE BURROWS HORTON and TRACY K. CRUISE

Traumatic Brain Injury in Children and Adolescents:
Assessment and Intervention
MARGARET SEMRUD-CLIKEMAN

Schools and Families: Creating Essential Connections for Learning
SANDRA L. CHRISTENSON and SUSAN M. SHERIDAN

Homework Success for Children with ADHD:
A Family–School Intervention Program
THOMAS J. POWER, JAMES L. KARUSTIS, and DINA F. HABBOUSHE

Assessment for Intervention
A PROBLEM-SOLVING APPROACH

◆ ◆ ◆

EDITED BY
Rachel Brown-Chidsey

FOREWORD BY
Jack A. Cummings

◆

THE GUILFORD PRESS
New York   London

Library of Congress Cataloging-in-Publication Data

Assessment for intervention: a problem-solving approach / edited by Rachel Brown-
Chidsey; foreword by Jack A. Cummings.
     p. cm. — (The Guilford school practitioner series)
   Includes bibliographical references and index.
   ISBN-10: 1-59385-140-5   ISBN-13: 978-1-59385-140-8 (cloth)
   ISBN-10: 1-59385-690-3   ISBN-13: 978-1-59385-690-8 (paper)
   1. School psychology—United States. I. Brown-Chidsey, Rachel. II. Series.
   LB1027.55.A77 2005
   371.4—dc22
                                                              2004029886

To David and Ellie

About the Editor

♦

Rachel Brown-Chidsey received her PhD in school psychology from the University of Massachusetts–Amherst. She is program coordinator and assistant professor of school psychology at the University of Southern Maine. Prior to obtaining her doctorate, Dr. Brown-Chidsey worked for 10 years as a general and special education teacher. Her publications and research address solution-focused assessment for intervention, including applications of curriculum-based measurement and response-to-intervention (RTI) methods. Dr. Brown-Chidsey was an on-site participant in the 2002 Multi-Site Conference on the Future of School Psychology in Indianapolis, Indiana. This book is a product of the collaboration and idea-sharing fostered by the conference.

Contributors

♦

Craig A. Albers, PhD, Department of Educational Psychology, University of Wisconsin–Madison, Madison, Wisconsin

Lauren A. Arbolino, MA, Department of Psychology, Syracuse University, Syracuse, New York

Mary Lynn Boscardin, PhD, Department of Education, University of Massachusetts–Amherst, Amherst, Massachusetts

Carolyn V. Brown, MD, MPH, Bartlett Memorial Hospital, Juneau, Alaska

George W. Brown, MD, Bartlett Memorial Hospital, Juneau, Alaska

Rachel Brown-Chidsey, PhD, School Psychology Program, University of Southern Maine, Gorham, Maine

R. T. Busse, PhD, School of Education, Chapman University, Orange, California

Nathan H. Clemens, MEd, Department of Education and Human Services, Lehigh University, Bethlehem, Pennsylvania

Peg Dawson, EdD, Center for Learning and Attention Disorders, Portsmouth, New Hampshire

Stanley L. Deno, PhD, Department of Educational Psychology, University of Minnesota, Bloomington, Minnesota

Beth Doll, PhD, Department of Educational Psychology, University of Nebraska–Lincoln, Lincoln, Nebraska

Tanya L. Eckert, PhD, Department of Psychology, Syracuse University, Syracuse, New York

Stephen N. Elliott, PhD, Peabody College, Vanderbilt University, Nashville, Tennessee

Mary Kelly Haack, PhD, Department of Educational Psychology, University of Nebraska–Lincoln, Lincoln, Nebraska

Ryan J. Kettler, MS, School of Education, University of Wisconsin–Madison, Madison, Wisconsin

Thomas R. Kratochwill, PhD, Department of Educational Psychology, University of Wisconsin–Madison, Madison, Wisconsin

Merilee McCurdy, PhD, Department of Educational Psychology, University of Nebraska–Lincoln, Lincoln, Nebraska

Mary Jean O'Reilly, PhD, Pittsfield Public Schools, Pittsfield, Massachusetts

Andrew T. Roach, MS, Peabody College, Vanderbilt University, Nashville, Tennessee

Lisa Hagermoser Sanetti, MS, Department of Educational Psychology, University of Wisconsin–Madison, Madison, Wisconsin

Edward S. Shapiro, PhD, Department of Education, Lehigh University, Bethlehem, Pennsylvania

Susan M. Sheridan, PhD, Department of Educational Psychology, University of Nebraska–Lincoln, Lincoln, Nebraska

Mark R. Shinn, PhD, National-Louis University, Evanston, Illinois

Mark W. Steege, PhD, School Psychology Program, University of Southern Maine, Gorham, Maine

Kevin Tobin, PhD, Pittsfield Public Schools, Pittsfield, Massachusetts

Foreword

♦

In the 1999 National Goals Panel report, *Lessons Learned, Challenges Ahead*, Richard Elsmore of Harvard University described a "seismic shift" in popular and political opinion on the role of states in education. Whereas the previous role of states had focused on inputs such as facilities and finances, the decade of the 1990s brought greater attention to monitoring how schools were performing. The focus shifted to students' achievement and performance as indicated by large-scale standardized testing.

Whether the race is for the governor's office or the office of the president, everyone is an "education" candidate. We live in a time of educational accountability, in which teachers and school administrators feel great pressure to have their students perform well on statewide examinations. Scrutiny is given at each level—the classroom or teacher, the school, the district, and the state. Classroom teachers are compared to their peers; each school's aggregate performance is published in the local newspaper, and all schools within a district are compared in what appear to be informative tables and graphs that indicate the good schools and the ones that need improvement. It is common for state departments of education to post summary test data by district and even by individual schools on their websites.

Gallup education polls repeatedly have indicated that the general public strongly endorses the recent calls for accountability. It is assumed that testing will have a positive influence on teachers' approaches to student learning and on individual students, who will work hard to "pass" the tests. The popular press has joined the call for greater accountability. Articles in news magazines highlight the failings of public schools and contribute to the public urgency to remedy the *problems* within contemporary education.

In 2001, Rod Paige was appointed U.S. Secretary of Education and given a mandate to change public education. No Child Left Behind (2001) was the first major education legislation of the new administration. The term "scientifically based research" appeared more than a hundred times in the text of the legislation. The Institute of Education Sciences was established in 2002 with the goal of cleaning up educational research by funding exclusively scientifically based research. The intent was to give greater prominence to the importance of educational research and, through the use of scientific methods, to achieve outcomes similar to the field of medicine, which had previously embraced random assignment to experimental groups. The overarching goal of the Institute of Education Sciences was to determine which educational interventions have merit. It was recognized that education has suffered from trends that have resulted from large-scale adoption of untested programs. Standardized testing was seen as a vehicle to bring accountability to public schools.

In contrast to the general public and the business community, educators have been less enthusiastic about the merits of high-stakes testing. Most K–12 teachers report that standardized test results provide little or no assistance in planning learning experiences for their students. Even when the lag between the testing sessions and learning the test results is reduced, insufficient information is provided on what the students know and don't know. The unintended consequence of high-stakes testing has been to limit teachers' freedom to design curricula they believe provide optimal experiences for the needs of their classes. Teachers often report that their curricula have narrowed and that much creativity has been lost. Teachers and school administrators feel tremendous pressure and urgency in their efforts to raise students' performance in academic domains. Unfortunately, high-stakes standardized tests have exacerbated the problem by adding to the stress placed on teachers and administrators.

With this current educational milieu as a backdrop, the Multi-Site Conference on the Future of School Psychology was held in November 2002. Seventy-three psychologists in Indianapolis and more than 650 at remote sites around the United States participated in the conference to examine contributions that school psychologists may make to address the needs of children, schools, and families. *Assessment for Intervention: A Problem-Solving Approach* is in part an outgrowth of the discussions at the conference. Rachel Brown-Chidsey served as the facilitator of the group that examined the issues associated with improved academic competence and school success for all children. Improving academic success emerged as one of the five priority outcomes as defined by the conference participants. More specifically, the practice objective associated with the improved academic competence priority was to ensure that assessment practices of school psychologists are linked to evidence-based strategies to improve academic performance and account for the influence of ethnicity. *Assessment for Intervention: A Problem-Solving Approach* explores the theoretical and practical aspects of what it means to use a problem-solving model. While there is a focus on improving educational attainment, the edited volume recognizes that meaningful changes in educational performance will require more than a strict focus on academic skill building.

In Chapter 2, Stanley L. Deno describes a problem-solving model that is not restricted to the needs of children typically referred to special education. Rather, Deno's focus is broader. He conceptualizes a problem-solving model that serves as a framework for reflecting on issues of schooling in general. This redefining of the definition of the problems to be addressed is consistent with Beth Doll and Mary Kelly Haack's population-based perspective in Chapter 5, which considers children's mental health needs on a schoolwide basis. Instead of waiting for referrals, the psychologist takes a multistage approach by starting with the entire population and then narrowing the focus. George W. and Carolyn V. Brown, likewise, describe an approach in Chapter 6, in which the first consideration is the whole population, as opposed to the individual.

Chapter 3, by Susan M. Sheridan and Merilee McCurdy, provides an illustration of how children's needs are conceptualized in broader terms than the conventional Wechsler, Woodcock–Johnson, and a behavior rating scale. Sheridan and McCurdy advocate using the strengths of the ecological and behavioral approaches to address children's needs. They emphasize the role of the home environment and how this critical domain interacts with the school. Both assessment and intervention occur across environments.

Consistent with the press from the U.S. Department of Education and the Institute of Education Sciences, the use of evidence-based interventions represents an underlying theme that permeates chapter after chapter. Lisa Hagermoser Sanetti and Thomas R. Kratochwill recognize that it takes more than a quality assessment to identify a child's needs and more than the selection of an intervention with a solid evidence base—it also requires ensuring that the intervention is implemented with fidelity. In Chapter 15, Sanetti and Kratochwill build a strong case that monitoring the progress of a child's behavior in response to an intervention should be supplemented with a determination of how faithfully it was implemented. Mary Lynn Boscardin's Chapter 14 further highlights the role that school administrators play in promoting a climate for the use of the problem-solving model and evidence-based interventions.

As one would expect in an edited volume that seeks to improve children's academic performance, curriculum-based measurement (CBM) receives frequent attention. Unlike standardized tests that lack utility for classroom teachers, CBM provides a sensitive measure of students' progress tied to the curriculum. In Chapter 13, Rachel Brown-Chidsey and Mark W. Steege describe a solution-focused report where stakeholders collaborate by contributing different portions of the report. Unlike conventional reports, the solution-focused report is dynamic in that progress monitoring continues over time.

The final chapter, by Mary Jean O'Reilly and Kevin Tobin, provides the real-world perspective of implementing a problem-solving approach in schools. It recounts a success story, but also tells of the obstacles and challenges that were faced in order to effect change on a districtwide basis. Again, O'Reilly and Tobin go beyond the conventional focus where assessment is done in response to a referral and an individual educational plan is constructed for a single referred student.

In conclusion, Rachel Brown-Chidsey has mounted an impressive assault on traditional individual testing. *Assessment for Intervention: A Problem-Solving Approach* goes beyond criticizing current practice by exploring thoughtful, well-researched alternatives. School psychology practitioners and university faculty will profit from the erudite discussions of the multiple dimensions to consider when implementing a problem-solving model.

JACK A. CUMMINGS, PhD
Professor, Indiana University
Co-Chair, 2002 Future of School
Psychology Conference

Contents

♦

PART III
Assessing School-Related Problems and Situations

PART IV
Identifying Solutions for School Problems

PART V
Implementing and Monitoring Solutions

PART I

◆ ◆ ◆

Introduction

◆

CHAPTER 1

◆ ◆ ◆

Introduction to Problem-Solving Assessment

◆

RACHEL BROWN-CHIDSEY

The context for this book springs from the expanding needs of children in schools. U.S. schools once possessed a fairly narrow mission of teaching children with average to above-average abilities how to read, write, and do arithmetic. Over time the mission of U.S. schools has grown and now includes the mandate to provide every child with a free appropriate public education. The wide-sweeping mandate to educate all children is based on the idea that there is a universal public benefit in providing all children with a basic education (Benner, 1998). Despite widespread efforts to improve the quality of educational services for all children (e.g., No Child Left Behind Act of 2001), numerous research studies have shown that educational outcomes vary considerably across the United States (National Center for Education Statistics, 2003). Current reform efforts such as No Child Left Behind (NCLB) have placed a heavy focus on specific outcome standards that virtually all children are expected to meet. Notably, all children, including those with disabilities, are expected to participate in the same educational experiences and assessment activities, and evidence of all students' progress toward specified standards must be reported at least annually.

While the standards and expectations for each school-age student have become more narrow and precise, the diversity of the student population has increased. Data published by the National Center for Education Statistics (2003) shows that the cultural, linguistic, and racial diversity of U.S. schools has increased steadily over time. For some students, the new standards for educational outcomes are too challenging relative to the knowledge and skills they possess upon entering school. In essence, there is too big a gap between what they know upon arriving at school and what they are expected to know on state-mandated exams. For these students, participation in and attainment of the education offered them is very difficult. Since 1975, the system in place to support and assist students with significant school difficulties has been special education. For some students, special education has allowed them to obtain a high-quality education and move on to postsecondary pursuits. Unfortunately, special education services have not been uniformly successful in supporting all students identified as having a disability and needing specialized education services (Kavale, 1990).

A large number of researchers have investigated the reasons for disparities in educational outcomes and how best to assess and teach students with special needs. One of the most successful research programs related to helping students achieve school success has been that related to problem-solving assessment and intervention methods. Stanley L. Deno and his colleagues at the University of Minnesota have produced a substantial amount of work on improving assessment and instruction for students with disabilities (Deno, 1985, 1989). Other problem-solving approaches to school-based decision making have also been published (Bergan, 1977; McClam & Woodside, 1994; Reschley & Tilly, 1998). Problem-solving methods have since been applied and evaluated by many educators and school systems across the country (Deno, 1986; Marston, Muyskens, Lau, & Canter, 2003; Reschly, Tilly, & Grimes, 1999; Tilly, 2002; Weishaar, Weishaar, & Budt, 2002) and are recognized as a "best-practice" approach to assessment and intervention (Deno, 2002).

Despite widespread evidence that application of a problem-solving approach to identifying and addressing the needs of school children is very effective, the number of schools and districts where such methods are used is still in the minority (Reschly & Tilly, 1998; Reschly & Ysseldyke, 2002; Ysseldyke & Marston, 1998). Reschly and Tilly (1998) identified a number of systems-based variables related to why problem-solving methods have not been more widely adopted in the United States, including legal requirements related to special education services, how such services are funded, and differences between medical and social models of disabilities. The legal requirements of the dominant approach to identifying which students are eligible and in need of special education services are often cited as a reason why problem-solving-based practices cannot be used. According to this argument, the requirement by the U.S. Department of Education that school districts cannot have access to federal special education funds unless they identify students according to one of 13 approved disability categories means that problem-solving-based, or "noncategorical," methods of helping students are not acceptable under federal standards. This is actually not the case, as seen in Iowa and other jurisdictions where problem-solving-based methods for identifying and helping students have been used for many years (Reschley & Tilly, 1998). Importantly, the U.S. Department of Eduacation will allow states and local educational agencies (LEAs) to access federal special education funds under problem-solving-based assessment and intervention methods.

Reschly and Tilly (1998) identified major differences between medical and social models of understanding disabilities as the major reason why more schools have not adopted problem-solving approaches to meeting students' educational needs. According to a medical model of disability, the "problem" underlying a student's lack of school achievement is within the child. This model posits that the child's disability is lifelong, will be manifest in all settings, and needs to be dealt with through individualized programming for the student. In contrast, a social understanding of disability views students' school-related problems as the result of differences between what is expected of the student and what is actually happening. According to the social model, all school "problems" are related and defined by the social environment and must be addressed by evaluating and understanding the expectations placed on children in school settings. As noted by Reschly and Tilly (1998), the medical and social models of disability have coexisted for many years, and few practitioners see them as mutually exclusive. Nonetheless, most school personnel still view the medical model as dominant and, when pressed to decide on what basis decisions about children's educational futures will be made, resort to the medical model.

The application of problem-solving-based methods in school settings has increased somewhat over time. For example, research into the use of curriculum-based assessment (CBA), a set of evaluation methods rooted in problem-solving methods, showed a steady rise among school psychologists (Shapiro, Angello, & Eckert, 2004; Brown-Chidsey & Washburn, 2004; Shapiro & Eckert, 1993). Shapiro et al. (2004) showed that use of CBA among school psychologists rose from 46% in 1991 to 54% in 2000. Brown-Chidsey and Washburn (2004) found that 81% of special education teachers and 76% of special education administrators used CBA routinely. These data suggest that problem-solving methods are not unknown, yet the variables contributing to their use have not been specifically identified. Importantly, Shapiro et al. (2004), Brown-Chidsey and Washburn (2004), and Shapiro and Eckert (1993) found that both special educators and school psychologists indicated a need for more specific training in problem-solving assessment methods.

This book offers a comprehensive discussion of problem-solving assessment and intervention methods. The volume is organized into five parts that reflect the five stages of Deno's problem-solving model. Part I (this chapter and Chapter 2) includes information about problem identification as well as the historical context of problem-solving-based assessment in special education and school psychology. Part II (Chapters 3–6) reviews information related to problem definition, including chapters related to specific assessment settings and situations. Part III (Chapters 7–12) covers the core assessment methods used in exploring solutions during problem-solving assessment. Part IV (Chapters 13–15) covers information important for monitoring solutions. Part V of the book (Chapters 16 and 17) includes chapters on program evaluation and case studies from a low-socioeconomic-status urban school district where problem-solving methods have been used for more than 10 years to improve student learning outcomes.

Each chapter is organized using a common framework. First, the background and context of the chapter's topic is reviewed. Next, the principles and procedures related to the use of problem-solving assessment practices are covered. These sections may overlap with information covered in book-length treatments of the topics; however, they provide comprehensive overviews of such methods. Each chapter concludes with one or more case studies in which problem-solving assessment methods are demonstrated. Some chapters include reproducible forms that readers can use in their assessment activities.

THE CONTEXT OF PROBLEM-SOLVING ASSESSMENT

One of the core models integrated throughout all the chapters is Stanley Deno's model of problem-solving assessment (Deno, 1985, 1989, 2002). Deno's work has had a strong influence on special education and school psychology for many years. Through seminal research, collaboration with schools, mentoring of doctoral students, and publications, Deno has contributed to a major paradigm shift in how school-based assessments are conceptualized. Chapter 2 was written by Deno and offers an up-to-date perspective on his important model. Deno's five-stage problem-solving assessment model is integrated into the remaining chapters of the book to illustrate how these five stages can be implemented in schools. The authors of the other chapters all provide their own interpretation and understanding of Deno's model.

In Chapter 3 Susan Sheridan and Merilee McCurdy provide insights into the many ecological variables that contribute to a student's school experience. Taking into account students' home, community, and school experiences, Chapter 3 shows how a student brings many cultural, linguistic, ethnic, and belief traditions to school every day. Tanya Eckert and Lauren Arbolino build on Chapter 3 and offer specific insights and perspectives on the unique role of classroom teachers in recognizing and addressing students' school difficulties. Eckert and Arbolino go beyond mere recognition of teacher participation in assessment and explore the many facets of how teachers can participate in facilitating school success.

Chapters 5 and 6 include information drawing from a public health model of wellness. Specifically, Beth Doll and Kelly Haack (Chapter 5) offer a population-based understanding of how any given subset of school students is likely to have manifest health problems that will affect school success. In Chapter 6, George and Carolyn Brown (both physicians) have integrated Deno's model with a more traditional medical understanding of student wellness, with a discussion of the five major physiological conditions common among school-age students. This chapter documents how physical and environmental variables can have a lasting effect on a student's school success, which can be enhanced or diminished according to whether school personnel appreciate the extent to which health complications affect school outcomes.

Chapters 7 through 12 include descriptions and details about how functional behavioral assessment (FBA), interviews, classroom observations, curriculum-based measurement (CBM), rating scales, and cognitive instruments can enhance and support problem-solving-based assessment. This section starts with a chapter by Mark Steege and Rachel Brown-Chidsey about FBA. This topic was chosen to begin the methods section because FBA offers a methodology for identifying and defining students' school problems. Chapter 8, by Peg Dawson, includes discussion of the important role that interviews of students, parents, teachers, and others can play in problem-solving assessments. Ed Shapiro and Nathan Clemens (Chapter 9) have compiled a concise description and primer of observation methods. Chapter 10, written by Randy Busse, offers information about rating scales and how they can play a role in assessment activities. Mark Shinn (Chapter 11) has provided an updated discussion about how to use CBM in problem-solving assessment activities. Chapter 12 offers insights on what role published norm-referenced tests might play in problem-solving assessments. Together, these six chapters cover the core assessment methods that can inform and shape problem-solving assessment activities.

The last five chapters of the book cover report writing, administrative issues, intervention integrity, methods for evaluating interventions, and examples of student success when problem-solving methods were used. Writing problem-solving-based reports is an important but new topic. Few resources on report writing exist, and fewer still cover problem-solving assessment methods. Chapter 13 offers a specific template for report writing that integrates all components of the problem-solving model. Mary Lynn Boscardin (Chapter 14) provides important information about how administrative support is crucial to full-scale implementation of problem-solving assessment practices. Related to the importance of administrative support are the twin topics of intervention integrity and evaluation. Lisa Hagermoser Sanetti and Tom Kratochwill provide a thorough description of how to increase the likelihood that interventions will be implemented correctly. Craig Albers, Stephen Elliott, Ryan Kettler, and Andrew Roach (Chapter 16) offer specific methods for evaluating interventions and determining whether the original problem has been solved. Finally, Chapter 17, by Mary Jean O'Reilly and Kevin Tobin, includes several case studies that document the effectiveness of problem-solving methods for individual students.

SUMMARY

This book evolved from the 2002 Future of School Psychology conference. This interactive and dynamic sequence of events offered the school psychology community the chance to take stock of the state of school psychology practice and set an agenda for the future. The conference agenda included five core components, including action plans to improve student academic outcomes, create access to mental health resources, and empower families as they support and nurture their children. This volume is designed to address the action plan for improving academic outcomes for all children.

By putting together chapters written by many of the senior scholars in school psychology and special education, this book is designed to help present and future assessment professionals learn and use assessment practices that close the gap between students' current school performance and those that are needed for them to graduate from high school and enter the adult workforce. Covering the history, development, components, and success of problem-solving assessment methods, the volume includes a comprehensive treatment of the emerging standards for "best practices" in schools. As the chapters unfold, readers are invited to consider, reflect, and integrate problem-solving practices into all aspects of their professional duties.

REFERENCES

Benner, S. M. (1998). *Special education issues within the context of American society.* Belmont, CA: Wadsworth.

Bergan, J. R. (1977). *Behavioral consultation.* Columbus, OH: Merrill.

Brown-Chidsey, R., & Washburn, K. R. (2004). *Are we on the same page? Comparison of curriculum-based assessment use by school psychologists and special educators.* Manuscript submitted for publication.

Deno, S. L. (1985). Curriculum-based measurement: The emerging alternative. *Exceptional Children, 52,* 219–232.

Deno, S. L. (1986). Formative evaluation of individual student programs: A new role for school psychologists. *School Psychology Review, 15,* 348–374.

Deno, S. L. (1989). Curriculum-based measurement and special education services: A

disagree on the outcomes, there should be no question that the primary purpose of schooling is to intervene in children's lives to produce those outcomes. As extensions of our society, then, educators are required to accept the developmental outcomes around which schools are organized, and work toward their attainment. Teachers and parents often do not like or agree with the outcomes that have been specified, but those whose children attend the public schools and those who are public employees are bound by the law and regulations. In the public schools, parents must accept that the state will direct their children toward the state's preferred outcomes, and educators must accept the responsibility to organize activities in the direction of those outcomes. Given these circumstances, the "problems" to be solved by educators ultimately are derived from the schools' responsibilities to promote growth and development in the direction of societally mandated outcomes. The term *intervention* underscores the fact that schools are designed to have an impact on what otherwise might be unstructured development.

Problems

In a problem-solving model of schooling, the focus of educational intervention is how to eliminate the difference between students' level of development at any point in time and the level of development expected by society in the future. The current emphasis on "standards" and high-stakes assessment clearly underscores this emphasis on solving the problem of where students *are* and where society *wants them to be*. With full implementation of the No Child Left Behind Act (NCLB, 2001), considerable pressure is being applied to both schools and students to assure that any discrepancies between societal standards and students' performance are eliminated. Whether or not this is realistic is not the issue here, of course. As stated previously, what is relevant is the public perception—articulated through federal and state governments—that problems with school achievement exist.

Outcomes

An examination of the standards set by state and federal governments easily leads to the conclusion that literacy and numeracy are the most fundamental outcomes toward which schooling is to be directed. This conclusion is supported by observation of time allocation to subject matter during the school day. Particularly in the elementary school years, far more time is allocated to fostering development in reading, writing, and arithmetic than other subjects. At the secondary level, language, literature, and mathematics are consistently required of all students, especially those who plan to attend college. In addition to the prominence of literacy and numeracy in curriculum organization, evidence of the primary nature of these two sets of outcomes can be obtained from emphasis in national assessments of student achievement. For example, the National Assessment of Educational Progress (NAEP), contracted for by the federal government, focused first on national trends in reading, writing, and math achievement. As greater attention has been given to setting standards, science has been added to the outcome emphasis placed on literacy and mathematics (National Center for Education Statistics, 1993).

Under the guidelines of NCLB and related state requirements, outcomes related to personal, social, and physical development, apparently, will be left to families and schools as secondary considerations. Standard-setting, then, is the process of making the public's values explicit. In doing so, standards setting clarifies and establishes the priorities that will be assigned to the problems of ordinary educational intervention. In the model presented in this book, the term *problem solving* is not reserved solely for efforts to promote change in atypical development. Instead, problem solving, or the problem-solving model, provides a framework for reflecting on the nature of schools, the purpose of schooling, and the nature of professional work in the schools.

Problem Solving through General and Compensatory Education

Two major types of intervention occur in education. The first, which we call general education, has been described previously as the mainstream instructional program created for all children. A second, smaller set of interventions consists of the various special and compensatory education programs created for students from diverse cultural and economic backgrounds and for students with disabilities. Different from the general education interventions, this second set of interventions is intended for smaller subsets of the student population. These two general types of intervention create somewhat different roles and responsibilities for psychologists and educators who engage in school-based problem solving. Much of that difference stems from the fact that interventions in special and compensatory programs are characterized by increased intensity since they occur when a student's response to the ordinary interventions of the general program is not satisfactory.

Intensification of Educational Intervention

Until quite recently, the idea that educators functioned as problem solvers would have seemed inappropriate. The primary reason for this is that schooling was viewed as an "opportunity" for students to learn and grow rather than a place where educators deliberately engineered environments to increase growth. In such an "agrarian" model of education the emphasis in teaching was on the teacher's responsibility to create the climate for growth. The general education program was to function as the fertile field prepared to nourish children's growth. The assumption was that students grew at different rates because it was "in their nature," not because educators were failing to prevent or overcome those differences. The classroom was a place where children were "free" to learn at their own rate, achieving to the level of their individual capabilities. Once the field was prepared teachers were expected to "weed and feed," but differences in growth rates were assumed to be the natural outcome of organic differences. In this model, the expectation was that the distribution of academic achievement would inevitably result in an approximation of the normal bell curve. In the agrarian model, assessment is used to identify which students are the "best" and the "brightest" fruits of the field who merit further academic nurturing. While it might be possible to see the role of educators as problem solvers in the agrarian model, accepting a normal distribution in achievement as appropriate—even inevitable—is not compatible with standards-based education policies under which all students are expected to learn certain skills to at least a minimum criterion.

Over the past several decades, a "sea change" has occurred in society's charge to America's schools. Beginning with a report entitled *A Nation at Risk*, published in 1983 by the Reagan administration, specific deficits in U.S. schools were identified. The change was made explicit toward the end of the century by the "Education 2000" challenge introduced during the administration of President George H. W. Bush (National Center for Education Statistics, 1993). In that document, and in many state initiatives since that time, the challenge presented to American educators was to create schools in which "all children" would learn. The assumption was that schools should be a place where "equity and excellence" could be expected for all students. This idea that "all" students could achieve at a high level if the schools would function properly led to "standards-based" reform efforts in virtually all states. Standards-based reform begins with the setting of criterion-referenced outcomes by political entities—typically state legislatures. Once the outcomes are specified, mandates are established compelling school districts to assure attainment of those outcomes for "all" of their students. Often, positive and negative incentives are attached to success and failure for both school districts and students. These same ideas have now been codified in law through the No Child Left Behind legislation passed in 2001 during the administration of George W. Bush. The original regulations that flowed from NCLB offered no surcease from the demand that the schools educate all children to a high standard of proficiency. Further, the assessment requirements were designed to assure that educators would regard achievement of less than high standards by all students as a problem.

An important effect of this sea change for American education was to alter the roles, responsibilities, and expectations for everyone working in the schools. The pressure of meeting existing standards replaced the luxury of a relaxed approach where it was possible to sit back and "watch the garden grow." Educators everywhere are now pressured to find those "evidence-based practices" that will provide them with the means to overcome inadequate growth rates. The idea that all students are capable of meeting the same standards and that educators are responsible for attaining that ideal represents a significant departure from the normal bell curve model that was the former basis of educational practice in the United States. In American education, the model of industrial engineering has replaced the agrarian approach to schooling. Problem solving is now a primary responsibility of all educators in the current educational environment.

Compensatory Programs as Intensified Problem Solving

Students do not grow at the same rate physically, nor do they grow at the same rates academically. When government agencies arbitrarily set standards for "acceptable" performance in different curriculum domains, the differences in students' rates of development inevitably result in some students failing to meet the standards. In response, schools create special and compensatory education programs designed to intensify problem solving beyond those organized as part of the general curriculum. Compensatory programs such as Title I and those for English language learners contain relatively large numbers of students, all receiving a common approach to improving their school success. As standards-based reform was implemented, additional remedial programs had to be created to intensify problem solving for those students who failed to meet standards. Beyond these compensatory programs, special education programs are provided for a smaller number of students whose developmental problems are even more intractable. During the 1960s, '70s, and early '80s, the efforts to solve the problems presented by this smaller number of students were organized through a continuum of options, or "Cascade of Services" (Deno, 1970). The levels described in this administrative model consisted of different types of programs where special educators served decreasing numbers of students. Since these special education programs added significantly to the cost of education, determining eligibility for special education programs has dominated the assessment responsibilities of school psychologists.

With the passage of NCLB, the demand increased for all educators to intensify problem-solving efforts. NCLB requirements have also heightened attention to the achievement problems for students in all types of compensatory programs. An increased focus on making adequate academic progress with even the lowest-achieving students has replaced the historic preoccupation with the procedural requirements that were necessary for determining eligibility for these programs. As a result of NCLB and related state policies, special and compensatory school programs now face the challenge of shifting their focus to demonstrating improved developmental outcomes for the students in those programs.

Societal Priorities in Problem Solving

In the problem-solving approach presented here, a "problem" is said to exist whenever expectations for performance exceed current capabilities. In this view, "problems exist in the eye of the beholder." Whenever the schools or teachers—or parents or politicians—are not satisfied with student achievement, a problem exists. At the simplest level a problem exists when a teacher expects a student to read a story and answer questions and some students do not do so. The problem exists regardless of whether the teacher's expectation is too high or the level of student performance is too low. No attribution of cause is necessary. Similar problems can be easily imagined for story writing when students do not have the necessary writing skills and for completing mathematical story problems when the student is unaware of the computation skills required for doing those problems. Whenever student performance is perceived to be discrepant from expectations, a problem is said to exist.

Person-Centered Disabilities and Situation-Centered Problems

Before considering how priorities are established among problems, an important distinction must be made between an academic disability and an academic problem. The term *academic disability* is used to refer to the relative incapability of a person to perform common academic tasks. In the foregoing examples, the students who are relatively unskilled in reading and computational math would be considered to have academic disabilities if their performance in these domains was extremely poor. In this sense, then, academic disabilities are centered in the individual. The term *academic problem*, in contrast, is used to refer to differences between what the person can do and what the environment requires of the person to be successful. In the reading and math examples previously described, problems exist because the conditions set by the teacher exceed what the students can do. From those examples, we cannot determine whether the students are academically disabled or whether the teacher's expectations are unreasonably high. Thus, we can say that an academic problem exists, but we cannot say that the appropriate solution for that problem lies in increasing student ability, altering the teacher's expectations, or making adjustments in both. In this perspective, we can see that problems are defined contextually in terms of the discrepancy between performance and environmental demands. Academic problems, then, are centered in the situation, while academic disabilities are centered in the person.

The Role of Cultural Imperatives

A useful approach for understanding how priorities among academic problems are established is the framework provided by the idea of "cultural imperatives" (Reynolds & Birch, 1977). Cultural imperatives are the implicit or explicit standards of conduct or performance imposed on anyone who would become a member of a culture. One example of an imperative in American culture that increasingly produces conflict is the requirement that all citizens speak English. As the United States becomes more culturally and linguistically diverse, the demand that citizens speak one language has been challenged. Even as the challenge has been raised, however, school districts in some states are legally required to provide all of their instruction in English. While imperatives such as speaking English are codified in law, other imperatives are not explicitly formal and legal. The expectation that adults should be independent, for example, is sanctioned socially but not legally. Inculcating many socially sanctioned, but not legally required, cultural imperatives is a primary charge of the public schools. Controversy has existed for some time over what constitute the cultural imperatives of American society that are to be transmitted by our schools (see Hirsch, 1987). As NCLB was implemented, and states were required to establish curriculum standards, political conflict ensued. Conflicts over what students should be required to learn may be interpreted as cultural struggles that derive from different value orientations over what the imperatives of American culture truly are.

One thing that becomes clear when conflict over cultural imperatives occurs is that, while agreement can be obtained at a general level, disagreement exists when specificity is required. For example, widespread agreement exists that "basic skills" should be given high priority in school instruction. Different viewpoints emerge, however, when efforts are made to specify the basic skills that must be learned by all students. One thing seems quite clear in examining the cultural imperatives toward which schooling is directed. Substantial instructional time has been, and is, allocated to teaching functional skills in reading, written expression, and arithmetic. At the very least, we can say that reading, writing, and arithmetic are cultural imperatives in the early school years.

Cultural Electives

As we attempt to establish priorities among academic problems, it is important to recognize that there are aspects of culture that may be valued by a majority of people in a society but are not required of all members. These valued, but optional, aspects of individual development are cultural electives. Playing a musical instrument is a good example of a cultural elective since it is widely valued but not required for successful membership in

American society. Since instrumental performance is an elective, opportunities to learn how to play an instrument are sometimes provided by the schools, but basic instrumental skill is not required for promotion through the grades. The distinction between reading as a cultural imperative and the playing of a musical instrument as a cultural elective is at the heart of establishing priorities among problems to be solved. The first consideration in problem solving is inevitably given to cultural imperatives. Clear evidence of this fact is the effect of the standards-based reform movement made explicit in NCLB. As outcomes become written into law, they serve to establish what the body politic views as cultural imperatives.

The Role of Normative Standards in Problem Definition

The distinction between cultural imperatives and cultural electives provides only a partial basis for identifying those problems important enough for organizing problem-solving efforts in the schools. A second criterion that must be added is the size of the difference between what a culture requires in its imperatives and what a member must do to be considered "at risk" for violating cultural expectations. How much must performance differ from the performance standards set by the culture for an individual to be considered seriously disabled? From an empirical, psychological point of view, the answer has been found in the normative behavior of the members of the culture. In this view, establishing important differences requires development of empirical norms that largely, but not exclusively, determine the performance standards imposed by the culture. For example, commercially developed achievement tests are based on the use of norms that provide a framework for judging performance in reading, written expression, and arithmetic. The standards are established by measuring student performance at different points throughout the school year to determine the distributions of performance for same-age cohorts. Students who widely diverge from their peers at the low end of these distributions are those typically thought of as disabled.

While academic *disabilities* are normatively defined, academic *problems* are situational and depend on the performance expectations in that situation. Thus, judgments that a discrepancy is serious reside in, and are conditioned by, the contexts within which a student's behavior occurs. This perspective means that teachers make judgments based not only on their experience with broad cultural norms but also on the behavior of students in the context of their classrooms and schools. The local frame of reference will always affect an individual's judgment. This point is important to remember when choices must be made among problems to be solved.

The standards-based reform movement clearly illustrates how standards other than those derived from prevailing norms influence problem identification. This call for reform was driven by the view that the normative performance of American students was markedly decreasing or inferior to the norms of other cultures. In the early 1980s, the schools were sharply criticized for apparent decreases in the national averages on the Scholastic Aptitude Test (SAT). Further, considerable alarm was created by evidence that students from Japan were superior in their mathematical performance to students in the United States. The result was a call to reject the normative criteria in favor of higher standards as cultural imperatives.

Academic disabilities contribute to the existence of academic problems, but they are not the sole basis for the existence of those problems. A lack of reading skill becomes a problem only when the standards for success in the environment require a level of reading skill not possessed by the individual. A reading disability becomes a problem when the teacher expects the students to study text they cannot read or when a person is required to read instructions in order to assemble a bicycle. Since these problems are created in relation to environmental demands, they are situation-centered rather than person-centered. Handicaps, then, are ecologically defined, since they can be described only in terms of the network of social and physical environmental relationships of which the individual is a part.

Establishing Priorities among Problems

Problems have been defined here as situation-centered performance discrepancies. Although such a definition is useful as a starting point for intensifying problem solving, two issues need to be addressed when allocating resources: (1) the situation-specific nature of problems and (2) the myriad expectations that define performance as discrepant. Since performance discrepancies are always defined with reference to a specific situation, people performing the same in two different situations might be viewed as having a problem in one situation (e.g., the school) but not the other (e.g., on the job). Students who do not compute well enough to complete word problems successfully in their math class may experience no difficulty in accomplishing the computation required for working in a fast-food restaurant. Indeed, most of us who might have been poor math students in school are not mathematically handicapped in our daily lives. It is also common to find differences in the acceptability of the same academic skills between schools or classrooms. For example, a student whose performance in reading might have led to eligibility for a compensatory education in a high-achieving suburban school district, upon transferring, might be placed in a top reading group in a low-achieving urban school. Even within the same school, a student's behavior is likely to be judged differently by different teachers from one grade to the next. Indeed, evidence exists that it is quite normal for a student to be identified as having a significant behavior problem during the elementary school years (Balow & Rubin, 1978). This situational character of educational problems makes it difficult to determine whether a problem is sufficiently important for precious supplementary time and money to be invested in its solution.

A second issue related to performance discrepancies in problem solving is the myriad, and seemingly arbitrary, academic and social–behavioral expectations faced by students. In general, teachers expect (1) compliance with reasonable requests, (2) attention and participation in class, (3) completion of independent classwork and homework, (4) self-direction on projects, and (5) development of accuracy and fluency in a variety of curriculum skills. When the specific expectations within this general set of expectations are identified, however, some seem less important than others. Students are often held accountable for completing activities that are included in curricula even when no clear empirical rationale can be developed for requiring the activity. When considering both the wide range of expectations and the situation-specific nature of many problems, it becomes clear that some set of criteria, or system, must be used to establish priorities among problems as efforts to intensify problem solving proceed.

Norms, Standards, and Consequences in Establishing Priorities

In the history of educational and psychological testing, norms have weighed heavily in the judgment of student performance. Indeed, "problems" have traditionally been identified through establishing the difference between an individual's level of performance and the mean performance for age and grade. When this normative perspective is used to define problems, the magnitude of a student's problem is established by scaling the normative difference. A subtext always missing in this approach to identifying problems, however, is a consideration of the consequences of the failure to achieve expectations. If nothing else, the standards-based school reform movement that relies on benchmark testing makes it abundantly clear that academic problems can be criterion-referenced as well as norm-referenced. Even more clearly, the movement has revealed that it is the magnitude of the consequences associated with failure to meet expectations that establishes the significance or importance of academic problems. High stakes have been attached to success and failure, and students can be denied grade promotion or even a high school diploma. Schools can be labeled as substandard and placed on probation, school districts can be required to pay for supplementary programs. In this climate, priorities among academic problems are a function of the consequences attached to prevention, elimination, and continuation of those problems. Priority for academic problems with less significant consequences gives way to priority for problems defined by law and regulation.

The raised stakes for schools and teachers have made it easier and more practical for teachers to establish collaborative priorities among academic problems. Though we might not all agree with the politics and the outcomes of the standards-setting process, arguments over priorities among problems decrease once standards have been established. Where standardized tests were once ignored, educators now are constrained to focus on achievement outcomes. Academic problems directly related to state standards now are given highest priority.

THE INCREASED NEED FOR PROGRESS MONITORING

The dramatic increase in pressure on the schools to document student attainment has resulted in a much sharper focus on assessment procedures. Without some means to establish that students are attaining the standards, of course, there can be no accountability. The key approach to establishing accountability has been to increase the number and types of assessments used to ascertain attainment of outcomes. Different states have taken different approaches to developing assessment procedures for establishing accountability. Initially, some states based their procedures on alternative approaches to assessment, such as performance sampling and portfolio assessment. With the broader range of assessment requirements introduced through NCLB, the emphasis on traditional objective test item formats for basic skills in reading, writing, and arithmetic have become more practically feasible. Now, many states have either developed or contracted for the development of new achievement tests that meet NCLB requirements. One remarkable aspect of this movement has been that, in many cases, the procedures developed to meet accountability standards were implemented without extensive technical work on their reliability and validity. Thus, many students, and many schools, are being held accountable through assessment procedures of uncertain technical adequacy (Ysseldyke, Dennison, & Nelson, 2004).

In addition to developing tests to meet the accountability requirements of high-stakes assessment, educational agencies have also recognized the need for, and potential of, regular and frequent progress-monitoring procedures. The need for progress monitoring stems from the fact that those being held accountable for student achievement on standards tests would like to be able to forecast likely student success on the standards tests. Obviously, being able to anticipate outcomes creates opportunities to make corrections to forestall or minimize any negative consequences. Thus, interest has increased in the potential of progress-monitoring procedures for formatively evaluating educational programs for the purpose of increasing the likelihood of program success.

The U.S. Department of Education has made educational agencies more aware of the importance of frequent progress monitoring by requiring its use in evidence-based programs. In its invitation to apply for the Reading First grants (NCLB, 2001) the Department required that all applications incorporate progress monitoring on the basis that sufficient evidence existed to show that success in attaining positive achievement outcomes in beginning reading increased when progress-monitoring data were used formatively to evaluate programs. Apparently, progress monitoring has achieved a status akin to the "well checks" conducted by health care providers to monitor children's health and development. In education, as in health, regular and early inspection enables detection of students whose growth rates place them at risk for failure to meet eventual standards.

Successful implementation of progress monitoring can create more and clearer occasions for educational professionals to engage in problem solving. The early identification of discrepancies between desired and projected levels of accomplishment indicate that risk exists and a need exists to intensify problem-solving efforts. To accomplish this, however, requires the availability of progress-monitoring procedures that provide data of sufficient reliability and validity that problem solvers can effectively use those data to formatively evaluate programs. It is in this environment that growth-monitoring procedures like curriculum-based measurement (CBM, Deno, 1985, 2003b) have become of particular interest.

INTENSIFIED PROBLEM SOLVING AS ACTION RESEARCH

In earlier writings on the role of school psychologists and special educators as problem solvers (Deno, 1986), the focus was on using single-case time-series research designs (Glass, Willson, & Gottman, 1975; Kazdin, 1982) as the basis for formatively evaluating individual student programs. The use of single-case research procedures to intensify problem solving adds systematic empirical evaluation of alternative interventions introduced into student programs. The primary assumption on which this systematic empirical problem-solving approach was recommended was that its application produces cumulative improvements in student programs. That improvement occurs because the evaluation procedures are formative rather than summative. The application of single-case research designs to evaluate programs formatively places educators squarely in the role of action researchers who are attempting to discover "what works" when they attempt to improve programs.

As with any idea, the roots for viewing educational reforms as experiments are old and deep. Donald Campbell (1969) advanced the empirical problem-solving approach presented here more than 35 years ago in his presidential address to the American Psychological Association. In that address, he proposed that societal reforms be conceived as experiments whose effects need to be tested rather than assumed. When that proposition is applied to education, it becomes clear that changes in students' programs implemented to prevent or eliminate problems can and should be carefully tested, using empirical procedures. In addition, empirically testing reforms helps to ensure that the precious resources allocated through compensatory programs do indeed lead to the reduction of those problems for which the resources have been allocated. Finally, the emphasis on empirical testing is consistent with one of the most desirable principles in NCLB—the need to use evidence to make educational decisions.

Problem Solving as Hypothesis Testing

Single-case research designs are created to test hypotheses regarding functional relationships (Steege, Brown-Chidsey, & Mace, 2002). Were we able to predict with certainty precisely what interventions would be successful, evaluation would be unnecessary. Unfortunately, and despite the call to use only "evidence-based programs" in education, we cannot say with certainty that any one program will be effective with all students. For that reason, we must recognize that any problem-solving alternative can never be more than an operational hypothesis about what will affect student performance. We owe it to the students into whose lives we are intervening that those operational hypotheses should be tested to either confirm or disconfirm our predictions.

The literature on problem solving is convincing in documenting that more effective problem solvers generate many possible plans of action prior to attempting a solution (Johnson & Johnson, 1982). Alternative plans of action are important for two reasons: first, selection of a "best solution" requires consideration of alternatives; second, our hypotheses regarding how to solve problems frequently are disconfirmed by the progress-monitoring data. Successful problem solvers are able to develop many action hypotheses directed toward solving the same problem. To solve academic problems, educators must generate and consider the application of alternatives. No "one size fits all" is possible nor should be assumed.

Perhaps the most obvious illustration of the need, and the opportunity, to consider problem solution alternatives occurs when students are declared eligible for special education and individualized education plans (IEPs) are developed. During the IEP development process, a problem-solving team should be able to reflect on potential alternative action hypotheses or reforms that could diminish the academic problems that have led to the student's being placed in special education. Unfortunately, limited resources too often now make it impossible to consider potentially effective alternatives. And, too often, pressures from well-meaning advocates result in conflict and rigid thinking in situations that require flexible thinking. When done right, compensatory programs like special education can become the basis for consideration, selection, and application of problem solution hypotheses intended to eliminate important performance discrepancies.

A PROBLEM-SOLVING MODEL
AND PROBLEM-SOLVING ASSESSMENT

Systematic efforts to intensify problem solving can benefit from the use of a problem-solving model. A clear and practical problem-solving model useful in education is the IDEAL problem-solving model described by Bransford and Stein (1984). That model consists of five steps: (1) *Identifying* the problem to be solved, (2) *Defining* the problem, (3) *Exploring* alternative solutions, (4) *Applying* the chosen solution, and (5) *Looking* at the effects. The basic steps are common to most problem-solving models. Its primary contribution to problem-solving assessment is that it clarifies and sequences the five major decisions that must be made in problem solving. Since assessment is conducted to provide information for decision making, educational problem solvers need to be aware of the problem-solving decision they are making and the types of information most helpful in making the decision.

Assessment and Evaluation

The IDEAL model presented in Table 2.1 illustrates the relationship problem-solving steps, the type of assessment required, and the evaluation decision that corresponds to each problem-solving step. In the model, assessment is distinguished from evaluation to clarify that the purpose of assessment is to provide descriptive information, typically numerical,

TABLE 2.1. A Data-Based Problem-Solving Model

Problem-solving steps	Assessment procedures	Evaluation decisions
1. Problem identification	Observing/recording student performance	Does a problem exist?
2. Problem definition	Quantifying the perceived discrepancy	Is the problem important?
3. Designing intervention plans	Exploring alternative goals and solution hypotheses	What is the best solution hypothesis?
4. Implementing intervention	Monitoring fidelity of intervention and data collection	Is the solution attempt progressing as planned?
5. Problem solution	Requantifying the discrepancy	Is the original problem being solved though this attempted solution?

whereas the purpose of evaluation is to make a decision. In assessing performance discrepancies, we seek objective, reliable, and precise data that can contribute to decision making. Evaluations of those discrepancies involve the consideration of data; however, they also require a weighing of values, laws, regulations, resources, and the probable personal and social consequences of selecting different courses of action. The point cannot be emphasized too strongly that while data from measurement can inform and direct decisions, they neither dictate nor determine those decisions. People will, and must, bring their values and their subjective judgments into decision making.

The Problem-Solving Model and Special Education

Although not central to this chapter, we can see that the problem-solving steps, assessment procedures, and evaluation activities represented in Table 2.1 correspond to the steps usually identified as requirements in providing special education service to students through special education. Typically, students are referred to special education; the referral is screened to determine the need for further assessment; if appropriate, assessment for determining eligibility follows; if the student is eligible for service, an IEP is developed including annual goals, short-term objectives, evaluation procedures, and the service to be provided; the IEP is then implemented and student progress toward IEP goals monitored; finally, the success of an IEP is reviewed periodically and annually to determine program success. The remaining chapters in this book will describe assessment methods compatible with the problem-solving steps found in Table 2.1. Such methods can be used for all students, not only those with disabilities.

SYSTEMS-LEVEL PROBLEM SOLVING USING CURRICULUM-BASED MEASUREMENT

Among the components of problem-solving assessment presented in this volume, CBM has the longest history and closest connection to problem-solving-based assessment practices. This chapter will illustrate how CBM can be used to solve a wide range of problems perceived in education. More information about CBM methods can be found in Chapter 10 of this volume.

Standardized Assessment Procedures

The curriculum-based measurement procedures advocated for use in problem-solving assessment were developed to quantify student performance in reading, written expression, spelling, and arithmetic. These procedures are the product of a systematic research and development program that established the technical adequacy of the data collected through applying these measurement procedures to student performance (see Deno, 1985, 1986, 2003a). The fact that these procedures are standardized rather than ad hoc assures a database for problem solving that is sufficiently reliable and valid. The issue of technical adequacy is especially important when comparisons are made between an individual student and the performance of that student's peers. The reliability and validity of data are also important when comparisons are made of the same student's performance at different times such as before, during, and after various attempts to solve a problem. In general, any time the data obtained from two or more measurements are compared, the reliability of those measurements is an important issue. Further, any time a question arises as to whether or not a performance discrepancy is important, the validity of a particular measurement or set of measurements must be established. It is not possible to be confident that any of the myriad performance discrepancies that could be identified through measuring a student's performance on somewhat arbitrarily selected curriculum tasks would be sufficiently important to attempt problem solution.

An Early Response to Intervention Model

In 1977, Deno and Mirkin presented a problem-solving assessment model entitled Data-Based Program Modification (DBPM). The basic premise of that model was that modifications in student programs could be tested by collecting progress-monitoring data reflecting student growth in relation to changes implemented to increase student academic and social development. The model was created as a tool for educators to evaluate the success of their interventions and to determine the level of special education service required to solve the problems precipitating referral and initial assessment. The DBPM model was complete in that it included specification of the observational data to be used for evaluating problem-solving efforts. At the same time, the technical adequacy of the assessment procedures had not been empirically investigated, nor had the potential effectiveness of using those procedures to improve programs been tested.

To address the issues of technical adequacy and the effectiveness of the DBPM model, a program of research was conducted between 1977 and 1983 through the Institute for Research on Learning Disabilities at the University of Minnesota. An important result of that program of research was the development of standardized procedures for monitoring student progress in reading, spelling, and written expression. The use of those procedures formatively to evaluate instruction was experimentally examined, leading to the conclusion that teachers could successfully increase achievement using those procedures (Fuchs, Deno, & Mirkin, 1984). At the same time, the progress-monitoring procedures became known as curriculum-based measurement (CBM; Deno, 1985). Subsequently, the use of CBM in assessment to conduct educational problem solving was presented as an alternative or supplementary approach to addressing problems using conventional standardized achievement testing (Deno, 1986, 1995, 2002; Minnesota Educational Effectiveness Project, 1987; Shinn, 1989).

The technical adequacy of the CBM approach to progress monitoring distinguishes it from other curriculum-based assessment (CBA) models. The technical adequacy of CBM has enabled problem solvers to use the data derived from CBM with confidence in both their reliability and validity. To achieve technical adequacy, the procedures have been standardized to the level that they include specification of *what to measure, how to measure,* and *how to score and interpret* the data on student growth. While it is beyond the scope of the present chapter to describe all of studies documenting the technical adequacy and development of the standardized CBM procedures, an illustration of the *core skills* used for standardized CBM in reading immediately follows.

Core Skill: Reading

The primary skill used to monitor progress and make instructional modifications in reading is *reading aloud from text.* Often, this is referred to as "oral reading fluency"; however, the use of that term confuses the purpose of that task for evaluating intervention effects with a characteristic of good readers (i.e., oral reading fluency). Nonetheless, CBM oral reading fluency has been shown to be a highly reliable and valid way to measure overall reading skills. More recently, *recognizing words deleted from text* (the "maze" procedure) and, for beginning readers, *reading isolated words* have been added as core skills for reading measurement. The core reading tasks are used with standardized administration procedures to obtain samples of performance on those tasks. The performance samples are then scored to produce data with known technical adequacy (Shinn, 1989).

Standardized CBM data can be used to inform key decisions in the problem-solving model. For example, stages 1 and 5 of the problem-solving model require decisions regarding the existence of a problem. As illustrated in Table 2.2, each of these questions can be informed by CBM data. At stage 1, the existence of a problem is evaluated. In order to determine the existence of a reading problem, an individual student's CBM reading scores could be compared with benchmark score ranges representing the average reading performance of all the students in a certain grade level. If the individual student's scores are lower than average for his or her grade, a problem could be identified. Again, at stage 5 of the model, the continuing existence of the problem is at question. Are the student's reading scores still below what is expected for his or her grade? If not, then it would make sense to conclude that the problem was solved.

TABLE 2.2. Application of Problem-Solving Stages 1 and 5 for Evaluation of Reading Skills

Stage	Questions	CBM components
1	Does a problem exist (in reading)?	Data reflecting the difference between current level and slope in reading aloud from text, and the desired level and slope in reading from that text
5	Is the original problem being solved through the attempted solution?	Data on the degree to which the current level and slope in reading aloud from text indicate that the original discrepancy is being reduced or will be eliminated

PROBLEM-SOLVING ASSESSMENT WITH CURRICULUM-BASED MEASUREMENT

CBM has been used to solve a wide range of educational problems. CBM offers a methodology for systems-level problem-solving applications. Those applications are illustrated in the paragraphs that follow. The illustrations begin with the more common applications of CBM and move to more recent applications and extensions of its use.

Improving Individual Instructional Programs

The primary purpose of developing CBM was to create a simple set of assessment procedures that teachers could use formatively to evaluate the instruction they were providing to individual students. The hypothesis that drove this development was that teachers using formative evaluation procedures would manifest higher rates of achievement than teachers who did not. The formative evaluation model using CBM as the database is represented graphically in Figure 2.1. As can be seen in the figure, individual student performance during an initial baseline phase is plotted, and a goal is established. A progress line connecting the initial level and the goal establishes the rate of improvement necessary for the student to achieve the goal. A change in the student's program is introduced and indicated by the first vertical line. Continued measurement of that student's performance after the intervention reveals that a leveling-off of performance follows the initial improvement. A second change is made in the program, and improvement occurs. This systematic approach to setting goals, monitoring growth, changing programs, and evaluating the effects of changes is the formative evaluation model. Research on the achievement effects of using this approach has revealed that teachers using systematic formative evaluation based on CBM produce greater achievement of their students (Fuchs, Deno,

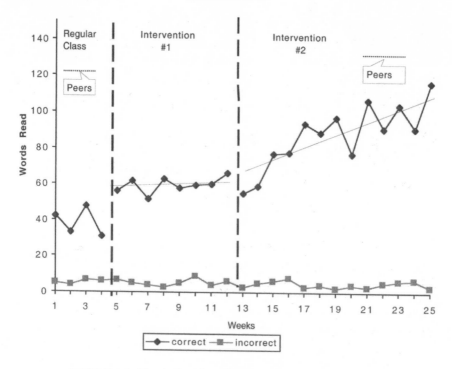

FIGURE 2.1. Curriculum-based measurement progress graph.

& Mirkin, 1984; Fuchs, Fuchs, & Hamlett, 1989; Fuchs, Fuchs, Hamlett, & Stecker, 1991; Shinn & Hubbard, 1992; Espin, Wallace, Lembke, Campbell, & Long, 2003).

Increased Ease of Communication

While the effectiveness of CBM in increasing both teacher and student awareness of goals has already been discussed, it is important to point out that the CBM graph with its multiple references creates opportunities for clearer communication. It has now become common practice for teachers to use the CBM data in parent conferences and at multidisciplinary team meetings to provide a framework for communicating an individual student's status. Professional educators and parents easily use the CBM data graph, since little or no interpretation of the scores is necessary (Shinn, Baker, Habedank, & Good, 1993). This contrasts sharply with the complexities related to communicating the results of commercially available standardized test scores. A simple illustration of both the ease and effectiveness of communicating around CBM data can be found in the results of the teacher planning study mentioned earlier (Fuchs et al., 1984). In that study students as well as teachers were asked whether they knew their annual reading goals and were asked to specify those goals. Those students whose teachers were using CBM and formative evaluation not only expressed that they knew those goals but were able to accurately specify their target reading scores.

Screening to Identify Students Academically "at Risk"

An increasingly common use of CBM is to screen students who are "at risk" for academic failure. As mentioned previously, since CBM procedures are standardized they can be used to contrast an individual's performance to that of the group. The use of local norms is common for this purpose, but norms are not required. CBM can be easily and quickly used to assess the performance of a group of students and to identify the lowest-achieving at-risk students in the group (Marston & Magnusson, 1988; Shinn, 1995) in the area of reading with the inclusion of the maze task that allows for group administration (Deno, Reschly-Anderson, Lembke, Zorka, & Callender, 2002). In the study by Deno and colleagues all of the students in a large urban elementary school were given three standard CBM maze passages, and their performance was aggregated within and across grades. The lowest 20% of the students on the CBM maze measure in each grade were considered sufficiently at risk to require progress monitoring every other week with the more conventional CBM oral reading measure. Identification of high-risk students in this manner has now become commonplace among schools practicing CBM.

Evaluating Classroom "Prereferral" Interventions

The cost and the consequences of special education are recurring issues in the literature of special education. Of particular concern is the possibility that students are being referred and placed in special education when they might succeed in regular class programs with different instruction by classroom teachers. One approach to addressing this issue is to require that classroom teachers conduct prereferral interventions to establish that such accommodations are insufficient. One problem with this approach has been that little useful data has been available to appraise the effects of those prereferral data. Since CBM data are sensitive to the effects of program changes over relatively short time periods, they can be used to aid in the evaluation of prereferral interventions. The use of CBM in evaluating prereferral academic interventions is the first component of the "problem-solving model" (Deno, 1989) that has been implemented at both the state and district levels (Shinn, 1995; Tilly & Grimes, 1998). The problem-solving model enables general and special educators to collaborate in the early stages of child study to determine with some validity that the problems of skill development faced by a student are more than "instructional failures." Documentation that the problem is not readily solvable by the classroom teacher becomes the basis for special education eligibility assessment.

Alternative Special Education Identification Procedures

Widespread dissatisfaction exists with traditional approaches to identifying students for special education that rely on standardized tests of either ability, achievement, or both (Reschly, 1988). Despite this dissatisfaction, few alternatives have been offered to replace those more conventional procedures. Over the past 20 years, the use of CBM within a systematic decision framework has been explored as a basis for developing alternative identification procedures (Marston, Mirkin, & Deno, 1984; Marston & Magnusson, 1988; Shinn, 1989). Recently, the use of CBM to test student's "responsiveness to intervention" (RTI) (Fuchs & Fuchs, 1998) has gained favor recently within policymaking groups. The RTI approach is an extension of prereferral evaluation and the problem-solving model to evaluate increased levels of intensity in instructional intervention. As each level of an academic intervention is introduced, CBM data are continually collected to examine the responsiveness of a student to that intervention. For example, if a student fails to increase his rate of growth in response to several regular classroom interventions, then a period of "pull-out" instruction from a special education resource teacher might be instituted and evaluated. If a student succeeds when receiving instruction from the resource teacher, then his responsiveness to that treatment establishes his need for special education. Some evidence has now begun to emerge that the alternative approaches to eligibility determination that are rooted in the problem-solving model have created an entirely different perspective on the concept of disability (Tilly, Reschly, & Grimes, 1999).

Recommending and Evaluating Inclusion

As increased emphasis has been placed on inclusion of students with disabilities in regular classrooms, and as laws and regulations have required schools to assure access to the regular class curriculum, the need to evaluate the effects of these changes on the academic development of students with disabilities has increased. CBM has proved to be a very useful tool for those accountable for the progress of students with disabilities as they seek to provide education of these students in the mainstream curriculum. The general strategy employed when using CBM to evaluate inclusion has been to collect data before and after integration into regular class instruction, and then to continue monitoring student progress to assure that reintegration of students is occurring "responsibly" (Fuchs, Roberts, Fuchs, & Bowers, 1996; Powell-Smith & Stewart, 1998). The results of the research in this area provide clear evidence that both special educators and classroom teachers can use CBM to provide ongoing documentation of student progress and signal the need for increased intensification of instruction when inclusive programs are unsuccessful.

Assessing English Language Learning Students

A particular problem confronting schools in the United States is the dramatically increasing proportion of students whose first language is not English and who are still learning to speak English while already learning to read and write in English. Commercially available standardized tests have not been useful because they have not included the full range of languages represented in English language learning (ELL) students within their norm samples. More significantly, many achievement tests draw heavily on background knowledge of the American culture in structuring questions. Among other problems that exist because of the lack of technically adequate procedures is how to distinguish ELL students who are having difficulty learning because of their lack of proficiency in English from ELL students whose struggles also stem from special disabilities. Several studies have explored the use of CBM to overcome the problems of assessing ELL students and to monitor their growth in mainstream classrooms. Baker and others (Baker & Good, 1995; Baker, Plasencia-Peinado, & Lezcano-Lytle, 1998) have focused primarily on using CBM reading scores of Spanish-speaking ELL students to evaluate their progress in regular class programs.

That research established levels of reliability and validity for the CBM procedures with ELL students in both their native and English languages that are comparable to native speakers of English. Further, longitudinal analyses revealed that students who begin with comparable proficiency in English often grow at very different rates. The apparent technical adequacy of CBM has led at least one urban school system to use CBM procedures for developing norms across reading, writing, and arithmetic on its ELL students (Robinson, Larson, & Watkins, 2002). CBM also has been used to predict differences in the success rates of middle school ELL students on state assessments as a function of their level of reading proficiency (Muyskens & Marston, 2002). Additionally, research has been conducted using CBM with students in countries where languages other than English are spoken. The evidence from that research indicates that the procedures and tasks to be used for measurement need to be consistent with formal differences in the language. For example, oral reading can be used to measure growth in other phonetic languages like Korean, but the maze procedure appears to be more appropriate for measuring growth in an iconic language like Chinese (Yeh, 1992).

Predicting Success in Early Childhood Education

The criterion validity of CBM oral reading scores has been sufficiently established to become an important criterion for establishing the predictive validity of prereading measures and the effectiveness of early literacy interventions. With the ascendant interest in the role played by phonological skills in learning to read, the utility of scores from measures of phonological skill has been established by examining their accuracy in predicting beginning oral reading scores (Kaminski & Good, 1996). As cited earlier (Good, Simmons, & Kame'enui, 2001), evidence has developed that CBM oral reading performance at the end of first grade is a significant indicator of subsequent reading success. Research in this area has established important linkages between measures of phonological skill in kindergarten, oral reading performance in grades 1–3, and success on state assessments. The evidence has become sufficiently persuasive that the federal government has, essentially, required projects funded under the Reading First grant program to include CBM oral reading data as a requirement for monitoring program effects. Finally, similar growth measures have been developed to assess preschool development and predict early literacy (McConnell, Priest, Davis, & McEvoy, 2002).

Assessing Students Who Are Deaf

A problem paralleling the problems associated with assessing ELL students is the problem faced by educators seeking to assess deaf students' progress at developing competence in written English. As with ELL students, deaf students must learn to read and write English despite the fact that they do not speak English. The problems differ, however, in that deaf students, generally, never learn to speak English and will not be able to use sound–symbol correspondence in learning to read and write. For that matter, they will not be able to use spoken English vocabulary referents to assist in comprehending text. In general, commercially available standardized tests have been of no use in assessing the achievement of deaf students.

Recently, research using the CBM written expression measure that was developed for hearing students has revealed that the same measure can be used to assess the written expression competence of deaf students, as well (Chen, 2002). Assessing the competence of deaf students reading English has required a different approach. Oral reading is not possible with deaf students who do not speak English, and using American Sign Language (ASL) is not an option because the ASL signs do not correspond word for word to English. An effort has been made to have students sign Exact English rather than ASL, but this has not proved to be useful. More promising has been the use of the CBM maze task to measure the reading of deaf students. Since that task requires only that students read text silently and make correct maze choices, the requirements for deaf and hearing students on this task are the same. Recent research on using the maze task with deaf students has provided evidence of the validity and utility of the measure (Chen, 2002; Deno et al., 2002).

SUMMARY

The perspective on problem solving provided in this chapter establishes the following:

- Problem solving is a characteristic of professional behavior.
- Problems are defined by the discrepancy between what someone wants and what someone gets.
- Schooling is an intervention organized to reduce the discrepancy between what society wants children to become and where children are when they come to school.
- Compensatory programs are created to intensify interventions for groups and individuals whose rates of development do not meet societal standards.
- Progress monitoring can be a useful mechanism for increasing the success of educational interventions.
- Federal and state mandates have clarified priorities among problems by making cultural imperatives more explicit.
- Educational problem solving should be viewed as action research where interventions are hypotheses to be empirically tested.

The primary function of the schools is to affect student development, and the first responsibility of educators is to create environments that facilitate that development. Successful performance of those primary role functions will be defined by the extent to which students attain cultural competence in a timely manner. Problems occur when rates of growth and levels of attainment fall below what is expected. Increased efforts to assess students are a manifestation of intensified problem solving. Successful problem-solving assessment will always include a careful explication of the expectations for performance as well as the measured levels of that performance. Problems are always defined by this difference between actual and desired performance and exist in the "eye of the beholder" of that problem. The importance of any problem will be established only by examining the degree of difference between actual and desired performance. More complete determination of the priority to be given to a problem is obtained by examining the immediate and long-term consequences to the student should the problem continue or fail to be resolved.

Identifying important problems that must be solved by the schools has become easier as federal and state legislative mandates have made societal expectations more explicit through high-stakes testing. One rational response to the accountability demands has been to increase the development and use of progress-monitoring procedures that enable educators to anticipate and prevent problems. CBM exists as one technically adequate approach for taking a more functional problem-solving approach to the prevention and solution of educational problems. Evidence exists that professional educators can increase their problem-solving effectiveness through the use of progress monitoring of student development and by systematically responding to those data as they reflect student growth.

REFERENCES

Baker, S. K., & Good, R. H. (1995). Curriculum-based measurement of English reading with bilingual Hispanic students: A validation study with second-grade students. *School Psychology Review, 24*, 561–578.

Baker, S. K., Plasencia-Peinado, J., & Lezcano-Lytle, V. (1998). The use of curriculum-based measurement with language-minority students. In M. R. Shinn (Ed.), *Advanced applications of curriculum-based measurement* (pp. 175–213). New York: Guilford Press.

Balow, B., & Rubin, R. (1978). Prevalence of teacher identified behavior problems: A longitudinal study. *Exceptional Children, 45*, 102–111.

Bransford, J. D., & Stein, B. S. (1984). *The IDEAL problem solver.* New York: Freeman.

Campbell, D. T. (1969). Reforms as experiments. *American Psychologist, 24*, 409–429.

Chen, Y. (2002). *Assessment of reading and writing samples of deaf and hard of hearing students by curriculum-based measurements.* Unpublished doctoral dissertation, University of Minnesota, Minneapolis.

Deno, E. (1970). Special education as developmental capital. *Exceptional Children, 37*, 229–237.

Deno, S. L. (1985). Curriculum-based measurement: The emerging alternative. *Exceptional Children, 52*, 219–232.

Deno, S. L. (1986). Formative evaluation of individual student programs: A new role for school psychologists. *School Psychology Review, 15*, 348–374.

Deno, S. L. (1989). Curriculum-based measurement and alternative special education services: A fundamental and direct relationship. In M. R. Shinn (Ed.), *Curriculum-based measurement: Assessing special children* (pp. 1–17). New York: Guilford Press.

Deno, S. L. (1995). The school psychologist as problem solver. In J. Grimes & A. Thomas (Eds.), *Best practices in school psychology III* (pp. 471–484). Silver Spring, MD: National Association of School Psychologists.

Deno, S. L. (2001). *The key role of fluency in curriculum-based measurement (CBM).* Presentation at the annual Interventions Conference, Utah State University, Logan, UT.

Deno, S. L. (2002). Problem-solving as best practice. In A. Thomas & J. Grimes (Eds.), *Best practices in school psychology IV* (pp. 77–99). Washington, DC: National Association of School Psychologists.

Deno, S. L. (2003a). Developments in curriculum-based measurement. *Journal of Special Education, 37*(3), 184–192.

Deno, S. L. (2003b). *Developing a school-wide progress monitoring system.* Paper presented at the Pacific Coast Research Conference, La Jolla, CA.

Deno, S. L., & Mirkin, P. K. (1977). *Data-based program modification: A manual.* Reston, VA: Council for Exceptional Children.

Deno, S. L., Reschly-Anderson, A., Lembke, E., Zorka, H., & Callender, S. (2002). *A model for schoolwide implementation of progress monitoring: A case example.* Presentation at the National Association of School Psychology Annual Meeting, Chicago, IL.

Espin, C. A., Wallace, T., Lembke, E., Campbell, H., & Long, J. (2003). *Creating a progress monitoring system: Preparing secondary-school students for success on the Minnesota Basic Skills Tests.* Presentation at the Pacific Coast Research Conference, La Jolla, CA.

Fuchs, D., Roberts, P. H., Fuchs, L. S., & Bowers, J. (1996). Reintegrating students with learning disabilities into the mainstream: A two-year study. *Learning Disabilities Research and Practice, 11*, 214–229.

Fuchs, L., Deno, S., & Mirkin, P. (1984). Effects of frequent curriculum-based measurement and evaluation on pedagogy, student achievement, and student awareness of learning. *American Educational Research Journal, 21*, 449–460.

Fuchs, L. S., & Fuchs, D. (1998). Treatment validity: A unifying concept for reconceptualizing the identification of learning disabilities. *Learning Disabilities Research and Practice, 13*, 204–219.

Fuchs, L. S., Fuchs, D., & Hamlett, C. L. (1989). Effects of instrumental use of curriculum-based measurement to enhance instructional programs. *Remedial and Special Education, 10*, 43–52.

Fuchs, L. S., Fuchs, D., Hamlett, C. L., & Stecker, P. M. (1991). Effects of curriculum-based measurement and consultation on teacher planning and student achievement in mathematics operations. *American Educational Research Journal, 28*, 617–641.

Glass, G. V., Willson, L. L., & Gottman, J. M. (1975). *Design and analysis of time series experiments.* Boulder, CO: Laboratory of Educational Research, University of Colorado.

Good, R. H., III, Simmons, D. C., & Kame'enui, E. J. (2001). The importance and decision-making utility of a continuum of fluency-based indicators of foundational reading skills for third-grade high stakes outcomes. *Scientific Studies of Reading, 5*, 257–288.

Hirsch, E. D. (1987). *Cultural literacy.* Boston: Houghton Mifflin.

Johnson, D. W., & Johnson, F. P. (1982). *Joining together* (2nd ed.). Englewood Cliffs, NJ: Prentice-Hall.

Kaminski, R. A., & Good, R. H. (1996). Toward a technology for assessing basic early literacy skills. *School Psychology Review, 25*, 215–227.

Kazdin, A. E. (1982). *Single-case research designs.* New York: Oxford University Press.

Leinhardt, G., Zigmond, N., & Cooley, W. (1981). Reading instruction and its effects. *American Educational Research Journal, 18*, 343–361.

Marston, D. B., & Magnusson, D. (1988). Curriculum-based assessment: District-level implementation. In J. Graden, J. Zins, & M. Curtis (Eds.), *Alternative educational delivery systems: Enhancing instructional options for all students* (pp. 137–172). Washington, DC: National Association of School Psychologists.

Marston, D. B., Mirkin, P. K., & Deno, S. L. (1984). Curriculum-based measurement:

An alternative to traditional screening, referral, and identification. *Journal of Special Education,18*, 109–117.

McConnell, S., Priest, J., Davis, S., & McEvoy, M. (2002). Best practices in measuring growth and development for preschool children. In A. Thomas & J. Grimes (Eds.), *Best practices in School Psychology IV* (pp. 1231–1246). Washington, DC: National Association of School Psychologists.

Minnesota Educational Effectiveness Project. (1987). *Program components* (Technical Report). St. Paul: Minnesota State Department of Education.

Muyskens, P., & Marston, D. B. (2002). *Predicting success on the Minnesota Basic Skills Test in Reading using CBM*. Minneapolis Public Schools. Unpublished Manuscript.

National Center for Education Statistics. (1993). *The national education goals report— 1993: Building a nation of learners*. Retrieved July 25, 2004, from *www.ed.gov/ pubs/goals/report/goalsrpt.txt*.

Powell-Smith, K. A., & Stewart, L. H. (1998). The use of curriculum-based measurement on the reintegration of students with mild disabilities. In M. R. Shinn (Ed.), *Advanced applications of curriculum-based measurement* (pp. 254–307). New York: Guilford Press.

Reynolds, M. C., & Birch, J. W. (1977). *Teaching exceptional children in all America's schools*. Reston, VA: Council for Exceptional Children.

Reschly, D. (1988). Special education reform: School psychology revolution. *School Psychology Review, 17*, 459–475.

Robinson, M., Larson, N., & Watkins, E. (2002). *What if they don't speak Spanish?: Assessing low incidence speakers for SLD*. Denver, CO: Council for Learning Disabilities International Conference.

Shinn, M. R. (Ed.). (1989). *Curriculum-based measurement: Assessing special children*. New York: Guilford Press.

Shinn, M. (1995). Best practices in curriculum-based measurement and its use in a problem-solving model. In J. Grimes & A. Thomas (Eds.), *Best practices in school psychology III* (pp. 547–568). Silver Spring, MD: National Association of School Psychologists.

Shinn, M. R., Baker, S., Habedank, L., & Good, R. H. (1993). The effects of classroom reading performance data on general education teachers' and parents' attitudes about reintegration. *Exceptionality, 4*, 205–229.

Steege, M., Brown-Chidsey, R., & Mace, F. C. (2002). Best practices in evaluating interventions. In A. Thomas & J. Grimes (Eds.), *Best practices in school psychology IV* (pp. 517–534). Washington, DC: National Association of School Psychologists.

Tilly, W. D., & Grimes, J. (1998). Curriculum-based measurement: One vehicle for systematic educational reform. In M. R. Shinn (Ed.), *Advanced applications of curriculum-based measurement* (pp. 32–88). New York: Guilford Press.

Tilly, W. D., Reschly, D. J., & Grimes, J. (1999). Disability determination in problem-solving systems: Conceptual foundations and critical components. In D. J. Reschly, W. D. Tilly, & J. Grimes (Eds.), *Special education in transition: Functional assessment and noncategorical programming* (pp. 221–254). Longmont, CO: Sopris West.

Yeh, C. (1992). *The use of passage reading measures to assess reading proficiency of Chinese elementary school students*. Unpublished doctoral dissertation, University of Minnesota, Minneapolis.

Ysseldyke, J., Dennison, A., & Nelson, R. (2003). *Large-scale assessment and accountability systems: Positive consequences for students with disabilities* (Synthesis Report 51). Minneapolis: University of Minnesota, National Center on Educational Outcomes. Retrieved July 26, 2004, from *education.umn.edu/NCEO/OnlinePubs/ Synthesis51.html*

SUGGESTED READINGS

Deno, S. L. (1985). Curriculum-based measurement: The emerging alternative. *Exceptional Children, 52*, 219–232.

The original article on the development of CBM. The article includes a rationale for CBM development, a description of its use with individual students, and the empirical evidence on its reliability and validity.

Deno, S. L. (1989). Curriculum-based measurement and alternative special education services: A fundamental and direct relationship. In M. R. Shinn (Ed.), *Advanced applications of curriculum-based measurement* (pp. 1–17). New York: Guilford Press.

The problem-solving model that subsequently became the basis for the problem-solving approaches to assessment described in this chapter. The author describes the relationship between CBM data and a reconceptualization of the nature and purpose of special education programs.

Deno, S. L. (1997). "Whether" thou goest: Perspectives on progress monitoring. In E. Kame'enui, J. Lloyd, & D. Chard (Eds.), *Issues in educating students with disabilities* (pp. 77–99). Mahwah, NJ: Erlbaum.

The chapter includes a description of two alternative approaches to progress monitoring that are used to track growth in basic skills. A distinction in made between the utility of the two approaches for use in evaluation interventions and making educational decisions.

Deno, S. L. (2003). Developments in curriculum-based measurement. *Journal of Special Education, 37*(3), 184–192.

The paper provides an extensive summary of the past developments and current research on CBM. Included is a discussion of the unique contribution of CBM to special education practices.

Fuchs, L., Deno, S., & Mirkin, P. (1984). Effects of frequent curriculum-based measurement and evaluation on pedagogy, student achievement, and student awareness of learning. *American Educational Research Journal, 21*, 449–460.

This article summarizes an experimental field test of the use of CBM in formative evaluation of special education student progress. Data are provided revealing the positive effects on student achievement, student knowledge of progress and goal attainment, and teacher practice.

Fuchs, L. S., & Deno, S. L. (1994). Must instructionally useful performance assessment be based in the curriculum? *Exceptional Children, 61*, 15–24.

The issue of whether typical uses of CBM measurement procedures must include stimulus materials from the curriculum is discussed. Successful applications of the generic procedures with stimulus materials drawn from other sources are documented.

Fuchs, L. S., & Deno, S. L. (1991). Paradigmatic distinctions between instructionally relevant measurement models. *Exceptional children, 57*, 488–501.

This article makes the distinction between typical approaches to curriculum-based assessment (CBA) that are based on a task-analytic mastery monitoring approach to progress assessment and the CBM approach that is rooted in general outcome measurement (GOM) approach to progress monitoring. The relative advantages and disadvantages are considered.

Fuchs, L. S., & Fuchs, D., & Speece, D. L. (2002). Treatment validity as a unifying construct for identifying learning disabilities. *Learning Disability Quarterly, 25*, 33–46.

The article introduces the concept of student response to treatment as a basis for considering a student's eligibility for special education services.

Shinn, M. R. (Ed.). (1989). *Curriculum-based measurement: Assessing special children.* New York: Guilford Press.

This edited book contains chapters by original researchers summarizing the research and the procedures for using CBM in formative evaluation. The book serves as a resource for how CBM procedures are used in problem solving with students who have mild disabilities.

Shinn, M. R. (Ed.). (1998). *Advanced applications of curriculum-based measurement.* New York: Guilford Press.

This edited book contains chapters summarizing applications and extensions of CBM research and development to problems and issues not addressed in the original research on CBM.

PART II

♦ ♦ ♦

Defining Problems
Children Experience in Schools

♦

CHAPTER 3

◆ ◆ ◆

Ecological Variables in School-Based Assessment and Intervention Planning

◆

SUSAN M. SHERIDAN
MERILEE McCURDY

DEFINITION AND RATIONALE FOR ECOLOGICAL ASSESSMENT

Traditional assessment of child difficulties and disorders has permeated the fields of school psychology and special education for several decades. Traditional assessment activities have included individualized cognitive, academic, and psychological testing. For better or for worse, service models for children with atypical performance have required extensive assessment of a range of variables related to child functioning, including those within cognitive, academic, language, socioemotional, and behavioral domains. Following suit, funding streams in special education have been tied to numbers of children "qualifying" for special education services, which are often delivered via educational arrangements outside of the general educational classroom setting. Job positions for a plethora of "specialists" are thus created for professionals who can "staff" these pull-out programs by identifying children in need of legally determined special educational programming. In other words, the existence of special education services as programmatic service units with specialized staff is often dependent upon an appropriate number of qualifying children as determined by traditional, standardized, psychoeducational assessment methods. The degree to which the assessment methods inform service delivery within these settings is often secondary to the placement decision.

Recently, both special education and school psychology researchers have been vigilant in encouraging new models and alternative functional approaches to assist children with unique learning needs. Almost since the inception of the field, school psychologists have argued against "gatekeeper" functions and for assessment approaches that link directly to meaningful and effective interventions. The introduction of behavioral school psychology provided a fruitful and data-based opportunity to link assessment to intervention. However, even this approach in isolation fails to consider the breadth and depth of environmental and ecological complexities that interact with and relate to a child's learning and development.

We support an ecological–behavioral approach to assessment and intervention that blends the strengths of both ecological and behavioral theories. With this approach, children's learning and behavior are conceptualized as a function of ongoing interactions between the characteristics of the individuals and the multiple environments within which they function (Sheridan & Gutkin, 2000). Ecological–behavioral theory demands attention to the child and his or her behaviors, but only in relation to the systemic influences that surround the child when assessing concerns and developing interventions. This requires evaluating not only variables inherent in the child (e.g., aptitudes) but also environmental variables and the degree to which there is a "match" between the child and his or her environment (e.g., instruction, demands). The main objective of assessment from an ecological–behavioral perspective is to collect and use data that facilitate the development of solutions that can be effective long after the formal assessment procedures have been concluded. In other words, effective services within this paradigm build ecological systems that can support children, youth, schools, and families by linking assessment to intervention, addressing a mixture of ecological/contextual variables, using a problem-solving framework, and focusing on outcomes.

RATIONALE FOR ECOLOGICAL ASSESSMENT

The assessment of contextual variables in relation to student learning and achievement is essential from theoretical, empirical, and functional perspectives. Conceptually, it is clear that multiple ecological conditions support children's development. Ecological theory supports the notion that various factors within and across contexts influence learning (Bronfenbrenner,

1979). Microsystemic influences are those that relate to the immediate setting within which a child functions, such as the classroom *or* home. Instructional variables (e.g., the manner in which lessons are delivered) and the availability of reading materials in the home represent two forms of microsystemic influence. Mesosystemic factors include the multitude of relationships and interactions among the various microsystems (e.g., home *and* school), such as the relationships and communication frequency and patterns between parents and their child's teacher. Events in settings in which the child does not participate, but that affect his or her immediate microsystems, define the exosystem. Finally, the macrosystem is the overall cultural or subcultural patterns of which all the other systems are a part, such as federal legislation affecting instruction or specific economic forces affecting schools and families (e.g., the No Child Left Behind Act). For purposes of this chapter, we will focus on microsystems (i.e., classroom and home environments) and mesosystems (i.e., relationships among these microsystems) since they are most amenable to intervention.

Attention to ecological theory points to numerous reasons for the consideration of broad-based conditions when assessing a child's learning. Children do not learn in isolation; their development cannot be considered devoid of their rich and complex social and learning environments. Both home and school are contexts for learning; psychologists and assessors need to consider *both* to understand fully the range of factors that contribute to or impede their learning.

BACKGROUND: ECOLOGICAL SETTINGS FOR ASSESSMENT

School and Classroom Environments

Unequivocally, the school environment has a large impact on a child's life, and this impact can be positive or negative. Classrooms that benefit children and enhance academic performance share similar characteristics such as positive approaches to instructional planning, management, and delivery. Children succeed academically and behaviorally when schools and classrooms actively focus on and improve these components of a child's education (Ysseldyke & Elliott, 1999). Table 3.1 presents the ecological variables found in the school system that affect a student's academic performance.

Instructional Planning

For students to benefit from instruction, teaching strategies and individual academic interventions must match a student's achievement level. Students learn by first acquiring new information (i.e., accuracy) and then using the

TABLE 3.1. Ecological Variables Related to the School Environment and Assessment Indicators

Correlate	Indicators
Instructional planning	• Instruction matches the student's learning stage. • Instruction is individualized for each student. • Teachers have high and reasonable expectations regarding student progress. • Students are held accountable to meet expectations.
Instructional management	• Teachers are effective managers of child classroom behavior. • Classroom management is preventative and not reactive. • Rules are displayed in the classroom. • Consequences are available for meeting or breaking classroom rules.
Instructional delivery	• Teacher instruction is direct and clear. • Teacher uses examples and models expected academic skill use. • Instruction allows students to actively participate. • Instructional activities focus on increasing opportunities to accurately respond. • Students are provided guided practice and independent practice. • Corrective feedback is used. • Motivational strategies are employed to increase involvement.

information quickly (i.e., fluency). Upon mastery of these primary stages, newly learned information is applied across novel contexts (i.e., generalization) and in creative ways (i.e., adaptation). Specific interventions can be tailored to increase student proficiency in each stage by identifying where a student's abilities lie. For example, interventions that incorporate modeling, prompting, and error correction are known to increase accurate responding, while repeated practice and incentives are strategies that will increase fluent responding (Haring, Lovitt, Eaton, & Hansen, 1978). However, not all interventions are effective for all children. The application of an intervention that has been found generally to be effective through research (i.e., empirically validated interventions; Kratochwill & Stoiber, 2002) may not be effective for all students. The effectiveness of an intervention must be *individually* validated using brief experimental analysis, and the intervention must be demonstrated to increase accurate academic responding to be useful on an individual student basis (Daly, Martens, Hamler, Dool, & Eckert, 1999). Teachers should be cognizant of what information a student has mastered and what remains unknown to effectively match instruction to a student's position in the learning hierarchy (Ysseldyke & Elliott, 1999).

Regardless of student achievement level, high and realistic expectations are necessary components of effective instruction. Research reported in Bickel (1999) found that effective schools not only promoted high expectations regarding immediate student performance but also had high expectations for future performance. In general, classroom instructional activities should be found to be challenging by students but not confusing or frustrating (Brophy & Alleman, 1991). Additionally, students should be held accountable to these teacher expectations (Kagan, 1992).

Instructional Management

To meet academic expectations, students are most productive when they are supported by helpful teachers and instructed in a positive learning environment (Ysseldyke & Elliott, 1999). Effective teachers establish and enforce classroom rules and routines and monitor student behavior. Proactive teacher classroom management is one primary component of a positive learning environment (Berliner, 1988; Gettinger, 1988). Accordingly, teachers should use behavior management strategies to prevent classroom problems rather than react to inappropriate classroom behaviors. Additionally, the identification and teaching of classroom rules and expectations is a key component of effective instructional management.

Instructional Delivery

The majority of research on teacher behavior is focused on instructional presentation and delivery. Instructional presentation and delivery should be clear and organized, include activities that increase a child's academic engaged time and accurate responding, and provide corrective feedback in response to errors. The goal of effective teaching strategies and instructional delivery is to increase students' academic engaged time, which is the time a student spends accurately responding to academic materials (Skinner, 1998). Teacher presentation of information using clear and defined instructions is essential in increasing student academic performance. Clear and well-defined instructions are those in which "explanations of content proceed in a step-by-step fashion, illustrations and applications of the content are provided, and questions are posed to gauge and extend students' understanding" (Gettinger & Stoiber, 1999, p. 942).

Students with learning concerns require additional learning trials to master academic material, including more trials on which the child responds accurately (Skinner, 1998). To increase accurate responding, teachers should use procedures such as demonstration, modeling, cueing, and routine drills (Haring et al., 1978). Demonstration, modeling, and cueing are teaching procedures that increase the probability of accurate student responding. Additionally, routine drills (i.e., practice) will increase a child's opportunity to respond to instructional materials. Following the completion of an academic task during identified practice activities, students should be provided immediate feedback from teachers, parents, or peers

(Greenwood et al., 1987) regarding their performance. Additionally, self-monitoring procedures (Skinner, Turco, Beatty, & Rasavage, 1989; Vargas & Vargas, 1991) are effective in increasing feedback and can be useful in highly populated classrooms when immediate feedback from teachers is impossible.

Along with the classroom and school environments, another system that constitutes a major learning context in a child's life is the child's home environment. Additionally, constructive interactions among these environments are essential for a child with learning and academic concerns (Christenson & Sheridan, 2001).

The Home Environment as a Learning Environment

Decades of research have yielded unequivocal findings: variables within the home environment influence learning. There are many characteristics of home settings that create contexts for learning, thus emphasizing the importance of including the home as a focus of assessment and intervention. According to Walberg (1984), variables within the home environment (i.e., encouragement and discussion of reading, monitoring of television viewing, expression of affection, interest in children's academic and personal growth, delay of immediate gratification to achieve goals) constitute the curriculum of the home and have the potential for facilitating children's educational success. Process variables within the home—that is, what parents do with their children in relation to their education and learning—have been shown to predict achievement. Similarly, Clark (1983) identified home variables that differentiated high and low achievers. In particular, high achievers experienced home characteristics such as frequent parent–child dialogue, strong parental encouragement about academic pursuits, warm and nurturing interactions, clear and consistent limits, and consistent monitoring of how students spend their time.

Numerous factors within the home environment collectively constitute its potential to serve as a learning environment. So far, the only researchers to identify a specific set of requisite variables most influential to learning have been Peng and Lee (1992). These researchers identified the following as having the greatest relationship with student achievement in grades K–8: parental educational expectations, talking with children about school, providing learning materials, and providing learning opportunities outside of school. Furthermore, both parental attitudes and actions toward schooling are variables that appear related to learning and achievement. Parents of high achievers have been shown to feel personally responsible to help their children gain knowledge and literacy skills, communicate regularly with school personnel, and become involved in school functions and activities (Clark, 1983; Kellaghan, Sloane, Alvarez, & Bloom, 1993).

Early language and literacy experiences have been shown consistently to support learning and development (Hart & Risley, 1995; Ramey & Ramey, 1998). There now exists unequivocal support for the strong and positive relationships between language-rich early environments and academic success. Reading to young children, which often occurs in the home, promotes language acquisition and correlates with literacy development, achievement in reading comprehension, and general school success (Wells, 1985). Being read to has been identified as a source of children's prerequisite skill development, including knowledge about the alphabet, print, and characteristics of written language (Bus, van IJzendoorn, & Pellegrini, 1995; Snow, Burns, & Griffin, 1998).

Table 3.2 presents a number of home variables that are positively correlated with student learning, with common indicators that may be included in a comprehensive ecological assessment. Given the extensive range of variables within home environments that contribute to learning, attention to these and related school/classroom variables is essential to understand ecological environments and their relationship to achievement.

Home and School (Cross-Setting) Variables

Consistent with an ecological approach, mesosystemic (i.e., cross-setting) factors are important for understanding the complex nature of a child's performance. In addition to microsystemic influences, interactions between systems present contexts for learning. Given that children spend the majority of their waking hours in the home and school settings, the connections and relationships among them are central. The degree of continuity, or match, among systems is an important contributor to students' school success (Christenson & Sheridan, 2001). Continuity among home and school environments has been shown to be related to positive outcomes for students. Low-achieving students have been reported to experience discordance between the home and school systems (Phelan, Davidson, & Yu, 1998), with greater discontinuity among systems leading to declines in academic grades (Hansen, 1986). In a seminal study, Hansen (1986) demonstrated greater achievement gains from third to fifth grades for students who experienced congruence in rules and interaction styles between the home and school environments.

Related research has demonstrated the importance of cross-system coordination in interventions. Gains in student performance are greater when programs are implemented across home and school settings rather than in isolation. Research in conjoint behavioral consultation has yielded consistent findings pointing to the effectiveness of home and school continuity in intervention implementation. For example, Galloway and Sheridan (1994) reported a study in which students with inconsistent academic

TABLE 3.2. Ecological Variables Related to the Home Environment and Assessment Indicators

Correlate	Indicators
Structure and discipline orientation	• Priority is given to schoolwork, reading, and learning. • There is consistent parental monitoring of how time is spent. • Parents engage in an authoritative parenting style. • A reflective problem-solving style is used with children. • Children are encouraged to delay immediate gratification to accomplish long-term goals. • There is a routine for completing home tasks.
Support for learning	• Parents take responsibility for assisting children as learners. • Leisure reading is encouraged and discussed. • Learning is modeled by parents as they read and use math. • Parents attend school functions. • Television viewing is monitored and jointly analyzed. • Parents have knowledge of their child's current schoolwork and strengths and weaknesses in learning.
Positive, realistic expectations	• Expectations for child success are clear, positive, and realistic. • Parents convey the importance of effort and ability as key attributes for learning, rather than skill or luck. • Parents demonstrate interest in children's schoolwork. • Standards for performance are established and communicated.
Enriching environment	• Children's attention is continuously oriented toward learning opportunities. • Parents read with their children. • Enriching learning experiences are provided. • Learning materials and a place for study are available in the home.
Communication	• There is frequent dialogue between parent and child. • Parent and child engage in conversations about everyday events. • Parents provide opportunities for the development of good language habits. • Parents communicate regularly with school personnel.
Positive affective environment	• There are positive emotional interactions between parent and child. • Parent is responsive to child's developmental needs/skills. • Parents express affection for their child.

Note. From Christenson and Sheridan (2001). Copyright 2001 by The Guilford Press. Reprinted by permission.

performance responded more favorably and more consistently when parents and teachers shared in problem solving and intervention implementation (i.e., conjoint consultation) than when parents were only peripherally involved (i.e., were provided a manual and told what to do). Similarly, Sheridan, Kratochwill, and Elliott (1990) found that when parents were involved actively in consultation-based decision making, students' demonstration of important social skills were greater and longer-lasting than when consultation occurred in the school setting only.

Connections between home and school settings represent an important variable related to learning. Mesosystemic variables, or home *and* school interrelationships, are important contexts for development, and thus represent areas for ecological assessment. Christenson and Christenson (1998) reviewed over 200 studies that examined the relationship between family, school, and community influences and positive school performance (e.g., standardized test scores, grades, teacher ratings of academic performance, measures of school adjustment such as motivation to learn and attendance) for students in grades kindergarten through 12. Extensive similarity was identified in the contextual influences that enhanced student learning from the family, school, and community literatures. That is, there emerged a common set of contextual influences important for learning regardless of the child's immediate home or school setting. The cross-setting (i.e., school *and* home) variables related to optimal student outcomes, defined in Table 3.3 included: standards and expectations, structure, opportunity to learn, support, climate/relationships, and modeling.

ECOLOGICAL ASSESSMENT METHODS

Although multiple methods exist for collecting information from parents, teachers, students, and classrooms, the goals of the assessment process should remain similar. The overall goals of the ecological assessment process are to (1) identify important learning environments within which a child functions, (2) identify and assess target concerns exhibited within or across these systems, and (3) use assessment data to develop intervention plans for target concerns found in each setting. Methods related to each of these goals are explored next.

Identify Important Learning Environments

As emphasized above, home and school systems are primary contexts for learning. The inclusion of family members and school personnel in the assessment process promotes understanding of broad ecological conditions affecting a child's performance and increases the likelihood of successful intervention planning. As a service delivery model, Conjoint Behavioral

TABLE 3.3. Home and School Cross-Setting Variables Related to Positive
Learning Outcomes

Cross-setting variable	Definition
Shared standards and expectations	The level of expected performance held by key adults for the student is congruent across home and school and reflects a belief that the student can learn.
Consistent structure	The overall routine and monitoring provided by key adults for the student have been discussed and are congruent across home and school.
Cross-setting opportunity to learn	The variety of learning options available to the youth during school hours and outside of school time (i.e., home and community) supports the student's learning.
Mutual support	The guidance provided by, the communication between, and the interest shown by adults to facilitate student progress in school is effective. It is what adults do on an ongoing basis to help the student learn and achieve.
Positive, trusting relationships	The amount of warmth and friendliness; praise and recognition; and the degree to which the adult–youth relationship is positive and respectful. It includes how adults in the home, in the school and in the community work together to help the student be a learner.
Modeling	Parents and teachers demonstrate desired behaviors and commitment and value toward learning and working hard in their daily lives to the student.

Note. From Ysseldyke and Christenson (2002). Copyright 2002 by Sopris West. Reprinted by permission.

Consultation (CBC; Sheridan, Kratochwill, & Bergan, 1996) provides a framework for the provision of consultation services in which the family and school are mutually involved. CBC involves parents and teachers as joint consultees (i.e., consultation occurs with parents and teachers serving as co-consultees in the same meetings) and other systems within the child's environment (i.e., medical professionals, day care providers, academic tutors). As a model that links ecological assessment to intervention, CBC can be adopted readily to fulfill the objectives of the problem-solving framework described in Chapter 2 of this volume.

Identify and Assess Target Concerns

In conducting an ecological assessment of a child's academic concerns, multi-informant, multimeasure, multisetting assessments are essential. "Best practice" assessment procedures require that data be collected using multiple formats across settings. Procedures such as interviews, observations, rating scales, curriculum-based measurements, and reviews of permanent product data should be used.

The most complete assessment package to date, the Functional Assessment of Academic Behavior (FAAB; Ysseldyke & Christenson, 2002), provides a thorough assessment of home and school factors that influence a child's academic performance. The FAAB, previously The Instructional Environment Scale (TIES-II; Ysseldyke & Christenson, 1993), incorporates multiassessment measures such as interviews, observations of classroom environments, and instructional environment checklists to complete an ecological assessment of home and school variables related to academic performance. Specifically, the FAAB evaluates the supports, such as instructional supports, home supports, and home–school supports, that impact a child's academic behavior and performance. The steps of the FAAB are consistent with a problem-solving assessment and ecological approach, and include (1) identifying and clarifying the referral concern, (2) understanding the student's instructional needs from the perspective of the teacher and the parents, (3) collecting data on the student's instructional environment, (4) prioritizing and planning interventions to meet the student's instructional needs, and (5) identifying ways for increasing home support for learning. The FAAB also incorporates detailed evaluation of the treatment plan, plan revisions if necessary, and documentation forms to report treatment effects. Among the assessment forms are the Instructional Environment Checklist, the Instructional Environment Checklist: Annotated Version, the Instructional Needs Checklist, Parental Experience with Their Child's Learning and Schoolwork, and the Intervention Documentation Record.

In addition to the FAAB, specific ecological assessment methods are available. Multiinformant *interview formats* are common across several ecological assessment models. For example, CBC utilizes the Conjoint Problem Identification Interview, the Conjoint Problem Analysis Interview, and the Conjoint Treatment Evaluation Interview to gather information on shared concerns from individuals related to different environmental systems. In CBC, consultants interact with consultees to operationally define target behaviors, analyze conditions surrounding behaviors, and evaluate outcomes and goal attainment across settings. Other interview instruments, such as the Teacher Interview Form for Problem Validation and the Teacher Interview Form for a Functional Academic Assessment (Witt, Daly, & Noell, 2000), are useful to validate the existence of an academic problem and to determine the cause of a problem.

Classroom/teacher observations and *parent observations* are essential components of an ecological assessment. Information on the classroom structure, instructional materials, presentation of instructional activities, child behavior, and peer behavior can be assessed via direct classroom observations. The Classroom Observation Checklist for a Functional Academic Assessment and the Classroom Observation Grid (Witt et al., 2000) are available to analyze the academic environment through direct observations. Likewise, observation systems such as the Behavioral Observation of Students in Schools (BOSS; Shapiro, 2003) and the Ecobehavioral Assessment Systems Software (EBASS; Greenwood, Carta, Kamps, & Delquadri, 1992) are available to examine student behaviors, teacher behaviors, instructional materials, and the interactions among these variables. Parents can also collect observation data regarding their child's academic performance at home. For example, parents can collect data on homework variables such as their child's homework routine, the amount of time spent on homework, and the correctness of homework completed.

To examine a child's academic performance, *curriculum-based measurement* (Shapiro, 1996; Shinn, 1989, 1997) evaluates a child's performance in multiple academic skill areas and the child's performance in comparison to other children with similar learning expectations (i.e., to facilitate the collection of local normative data). Once a general assessment determines that a performance or skill deficit exists and that the significance of this deficit requires intervention, more intensive assessment can identify the specific skill area in need of remedial services.

Use Assessment Data to Develop Intervention Plans

The identification of a skill deficit and the recognition of a need for services does not mark the end of an ecological assessment. The data collected through interviews, observations, and curriculum-based measurement are useful for constructing interventions in each setting and evaluating the effects of those interventions. The inclusion of a variety of measurement sources will increase the utility of the assessment and will allow for a careful analysis of academic skill performance in each system. Following the identification of a specific skill deficit, a brief experimental analysis (Daly et al., 1999; Daly, Witt, Martens, & Dool, 1997) should be conducted to examine several interventions that could be effective in remediating the academic concern. Interventions should be chosen based on availability of resources, ease of implementation, and effectiveness. Additionally, an ecological assessment may identify other service providers in the community available to provide remedial services. Continual progress monitoring is required to determine the effectiveness of interventions implemented within and across settings.

For example, consider the case of a 10-year-old student referred to a school psychologist due to difficulties in mathematics. Through an ecological assessment procedure involving the child's family and school personnel, curriculum-based assessments identify that a skill deficit in mathematics does exist. Parent and teacher verbal reports identify the skill deficit as related to lack of homework completion, and an observation of classroom behavior indicates the lack of clear homework guidelines affecting the rates of homework completion. Unless data are gathered in each setting, useful information will be neglected and the most effective intervention may be overlooked.

CASE SCENARIO

A case scenario of an 8-year-old third-grade student (Jenny) is reviewed next. Due to inattention and lack of follow-through on tasks at school and home, Jenny was referred to a doctoral-level school psychology student completing a consultation practicum. The consultant in this case followed the methods of ecological problem solving, which consisted of the following methods: (1) identify important learning environments, (2) identify and assess target concerns within or across settings, and (3) use assessment data to develop intervention plans. An evaluation of the intervention plans was included as an additional problem-solving component.

Identify Important Learning Environments

Upon initial referral, the consultant explored possible environments in which Jenny's lack of attention and follow-through may have been interfering with her learning. Initial discussions with Jenny's teacher identified concerns related to general work behaviors, difficulty with attention and focus in the classroom, and persistent lack of homework being completed and returned to school. Given the teacher's statements related to performance both within the classroom and her expectations for uncompleted work to be finished at home, both the classroom and the home were identified as essential learning environments to be included in assessment and consultation. Therefore, conjoint behavioral consultation (Sheridan et al., 1996) services were provided, with the school psychologist serving as a consultant and the parent and teacher serving as joint consultees.

Identify and Assess Target Concerns within and across Systems

A number of assessment methods were used to identify and assess target concerns at both home and school. The assessment process was conceptualized within a multimethod, multisource, multisetting framework, within the context of joint and collaborative problem solving. Specifically, structured conjoint behavioral interviews were conducted, followed by behavioral rating scales, direct observations, and work samples.

Conjoint Behavioral Interviews

A series of structured interviews were conducted, with Jenny's mother and teacher serving as joint consultees. The first was a conjoint Problem Identification Interview (PII), in which Jenny's strengths were identified, as were concerns about her academic performance. Through open-ended strategic questioning by the consultant, it was determined that Jenny's lack of attention and follow-through were areas in need of consideration. Specifically, at school Jenny was reported to have difficulty attending to tasks and completing work. At home, starting homework and completing it in a timely and focused manner was reportedly problematic. In addition, behaviors suggestive of noncompliance with work were beginning to emerge, such as arguing and lying about homework.

Observations

Several forms of observations were conducted to assess Jenny's attention to and follow-through with tasks. First, the Instructional Environment Checklist of the Functional Assessment of Academic Behavior (FAAB) system (Ysseldyke & Christenson, 2002) was completed by the consultant. Through this assessment, important contextual features of the instructional environment were revealed. Specifically, the consultant noted that Jenny had difficulties transitioning from one activity to the next. Reading instruction occurred following math periods, during which students often worked in small groups at stations with manipulable objects (e.g., stacking towers, play money) or worked independently in workbooks. Teacher directives to end math activities and begin reading tasks (i.e., take out books, wait for the reading group to be called) often required several minutes for Jenny. Instructions related to assignments, expectations, and other task demands occurred during this transition, when Jenny was searching for the appropriate books, looking for writing utensils, or otherwise engaging in behaviors to prepare herself for the task. Therefore, Jenny did not appear to be focused on learning or prepared for academic engagement during the transitional period.

Observations revealed that instructions provided to Jenny were of a verbal nature, with no modeling or demonstrations by the teacher. Directions on worksheets or reading materials were written, and no modifications were made to meet Jenny's needs. Unplanned modifications, such as peers reading directions for Jenny, assisted her in initiating and completing the tasks. Likewise, clear instructions regarding completion expectations (e.g., "you need to be finished before recess") appeared to provide structure and assist in work completion.

In addition to consultant observations, Jenny's teacher collected data daily on Jenny's on-task behavior. Specifically, she self-recorded the number of times Jenny had to be reminded to engage in an academic task during the selected setting of reading instruction. During a baseline period of 1 week, Jenny's teacher reported prompts to return to task an average of 4 times per day during reading.

Jenny's mother reported on expectations for homework and Jenny's behaviors during evening homework time. Her mother stated that there was inconsistency in establishing and maintaining rules around homework activities. That is, there did not appear to be a structured time or location to complete homework, and several distractions often interfered with homework completion (e.g., television shows, sibling conflicts). Arguments about homework were common between Jenny and her mother, with most discussions about school being negative.

Jenny's mother recorded her work behaviors during homework. First, she recorded how long it took Jenny to begin working on homework following the first prompt and how long it took for her to complete all assigned work. Similarly, she recorded the number of times Jenny needed to be reminded to work. During 1 week of baseline, Jenny's mother reported that she routinely failed to begin homework when given the instruction, with an average of 40 minutes elapsing between initial instruction and initiation of work.

Brief Curriculum-Based Assessment

A brief curriculum-based assessment (CBA; Shapiro, 1996) was conducted to assess Jenny's level of reading performance. Specifically, a reading passage from the third-grade curriculum was administered by asking Jenny to read for 1 minute. Words read correctly and errors were recorded. On this assessment, Jenny read 27 words correctly in 1 minute with two errors. The same probe was administered to a classroom peer exhibiting average reading performance and classroom behavior. The comparison peer read 64 words correctly per minute with 0 errors. The assessment indicated that although Jenny read the passage with accuracy she had difficulty reading the material quickly (i.e., reading fluency).

Rating Scales

To determine the extent of the concerns related to Jenny's inattentiveness and difficulties with work completion, the Behavioral Assessment Scale for Children (BASC), the Child Behavior Checklist—Parent Report Form (CBCL-PRF), and the Child Behavior Checklist—Teacher Report Form (CBCL-TRF) were administered to her mother and teacher. On these scales, Jenny was noted to exhibit clinically significant levels of attention problems. It was reported that she failed to finish things, couldn't concentrate or pay attention for long periods of time, couldn't sit still, produced poor schoolwork, gave up easily when learning something new, had a short attention span, forgot things, and was inattentive or easily distracted. Additionally, at school she was reported as having difficulty learning and talking out of turn. At home, she was reported to rarely complete homework from start to finish without breaks, and failed to complete work on time. In addition, clinically significant levels of learning problems were noted on the BASC. Items endorsed by her teacher included that Jenny did not complete tasks, made careless errors, received failing grades, had spelling and reading problems, and had poor handwriting and printing.

Use Assessment Data to Develop Intervention Plans

As part of the problem-solving process, a conjoint Problem Analysis Interview (PAI) was conducted with Jenny's mother and teacher. The purposes of the interview were to (1) evaluate the baseline data to determine the existence of a concern in need of intervention; (2) propose hypotheses related to the target behavior, which could lead to the development of an effective intervention; and (3) develop an intervention plan to be implemented across home and school settings.

Evaluate Baseline Data

The baseline data were evaluated, and it was noted that an average of four prompts were provided at school, requesting that she "get to work," or "get back to work." Similarly, at home, Jenny required an average of 40 minutes to begin homework. Homework took, on average, 2 hours to complete. She required approximately four redirections to "get back to work." If after 2 hours Jenny's homework was not completed, her mother typically allowed her to stop working.

Within reading instruction, two distinct activities were common: independent seat reading (including reading passages and completing worksheets), and small group reading instruction. Once independent work time began, it often took Jenny 10 minutes to initiate her work. Common behaviors during independent work time included looking at peers, searching in her desk, dropping objects, and walking across the classroom. During small group reading instruction, Jenny often looked at her peers or around the classroom. When instructed to read, she often did not know where to begin and then read slowly with several errors. An average of four prompts to return to work was required by Jenny's teacher during each reading period.

An analysis of Jenny's reading performance on the brief CBA revealed slow reading speed. Jenny was observed to read very slowly and hesitate when pronouncing words. She successfully sounded out words; however, she often required one to two seconds to decode unfamiliar words. At times Jenny lost her place in the passage and required redirection.

Develop Hypotheses

Given the interview, observation, CBA, and rating scale data, it was hypothesized that Jenny's inattention to tasks was related to several factors. Specifically, in analyzing the data jointly, the consultant, teacher, and parent identified three areas interfering with her performance: lack of skill in reading at the expected level, lack of organization related to work tasks (including not having the necessary tools in an organized and accessible manner, and lack of structure), and distractibility during instruction and work time (leading to a lack of knowledge and understanding about task expectations and demands). An intervention was needed that would ensure that she understood the tasks that were expected of her, had the necessary materials to complete the tasks, worked in a homework environment that was structured and free from distractions, and acquired the skills to complete the expected work (i.e., reading fluency).

Develop Intervention Plan

A multicomponent intervention package was developed to address these areas. First, the reading period was changed to the first class of the day, to minimize difficult transitions from an active math class. Second, clear instructions were provided at the beginning of reading after ensuring that Jenny was attending to the teacher (rather than looking for materials or engaging in other off-task behaviors). The reading activity instructions were modeled by the teacher, who demonstrated how to complete steps of the task for the entire class. A visual cue was placed on Jenny's desk, with clear expectations provided for the length of the task (e.g., page numbers) and time at which the task should be completed (e.g., before recess). Picture cues were provided on the chart to minimize reading demands.

During large group work, Jenny was paired with a peer to allow her to have directions re-read to her as necessary and to ask for help. The peer also modeled effective work behaviors and gave Jenny cues to return to work when necessary. Similarly, in small reading groups, directions were stated to Jenny, using eye contact and close physical proximity. Jenny was allowed to read first to minimize extraneous distractions. Praise was provided frequently for remaining on task and for her reading performance.

To increase fluent reading, a school volunteer read with Jenny four times per week for 20 minutes each day. The reading period incorporated increased repeated practice with classroom reading materials. While reading with the volunteer, Jenny was asked to read the daily story until she reached mastery levels (i.e., 60–70 correct words per minute). If she made any errors, the volunteer stated the word correctly and asked Jenny to repeat the word correctly three times. Jenny was then directed to re-read the entire sentence with the mispronounced word and continue reading the story.

At home, the intervention included three components. First, a structured homework time free from distractions was provided. A set homework time (i.e., 6:30–7:30 P.M.) was established, and Jenny sat at a desk in a room apart from family activities to complete her work. Her mother was in close proximity to provide assistance as necessary and to praise her for working on task during the homework time. Second, clear and positively stated directives were provided by her mother that clarified both expectations (e.g., "Finish the reading worksheet") and positive consequences (e.g., "You can go outside and play after finishing homework"). Finally, a contingency plan was developed wherein Jenny received a predetermined special privilege (i.e., game with mother, play outside with friends, ice cream dessert) each night that she completed her work with two or fewer redirections.

Plan Evaluation

Two weeks following the conjoint Problem Analysis Interview (PAI), a Treatment Evaluation Interview (TEI) was conducted with the consultant and Jenny's mother and teacher present. At home, Jenny's mother reported that the increased structure and attention to desired behaviors (via praise and a contingency plan) resulted in Jenny starting her homework within 5 minutes of her initial instruction and remaining on task without multiple prompts. Specifically, on average Jenny required only two prompts per night to return to task, and to complete homework within the allotted time. However, her mother noted that she continued to need assistance in reading assignment directions and various items on her worksheets.

Data that were collected by Jenny's teacher revealed that the number of prompts required to assist Jenny in returning to task were reduced by 50% at school. That is, Jenny's teacher reported that the intervention (i.e., changing the time of reading to reduce the need for transitions, providing clear instructions, allowing for peer support) resulted in a decrease in prompts to two per day. In small reading groups, Jenny was allowed to be the first to initiate reading, thus precluding the need for prompts and redirections. However, her teacher reported that Jenny continued to read slowly, and modifications to the plan were discussed. Specifically, school passages were re-read with Jenny's mother at home, and this task was added to the contingency plan. This was expected to increase Jenny's proficiency in reading and aid fluency.

SUMMARY

Ecological approaches to assessment, consultation, and intervention represent the present and future of service delivery in an increasingly evidence-based educational climate. Understanding school and home influences on learning, and the intersections among these and related systems in a child's life, remains at the cornerstone of the ecological model. The assessment of ecological variables represents "best practices" in educational planning and problem solving, with emphasis on evidence-based models of practice. Specifically, ecological practices support the (1) identification of important learning environments, (2) assessment of target concerns within or across settings, (3) use of assessment data to develop intervention plans consistent with data-based hypotheses, and (4) evaluation of interventions implemented across settings. Within this comprehensive framework, services can extend beyond child-focused "problems" and strengthen the multiple interconnected ecologies influencing learning and development.

ACKNOWLEDGMENTS

The preparation of this chapter was supported in part by a grant provided to Susan M. Sheridan by the U.S. Department of Education, Office of Special Education Programs. The opinions stated herein are those of the authors and do not reflect the funding agency. We would like to acknowledge M. Kelly Haack, who served as consultant in the case study and granted permission to include case information to illustrate ecological assessment and conjoint consultation in practice.

REFERENCES

Berliner, D. C. (1988). Effective classroom management and instruction: A knowledge base for consultation. In J. L. Graden, J. E. Zins, & M. C. Curtis (Eds.), *Alternative educational delivery systems: Enhancing instructional options for all students* (pp. 309–325). Washington, DC: National Association of School Psychologists.

Bickel, W. E. (1999). The implications of the effective schools literature for school restructuring. In C. R. Reynolds & T. B. Gutkin (Eds.), *The handbook of school psychology* (pp. 959–983). New York: Wiley.

Bronfenbrenner, U. (1979). *The ecology of human development.* Cambridge, MA: Harvard University Press.

Brophy, J., & Alleman, J. (1991). Activities as instructional tools: A framework for analysis and evaluation. *Educational Researcher, 20*(4), 9–23.

Bus, A. G., van IJzendoorn, M. H., & Pellegrini, A. (1995). Joint book reading makes for success in learning to read: A meta-analysis of intergenerational transmission of literacy. *Review of Educational Research, 65,* 1–21.

Christenson, S. L., & Christenson, C. J. (1998). *Family, school, and community influences on children's learning: A literature review* (Report No. 1, Live and Learn Project). Minneapolis: University of Minnesota Extension Service.

Christenson, S. L., & Sheridan, S. M. (2001). *Schools and families: Creating essential connections for learning.* New York: Guilford Press.

Clark, R. M. (1983). *Family life and school achievement.* Chicago: University of Chicago Press.

Daly, E. J., III, Martens, B. K., Hamler, K. R., Dool, E. J., & Eckert, T. L. (1999). A brief experimental analysis for identifying instructional components needed to improve oral reading fluency. *Journal of Applied Behavior Analysis, 32,* 83–94.

Daly, E., J., III, Witt, J. C., Martens, B. K., & Dool, E. J. (1997). A model for conducting a functional analysis of academic performance in the schools. *School Psychology Review, 26,* 554–574.

Galloway, J., & Sheridan, S. M. (1994). Implementing scientific practices through case studies: Examples using home-school interventions and consultation. *Journal of School Psychology, 32,* 385–413.

Gettinger, M. (1988). Methods of proactive classroom management. *School Psychology Review, 17,* 227–242.

Gettinger, M., & Stoiber, K. C. (1999). Excellence in teaching: Review of instructional and environmental variables. In C. R. Reynolds & T. B. Gutkin (Eds.), *The handbook of school psychology* (3rd ed., pp. 933–958). New York: Wiley.

Greenwood, C. R., Carta, J. J., Kamps, D., & Delquadri, J. (1992). *Ecobehavioral Assessment Systems Software (EBASS): Practitioners' manual.* Kansas City: Juniper Gardens Children's Project, University of Kansas.

Greenwood, C. R., Dinwiddie, G., Terry, B., Wade, L., Stanley, S. O., Thibadeau, S., & Delquadri, J. C. (1987). Teacher versus peer-mediated instruction: An ecobehavioral analysis of achievement outcomes. *Journal of Applied Behavior Analysis, 17,* 521–538.

Hansen, D. A. (1986). Family–school articulations: The effects of interaction rule mismatch. *American Educational Research Journal, 23,* 643–659.

Haring, N. G., Lovitt, T. C., Eaton, M. D., & Hansen, C. L. (1978). *The fourth R: Research in the classroom.* Columbus, OH: Merrill.

Hart, B., & Risley, T. R. (1995). *Meaningful differences in the everyday experience of young American children.* Baltimore: Brookes.

Kagan, D. M. (1992). Implications of research on teacher belief. *Educational Psychologist, 27,* 65–90.

Kellaghan, T., Sloane, K., Alvarez, B., & Bloom, B. S. (1993). *The home environment and school learning: Promoting parental involvement in the education of children.* San Francisco: Jossey-Bass.

Kratochwill, T. R., & Stoiber, K. C. (2002). Evidence-based interventions in school psychology: Conceptual foundations of the procedural and coding manual of Division 16 and the Society for the Study of School Psychology Task Force. *School Psychology Quarterly, 17,* 1–55.

Peng, S. S., & Lee, R. M. (1992, April). *Home variables, parent–child activities, and academic achievement: A study of 1988 eighth graders.* Paper presented at the annual meeting of the American Educational Research Association, San Francisco.

Phelan, P., Davidson, A. L., & Yu, H. C. (1998). *Adolescents' worlds: Negotiating family, peers, and school.* New York: Teachers College Press.

Ramey, C. T., & Ramey, S. L. (1998). Early intervention and early experience. *American Psychologist, 53,* 109–120.

Shapiro, E. S. (1996). *Academic skills problems: Direct assessment and intervention* (2nd ed.). New York: Guilford Press.

Shapiro, E. S. (2003). *Behavior observation of students in schools (BOSS).* San Antonio, TX: Harcourt Assessment.

Sheridan, S. M., & Gutkin, T. B. (2000). The ecology of school psychology: Examining and changing our paradigm for the 21st century. *School Psychology Review, 29,* 485–502.

Sheridan, S. M., Kratochwill, T. R., & Bergan, J. R. (1996). *Conjoint behavioral consultation: A procedural manual.* New York: Plenum Press.

Sheridan, S. M., Kratochwill, T. R., & Elliott, S. N. (1990). Behavioral consultation with parents and teachers: Delivering treatment for socially withdrawn children at home and school. *School Psychology Review, 19,* 33–52.

Shinn, M. R. (1989). *Curriculum-based measurement: Assessing special children.* New York: Guilford Press.

Shinn, M. R. (Ed.). (1998). *Advanced applications of curriculum-based measurement.* New York: Guilford Press.

Skinner, C. H. (1998). Preventing academic skills deficits. In T. S. Watson & F. M. Gresham (Eds.), *Handbook of child behavior therapy: Issues in clinic child psychology* (pp. 61–82). New York: Plenum Press.

Skinner, C. H., Turco, T. L., Beatty, K., & Rasavage, C. (1989). Copy, cover, compare: A method for increasing multiplication fluency in behavior disordered children. *School Psychology Review, 14,* 412–420.

Snow, C. E., Burns, M. S., & Griffin, P. (Eds.). (1998). *Preventing reading difficulties in young children.* Washington, DC: National Academy Press.

Vargas, E. A., & Vargas, J. S. (1991). Programmed instruction: What it is and how to do it. *Journal of Behavioral Education, 1,* 235–251.

Walberg, H. J. (1984). Families as partners in educational productivity. *Phi Delta Kappan, 65,* 397–400.

Wells, C. B. (1985). Preschool literacy-related activities and success in school. In M. P. Olson, D. N. Terrance, & A. Hildyard (Eds.), *Literacy, language and learning: The nature and consequences of literacy* (pp. 229–255). Cambridge, UK: Cambridge University Press.

Witt, J. C., Daly, E. M., & Noell, G. (2000). *Functional assessments: A step-by-step guide to solving academic and behavior problems.* Longmont, CO: Sopris West.

Ysseldyke, J. E., & Christenson, S. L. (1993). *The Instructional Environment Scale—II.* Longmont, CO: Sopris West.

Ysseldyke, J. E., & Christenson, S. L. (2002). *Functional Assessment of Academic Behavior (FAAB): Creating successful learning environments.* Longmont, CO: Sopris West.

Ysseldyke, J. E., & Elliott, J. (1999). Effective instructional practices: Implications for assessing educational environments. In C. R. Reynolds & T. B. Gutkin (Eds.), *The handbook of school psychology* (pp. 497–518). New York: Wiley.

SUGGESTED READINGS

Sheridan, S. M., Kratochwill, T. R., & Bergan, J. R. (1996). *Conjoint behavioral consultation: A procedural manual.* New York: Plenum.

This book provides a thorough summary of the procedures involved in Conjoint Behavioral Consultation (CBC), including models for working with parents, the stages of CBC process, and the research supporting the use of CBC. In addition, five case examples are provided to describe ecological models of service delivery.

Ysseldyke, J. E., & Christenson, S. L. (2002). *Functional Assessment of Academic Behavior (FAAB): Creating successful learning environments.* Longmont, CO: Sopris West.

The FAAB is a technical manual that provides step-by-step instructions for implementation of an ecological assessment including essential home and school variables that influence a child's academic performance. The FAAB incorporates multi-assessment measures such as interviews, observations of classroom environments, and instructional environment checklists necessary to complete an ecological assessment.

Ysseldyke, J. E., & Elliott, J. (1999). Effective instructional practices: Implications for assessing educational environments. In C. R. Reynolds & T. B. Gutkin (Eds.), *The handbook of school psychology, 3rd edition* (pp. 497–518). New York: Wiley.

This chapter provides a detailed review of components in the educational environment that influence student learning and academic performance. Additionally, it provides a rationale for the assessment of academic environments and provides examples of methodologies that are useful in the assessment of environmental factors affecting academic outcomes.

CHAPTER 4

◆ ◆ ◆

The Role of Teacher Perspectives in Diagnostic and Program Evaluation Decision Making

◆

TANYA L. ECKERT
LAUREN A. ARBOLINO

Valid and reliable assessments of students' academic skills have been identified as one of the most fundamental variables related to effective educational decision making and positive student outcomes (Fuchs & Fuchs, 1986; Shinn, 1989; Ysseldyke & Christenson, 1987). Given the importance of academic assessment, a variety of approaches and measures can be employed to evaluate students' academic skills. The role of teachers' perspectives relating to students' academic achievement plays a primary role in assessment and intervention activities. In this chapter, we describe how indirect and direct forms of academic assessment that incorporate teachers' perspectives can be used in a problem-solving model of assessment. Specifically, teachers' estimates of students' academic skills can provide information about students' general academic functioning (i.e., problem identification) as well as comparative information about students' academic functioning in relation to expected functioning (i.e., problem definition).

The purpose of this chapter is to review and evaluate a number of indirect and direct forms of academic assessment that incorporates teachers' perspectives. Specifically, general teacher estimates of students' academic achievement, standardized teacher estimates of students' academic achievement, and authentic assessment, which includes product assessment, portfolio assessment, and performance assessment, are reviewed. Information pertaining to the development and structure of each form of academic assessment is presented descriptively. The research evidence supporting the use of these forms of academic assessment is discussed. In addition, each assessment method is described in the context of a problem-solving model for assessment (Deno, 1989). Finally, we present a brief scenario to illustrate the use of indirect and direct forms of academic assessment that incorporates teachers' perspectives. Standardized teacher estimates of students' academic achievement and performance assessment are highlighted in this case scenario.

BACKGROUND

Approximately 40% of school-age children experience academic difficulties during their school experience, with a smaller percentage (10–12%) of school-age children experiencing academic difficulties severe enough to be considered eligible for special education services (National Institute of Child Health and Human Development, 2000). Typically, general education teachers are the foremost school personnel to recognize that a student is experiencing an academic problem (Salvia & Ysseldyke, 2004). For example, a teacher may notice that a student's skill level is declining or cannot be maintained in the classroom. As a result, the teacher may attempt to remediate the student's skills by providing additional instructional assistance in the general education classroom. If the teacher is unable to address the student's needs, he or she may seek formal assistance from school personnel or refer the student for special education consideration (Salvia & Ysseldyke, 2004). Regardless of the type of referral initiated by teachers (i.e., prereferral team, multidisciplinary evaluation referral), the role of teachers' perspectives relating to students' academic achievement plays a primary role in a problem-solving model of assessment.

Teachers' judgments of students' academic achievement are often based on repeated classroom observations that have been collected over time (Gerber & Semmel, 1984; Gresham, MacMillan, & Bocian, 1997). As a result, it has been argued that a teacher's judgment of students' academic achievement is one of the primary factors related to positive student outcomes (Gresham et al., 1997; Hoge, 1983; Hoge & Coladarci, 1989). For example, teachers often make daily decisions regarding the selection of instructional materials, teaching strategies, and student-learning groups based on their perceptions of how students are achieving in their classroom (Sharpley & Edgar, 1986). In addition, teachers' instructional decision making is often related to their perceptions of students' comprehension during classroom activities (Clark & Peterson, 1986; McNair, 1978). Furthermore, teachers are mainly responsible for identifying students with sufficiently severe learning difficulties to warrant consideration for special education services (Gresham et al., 1997; Salvia & Ysseldyke, 2004). For example, the first step in most school-based service delivery models is referral, which is generated by the classroom teacher (Shapiro & Kratochwill, 2000). Therefore, the role of teachers' perspectives related to students' academic achievement plays a primary role in diagnostic and program evaluation decision making (Feinberg & Shapiro, 2003).

Teachers' perspectives of students experiencing learning difficulties are largely the result of a perceived discrepancy between what constitutes acceptable and unacceptable academic performance (Merrell, 1999). This may be determined based on a student's performance in one core skill area, such as reading, or based on a comparative assessment of a student's level of functioning in relation to the peer group. For example, if a student cannot be successfully maintained in the lowest instructional group in a classroom, the teacher may determine that the student as experiencing a severe learning difficulty (Salvia & Ysseldyke, 2004). This decision is predominately based on teacher observations and assessments of the student's academic achievement.

A variety of assessment approaches and measures can be employed by a teacher to evaluate a student's academic achievement (Sattler, 2001). Based on the degree to which the assessment approach measures the target behavior and the manner in which the target behavior has been measured, assessment approaches can be conceptualized along a continuum, ranging from indirect to direct methods (Cone, 1978; Shapiro & Kratochwill, 2000). For example, teacher reports and interviews represent indirect forms of academic assessment, whereas self-observations or analogue assessments of students' academic achievement represent direct forms of academic assessment. In sum, teachers' perceptions of students' academic skills can incorporate indirect or direct assessment methods. Each of these assessment methods will be described in further detail.

Indirect Forms of Academic Assessment

Indirect forms of academic assessment require teachers to report their global perceptions of students' academic performance as it occurs in the natural environment or in an analogue setting (Kratochwill & Shapiro, 2000). This form of assessment is considered to be more circuitous, in that teachers are removed from the naturally occurring environment and responses are gathered at a point in time when the students' academic behaviors are typically not occurring. Examples of indirect forms of academic assessment include conducting an informal interview with a teacher regarding a student's academic skills (i.e., general teacher estimates of student performance) or asking a teacher to complete a standardized rating scale pertaining to a student's academic skills (i.e., standardized teacher estimates of student performance) (Shapiro, 1996). In both of these cases, indirect teacher judgments are obtained pertaining to a student's academic performance (Wright & Wiese, 1988).

General Teacher Estimates of Students' Academic Achievement

General teacher estimates of students' academic performance are commonly reported to parents and other school professionals in the form of grades or other evaluation standards (Feinberg & Shapiro, 2003) and are often mandated as part of the decision-making process (Gerber & Semmel, 1984). When teachers provide a general estimate of a student's academic achievement, it may be based on an informal examination of a student's achievement over a limited period of time (e.g., weeks) or it may be based on repeated observations of a student's achievement over an extended period of time (e.g., months) (Gerber & Semmel, 1984; Gresham et al., 1987). In addition, the manner in which a teacher provides a general estimate of student achievement may vary considerably. For example, teachers may provide a general estimate based on a student's skills relative to the peer group (Luce & Hoge, 1978) or based on a student's instructional level (Oliver & Arnold, 1978).

Standardized Teacher Estimates of Students' Academic Achievement

Standardized teacher estimates of students' academic achievement requires teachers to respond to a series of items or questions pertaining to student' academic achievement during a specified period of time. A number of different response formats may be used on a standardized measure. For example, a teacher may provide a proficiency rating, such as estimating whether a student's academic skill is "far below grade level" or "far above grade level." In other instances, a teacher may be required to provide a frequency rating for a student's academic skill that may range from "never" to "almost always." Furthermore, a teacher may be asked to provide a qualitative rating, such as "poor" or "excellent" relative to a student's academic skill level.

Indirect Forms of Academic Assessment: Research Evidence and Implications

Research examining the relationship between teacher estimates of students' academic achievement and standardized measures of student achievement demonstrates moderate to high levels of correspondence (Hoge, 1983;

Hoge & Coladarci, 1989). In a synthesis of 16 empirical studies examining the correspondence between teacher estimates of students' academic achievement and standardized measures of academic achievement, Hoge and Coladarci found the median correlation between ratings and achievement measures was .66. However, a stronger relationship between direct teacher judgments of student achievement (i.e., standardized teacher estimates; range, $r = .48$ to .92) as compared to indirect teacher judgments of student achievement (i.e., general teacher estimates; range, $r = .29$ to .86) was reported. Given that general teacher estimates were less strongly associated with actual student achievement than standardized teacher estimates, it appears that more reliable indications of students' academic skills are obtained when standardized teacher estimates are used as part of a problem-solving model of academic assessment.

Two recent studies have increased our knowledge and understanding of using teachers' perspectives as part of a problem-solving assessment. Kenny and Chekaluk (1993) examined the relationship between teacher ratings of students' reading skills and a battery of standardized reading measures with a sample of 312 elementary-age students in kindergarten through second grade. These researchers found that the strength of relationship between ratings and standardized measures increased from kindergarten to second grade. These results suggest that standardized teacher estimates of students' reading skills may be more reliable as the students' grade level increases. That is, more confidence can be placed in teachers' estimates of students' reading skills after second grade than during the early elementary grades.

In another study, Demaray and Elliott (1998) examined the relationship between two types of standardized teacher ratings and a standardized measure of academic achievement. Twelve teachers estimated the academic competence of 47 students using the Academic Competence Scale of the SSRS (Gresham & Elliott, 1990) and then rated each student's performance on an item-by-item basis on the Kaufman Test of Educational Achievement Brief Form (K-TEA; Kaufman & Kaufman, 1985). A high correlation between teachers' standardized ratings on the Academic Competence Scale of the SSRS and the K-TEA was obtained (.70) as well as between teachers' predictions of students' performance on individual items of the K-TEA (.79). These results suggest teachers' perspectives of students' academic skills can be slightly enhanced if more explicit information is provided regarding the specific content of the academic area targeted.

Finally, Gresham and colleagues (1997) examined the relationship between standardized teacher ratings on the Academic Competence Scale of the SSRS (Gresham & Elliott, 1990), general teacher ratings relating to special education disability categories, and actual student placement in special education disability categories. Teachers rated students in second through fourth grades who had been referred due to academic skills problems according to three categories: learning disabilities (n = 47), low achievement (n = 60), and low cognitive ability (n = 43). In addition, each teacher rated a comparison group of typical students who did not display academic skill problems (n = 90). The results of this study indicated that teachers were able to predict student group membership with 95% accuracy. However, the standardized ratings on the Academic Competence Scale of the SSRS did not distinguish among the three groups. As a result, these findings suggest that teachers' ratings may not be reliable in identifying specific educational disability categories among children experiencing academic skills problems.

Direct Forms of Academic Assessment

Direct forms of academic assessment necessitate the observation of a student's academic performance in the naturally occurring environment or in an analogue setting (Kratochwill & Shapiro, 2000). This form of assessment is considered to be more exact, in that teachers are requested to assess a student's academic performance in the naturally occurring environment while the student is engaging or has engaged in the relevant academic behaviors. Examples of direct forms of academic assessment include asking a teacher to evaluate a student's academic performance based on a sample of the student's classroom work or having a student compile a portfolio of work samples for teacher evaluation. Teachers' evaluations of classroom work samples provides a direct contrast between teachers' judgments and actual student achievement, and is considered to be one type of authentic assessment (Archbald, 1991).

Authentic Assessment

Authentic assessment involves teacher evaluation of original student work samples (Elliott, 1991; Radcliff, 2001) and can be divided into three subtypes: (1) product assessment, (2) portfolio assessment, and (3) performance assessment (Schurr, 1998). Product assessment requires a student to provide some type of concrete evidence that a specific ability or concept has been learned and applied. Generally, product assessment can be conceptualized as a form of criterion-referenced assessment. For example, a student could demonstrate that a science concept has been learned and applied by developing a videotape on the concept or writing a report on the concept. Conversely, portfolio assessment is defined as a cross-curricular collection of student work samples that demonstrates a student's achievement, creativity, and effort across a number of scholastic domains (Herman, 1998). For example, student portfolios may contain paper-and-pencil tests, writing assignments, graphs, worksheets, or drawings. Finally, performance assessment focuses on the process of student learning by observing student performance on an analogue task (Guskey, 1994). For example, specific tasks are identified, and a student's performance is observed and assessed by the teacher (Stiggins, 1997).

Each of these subtypes of authentic assessment can provide information that is useful during the problem-solving process. A product assessment can be used to explore whether a student is experiencing a specific skill deficit in the classroom. The extent to which a student can demonstrate that a skill has been mastered and can be applied in the classroom assists in providing information about students' general academic functioning. Portfolio assessment can be used to examine the processes of a student's learning in the classroom, and the final products included in the portfolio can be examined as part of a permanent product assessment. A performance assessment can be used to verify whether a student is experiencing academic difficulties and examining the extent to which the academic difficulties are interfering with other aspects of a student's educational experience. Of these three subtypes of authentic assessment, performance assessment has received the most attention within the context of a problem-solving approach to academic assessment (Fuchs & Fuchs, 2000; Shapiro & Elliott, 1999). Therefore, for the purposes of this chapter we will focus on performance assessment as one type of authentic assessment.

Historically, performance assessment has emphasized (1) specifying the area of performance that will be evaluated, (2) developing tasks to elicit the specified area of performance, and (3) creating an evaluation system for observing and recording performance (Stiggins, 1997). More recent applications of performance assessment have included (1) identifying tasks that are aligned to classroom instruction, (2) informing students of the evaluation system, (3) providing explicit models of acceptable performance, (4) promoting student self-evaluations of performance, and (5) comparing students' performance to normative standards (Elliott, 1998; Shapiro & Elliott, 1999). Many forms of performance assessment have been reported in the literature (Archbald & Newmann, 1988; Baker, 1991; Brewer, 1991; Sammons, Kobett, Heiss, & Fennell, 1992), and two specific models of performance assessment have recently emerged in the areas of spelling (Elliott & Bischoff-Werner, 1995; Olson, 1995) and mathematics (Fuchs & Fuchs, 2000).

Direct Forms of Academic Assessment: Research Evidence and Implications

Although many advantages associated with authentic assessment have been reported (Archbald, 1991; Christenson, 1991; Kamphaus, 1991), there is a lack of empirical evidence regarding the psychometric properties of authentic assessment methods (Baker, O'Neil, & Linn, 1993; Elliott, 1998;

Gettinger & Seibert, 2000, Gresham, 1991). In addition, there appears to be limited training of school-based professionals in developing and implementing authentic assessment methods (Jitendra & Kame'enui, 1995). Therefore, the extent to which reliable, valid, and generalizable findings can be obtained using authentic assessment methods remains tentative (Gettinger & Seibert, 2000, Gresham, 1991). Similar concerns have been raised regarding the use of performance assessment (Fuchs & Fuchs, 2000; Gettinger & Seibert, 2000; Shapiro & Elliott, 1999).

Relationship between Teachers' Perspectives and a Problem-Solving Approach to Assessment

Teachers' perspectives, obtained either through standardized ratings or performance assessment, can offer important supplemental information that can affect problem solving for educational intervention. Within the context of a data-based problem-solving model for assessment (Deno, 1989), teachers' estimates of students' academic skills can provide information about students' general academic functioning (i.e., problem identification) as well as comparative information about students' academic functioning in comparison to expected functioning (i.e., problem definition). For example, standardized ratings of students' academic performance can provide initial information regarding students' academic skills and identify specific academic skills that are of significant concern. Using standardized teacher estimates of students' academic skills and explicitly discussing the content area before teacher estimates are obtained can improve the reliability of indirect teacher judgments during the problem-solving process. Performance assessment can also be used to validate the standardized teacher ratings as well as obtain more specific assessments of students' performance on academic tasks that involve the application and integration of multiple skills. In certain cases, standardized teacher ratings and performance assessment can be used to identify specific target skills for intervention (i.e., exploring solutions) and determine whether interventions are effective (i.e., implementing solutions). However, the focus of this chapter will be on applying teacher ratings and performance assessment to the first two steps of a data-based problem-solving model for assessment (Deno, 1989).

METHODS

Teacher Estimates of Students' Academic Achievement: Standardized Measures

A number of standardized measures have been developed to assess students' academic performance. These measures include the teacher report form of the Social Skills Rating System (SSRS-T; Gresham & Elliott, 1990), the school competence scale from the Self-Perception Profile for Children (SPPC; Harter, 1985), and the school competence scale from the Child Behavior Checklist (CBCL; Achenbach, 1991). However, the aforementioned standardized measures focus on the broad construct of academic competence and provide minimal information regarding students' academic achievement or performance. To date, only three standardized measures have been developed to assess teachers' perceptions of students' academic skills in school settings. These measures include the Teacher Rating of Academic Performance (TRAP; Gresham, Reschly, & Carey, 1987), the Academic Performance Rating Scale (APRS; DuPaul, Rapport, & Perriello, 1991), and the Academic Competence Evaluation Scales (ACES; DiPerna & Elliott, 2000).

Teacher Rating of Academic Performance

The TRAP (Gresham et al., 1987) assesses teachers' perceptions of students' academic achievement and consists of five items that measure students' overall academic achievement as well as achievement in the content areas of reading and mathematics. Teachers are required to rate each item on a six-point Likert-type scale that ranges from "the lowest 10% or well below grade level" to "the highest 10% or well above grade level." Internal consistency estimates of the TRAP are good (alpha = .83). Furthermore the TRAP has yielded an overall accuracy rate of 91% when used to differentiate students without academic difficulties from students identified with specific learning disabilities.

Academic Performance Rating Scale

The APRS (DuPaul et al., 1991) was designed as a method of identifying academic skill deficits and monitoring changes in academic skills over time. The scale consists of 19 items evaluating students' academic skills and work performance in multiple academic areas such as reading, mathematics, spelling, and written language. Items are rated on a five-point Likert-type scale, ranging from "never" or "poor" to "very often" or "excellent." The scale has been shown to have high internal consistency (alpha = .95) and high test–retest reliability (r = .95). In addition, there is evidence to support the discriminant validity of the APRS.

Academic Competence Evaluation Scales—Teacher

The ACES—Teacher form (DiPerna & Elliott, 2000) was designed to assess the academic competence of students in kindergarten through grade 12. The ACES—Teacher, in conjunction with two other measures, Goal Attainment Scales (GAS; Kiresuk, Smith, & Cardillo, 1994) and the

Academic Intervention Monitoring Systems (AIMS, DiPerna, Elliott, & Shapiro, 2000), can be used to identify academic concerns, analyze academic concerns within the instructional environment, plan for interventions, implement interventions and monitor student progress, and evaluate the effectiveness of interventions. The ACES—Teacher includes two scales: Academic Skills (i.e., reading/language arts, mathematics, critical thinking) and Academic Enablers (i.e., motivation, study skills, engagement, interpersonal skills). The number of items on each scale varies as a function of the students' grade level, ranging from 66 to 73 items. For the Academic Skills scale, teachers provide two ratings on a 5-point scale of Proficiency (1 = Far Below Grade-level Expectations, 5 = Far Above Grade-level Expectations) and a 3-point scale of Importance (1 = Never, 3 = Critical). For the Academic Enablers scale, teachers provide two ratings on a 5-point scale of Frequency (1 = Never and 5 = Almost Always) and 3-point scale of Importance (1 = Never, 3 = Critical). The ACES—Teacher has been shown to have high internal consistency (alpha = .97 to .99), high test–retest reliability across a 3-week period (r = .88 to .97), and low to high interrater agreement (range, .31 to .99). Furthermore, there is evidence of the content validity and factor structure of the ACES—Teacher as well as substantial convergent and discriminant evidence (DiPerna & Elliott, 1999).

Teacher Estimates of Students' Academic Achievement: Performance Assessment

Although a number of models of performance assessment have been developed (Shapiro & Elliott, 1999; Fuchs & Fuchs, 2000), only two have been developed that fit within a problem-solving model of assessment. Both of these models of performance assessment are directly connected to the grade-level curriculum, require students to apply and integrate problem-solving strategies within the context of the performance assessment, and employ a standardized scoring system for assessing students' proficiency. The goal of these two models of performance assessment is to guide teachers and students toward important learning outcomes that reflect real-life problem-solving activities in the relevant content area (Fuchs & Fuchs, 2000).

Mathematics

One model of performance assessment that has recently been developed and tested is the Curriculum-Based Measurement (CBM) Problem-Solving Assessment System in mathematics (Fuchs & Fuchs, 2000). The goal of this model was to link CBM with performance assessment in the area of mathematics and extend the model to more complex applications (Fuchs & Fuchs, 2000). Four characteristics that were identified as essential in development include (1) repeated measurement of long-term goals, (2) standardized methods for describing student performance levels, (3) capacity to index growth, and (4) utility for instructional planning. Five performance assessments in mathematics for grades 2–6 were developed based on core mathematics skills that were systematically evaluated by school personnel. The resulting performance assessments require students to read a narrative describing a problem situation that involves the application of mathematics. A number of questions are raised, requiring students to apply core mathematics skills, discriminate between relevant and irrelevant information, generate additional information that is not explicitly contained in the narrative, and explain their responses in written form (Fuchs & Fuchs, 2000). Each performance assessment is scored based on an adapted scoring rubric that was extensively reviewed by school personnel (Fuchs et al., 1998; Fuchs et al., 2000).

The technical features of this model of performance assessment have been evaluated in a series of studies (Fuchs & Fuchs, 1986; Fuchs et al., 1998; Fuchs et al., 2000). These studies suggest that this model of assessment has high alternate form and test–retest reliability ($r = .66$ to $.76$), demonstrates adequate criterion validity with other standardized measures of mathematics ($r = .60$ to $.68$), and can be used to discriminate student growth over time.

Spelling

Performance in spelling (Elliott & Bischoff-Werner, 1995; Olson, 1995) is one form of performance assessment that was developed to assess students' use of spelling and writing skills. Ten spelling words (i.e., 5 student-selected words, 5 teacher-selected words) are identified each week and reflect content related to written assignments. Students study the words for 1 week and then are tested in their competency (i.e., spelling and writing proficiency). Prior to each examination, students are provided with the scoring requirements that will be used. For example, students' spelling and writing proficiency are scored in the areas of accuracy, usage, punctuation, and legibility using the following standards: (1) Exemplary = 90–100%, (2) Satisfactory = 70–89%, and (3) Inadequate = 0–69% (Shapiro & Elliott, 1999). No published studies have evaluated this approach to performance assessment; however, this model offers a real-time direct assessment of students' spelling skills that teachers might use.

CASE SCENARIO

We will illustrate the application of standardized teacher estimates of students' academic performance and an authentic assessment in the context of a problem-solving approach to academic assessment with a fictitious third-grade student. Specifically, we will review the case of a third-grade student,

Theo, in the area of mathematics, using the ACES—Teacher scale (DiPerna & Elliott, 2000) and performance assessment in mathematics as part of the problem-solving process.

Theo is an 8-year-old third-grade student in a general education classroom in a public elementary school in the northeastern United States. According to his parents, Theo experienced typical cognitive and physical development until he entered second grade. Prior school performance, as well as hearing, vision, health, and school attendance, were reported as normal. During Theo's second-grade year, his parents reported that he began to experience slight difficulties in the content area of mathematics, specifically completing independent assignments with poor accuracy. Theo's current teacher reports that his skill level in mathematics is significantly below that of his peers. His is currently performing at grade level in all other academic areas. Most recently, Theo has not been completing any of his homework assignments, has completed approximately 30% of assigned classroom work with 50% accuracy, and scores poorly on classroom tests. His teacher reports that Theo has become more visibly frustrated during mathematics and has become noncompliant with teacher directions.

Problem Identification

The first step in the problem-solving process involves collecting data to determine whether a problem exists and whether the problem is significant enough to warrant further investigation (Deno, 1989; Shinn, Collins, & Gallagher, 1998). In response to Theo's referral to the school district's multidisciplinary team, an extensive amount of information was collected regarding Theo's academic achievement, including standardized teacher ratings of his academic competence. Theo's classroom teacher was administered the ACES—Teacher form (DiPerna & Elliott, 2000) and ratings were obtained for both the Academic Skills and Academic Enablers scales. The results of this measure showed that Theo's Academic Skills total score indicates that his skills are currently in the Developing range, whereas Theo's Academic Enablers total score indicates that his enabling behaviors are falling in the Competent range. These results suggest that Theo is experiencing academic difficulty. Further inspection of Theo's Academic Skills subscales (i.e., Reading/Language Arts, Mathematics, Critical Thinking) indicate that his level of skill varies across the three subscales. In particular, Theo is functioning above grade-level expectations in Reading/Language Arts and Critical Thinking; however, he is functioning far below grade-level expectations in Mathematics. Examination of the Academic Enablers subscales indicates that his Interpersonal Skills, Engagement, and Motivation represent areas of strength. These results, in combination with additional academic assessment data, were used to determine that a significant skills discrepancy existed in the area of mathematics. Data obtained from the Academic Enablers Scale of the ACES—Teacher were used to rule out alternative explanations for the academic skills discrepancy.

Problem Definition

The second step in the problem-solving process involves collecting additional information to determine whether the problem is of sufficient importance to warrant supplementary educational resources (Deno, 1989; Shinn, Collins, & Gallagher, 1998). Using performance assessment procedures developed by Fuchs and Fuchs (2000), a set of core mathematics application concepts was developed to assess the long-term mathematics goals developed by the teachers in Theo's school district. The third- and fourth-grade classroom teachers identified core skills that they believed were compulsory or important for entry into fourth grade. Based on this teacher input, a three-page performance assessment in mathematics was developed (Fuchs & Fuchs, 2000) that allowed Theo the opportunity to apply the core set of skills identified by the teachers as well apply and integrate these skills to a real-life problem-solving situation. Theo's third-grade teacher read background information regarding performance assessment and was trained to use a scoring rubric (Fuchs et al., 1998; Fuchs et al., 2000). The performance assessment was administered to all of the students in third grade as well as all of the students in fourth grade. Examination of Theo's performance on the performance assessment indicated that he had not mastered the core mathematic skills or the supplemental mathematics skills that were deemed necessary for successful entry into fourth grade. In comparison to students in Theo's third-grade classroom, his performance assessment scores fell below the 15th percentile. These results, in combination with additional academic assessment data, were used to determine that Theo could be considered eligible for additional educational services, either available in the general education classroom or in a resource classroom. The data obtained from the performance assessment in mathematics were used to supplement additional academic assessment data and verify whether Theo's difficulties in mathematics were severe enough to warrant additional educational services.

SUMMARY

In this chapter we have discussed a number of approaches that may be useful to obtain reliable and valid teacher estimates of students' academic skills. Specifically, standardized teacher estimates that assess academic skills and competencies as well as one form of authentic assessment, performance assessment, were reviewed. Teacher estimates of students' academic performance serve an important role in assessment for individualized education. In addition, standardized teacher estimates are relatively brief and hence readily completed by teachers. Furthermore, teachers estimates of students' academic skills serve an important role in the context of a problem-solving model of assessment because they provide information about students' general academic functioning (i.e., problem identification) and comparative information about students' academic functioning in relation to expected functioning (i.e., problem definition). Furthermore, teacher estimates of students' academic performance have the potential to be used to identify specific target skills for intervention (i.e., exploring solutions) and determine whether interventions are effective (i.e., implementing solutions).

REFERENCES

Achenbach, T. (1991). *Manual for the child behavior checklist: 4–18 and 1991 profile.* Burlington: University of Vermont Department of Psychiatry.

Archbald, D. A. (1991). Authentic assessment: Principles, practices, and issues. *School Psychology Quarterly, 6,* 279–293.

Archbald, D. A., & Newmann, F. M. (1988). *Beyond standardized testing: Assessing academic achievement in the secondary schools.* Reston, VA: National Association of Secondary School Principals.

Baker, E. L. (1991). *Expectations and evidence for alternative assessment.* Paper presented at the annual meeting of the American Educational Research Association, Chicago.

Baker, E. I., O'Neil, H. F., & Linn, R. L. (1993). Policy and validity prospects for performance-based assessment. *American Psychologist, 48,* 1210–1218.

Brewer, R. (1991). *Authentic assessment: The rhetoric and the reality.* Paper presented at the annual meeting of the American Educational Research Association, Chicago.

Christenson, S. L. (1991). Authentic assessment: Straw man or prescription for progress? *School Psychology Quarterly, 6,* 294–399.

Clark, C. M., & Peterson, P. L. (1986). Teachers' thought processes. In M. C. Wittrock (Ed.), *Third handbook of research on teaching* (pp. 255–296). New York: Macmillan.

Cone, J. D. (1978). The behavioral assessment grid (BAG): A conceptual framework and a taxonomy. *Behavior Therapy, 9,* 882–888.

Demaray, M. K., & Elliott, S. N. (1998). Teachers' judgments of students' academic functioning: A comparison of actual and predicted performances. *School Psychology Quarterly, 13,* 8–24.

Deno, S. L. (1989). Curriculum-based measurement and special education services: A fundamental and direct relationship. In M. Shinn (Ed.), *Curriculum-based measurement: Assessing special children* (pp. 1–17). New York: Guilford Press.

DiPerna, J. C., & Elliott, S. N. (1999). The development and validation of the Academic Competence Evaluation Scale. *Journal of Psychoeducational Assessment, 17,* 207–225.

DiPerna, J. C., & Elliott, S. N. (2000). *Academic Competence Evaluation Scales.* San Antonio: Psychological Corporation.

DiPerna, J. C., Elliott, S. N., & Shapiro, E. S. (2000). *Academic Intervention Monitoring Systems.* San Antonio: Psychological Corporation.

DuPaul, G. J., Rapport, M. D., & Perriello, L. M. (1991). Teacher ratings of academic skills: The development of the Academic Performance Rating Scale. *School Psychology Review, 20*, 284–300.

Elliott, S. N. (1991). Authentic assessment: An introduction to a neobehavioral approach to classroom assessment. *School Psychology Quarterly, 6*, 273–278.

Elliott, S. N. (1998). Performance assessment of students' achievement: Research and practice. *Learning Disabilities Research and Practice, 13*, 253–262.

Elliott, S. N., & Bischoff-Werner, K. (1995). *Performance spelling*. Unpublished manual, University of Wisconsin–Madison.

Feinberg, A. B., & Shapiro, E. S. (2003). Accuracy of teacher judgments in predicting oral reading fluency. *School Psychology Quarterly, 18*, 52–65.

Fuchs, L. S., & Fuchs, D. (1986). Treatment validity: A unifying concept for reconceptualizing the identification of learning disabilities. *Learning Disabilities Research and Practice, 13*, 204–219.

Fuchs, L. S., & Fuchs, D. (2000). Analogue assessment of academic skills: Curriculum-based measurement and performance assessment. In E. S. Shapiro & T. R. Kratochwill (Eds.), *Behavioral assessment in schools: Theory, research, and clinical foundations* (2nd ed., pp. 168–201). New York: Guilford Press.

Fuchs, L. S., Fuchs, D., Karns, K., Hamlett, C. L., Katzaraoff, K., & Dutka, S. (1998). Comparisons among individual and cooperative performance assessments and other measures of mathematics competence. *Elementary School Journal, 98*, 3–22.

Fuchs, L. S., Fuchs, D., Kazdan, S., Karns, K., Calhoon, M. B., Hamlett, C. L., & Hewlett, S. (2000). The effects of workgroup structure and size on student productivity during collaborative work on complex tasks. *Elementary School Journal, 100*, 83–212.

Gerber, M. M., & Semmel, M. I. (1984). Teacher as imperfect test: Reconceptualizing the referral process. *Educational Psychologist, 19*, 137–148.

Gettinger, M. B., & Seibert, J. K. (2000). Analogue assessment: Research and practice in evaluating academic skills problems. In E. S. Shapiro & T. R. Kratochwill (Eds.), *Behavioral assessment in schools: Theory, research, and clinical foundations* (2nd ed., pp. 139–167). New York: Guilford Press.

Gresham, F. M. (1991). Alternative psychometrics for authentic assessment? *School Psychology Quarterly, 6*, 305–309.

Gresham, F. M., & Elliott, S. N. (1990). *Social Skills Rating System*. Circle Pines, MN: American Guidance Service.

Gresham, F. M., MacMillan, D. L., & Bocian, K. M. (1997). Teachers as tests: Differential validity of teacher judgments in identifying students at-risk for learning difficulties. *School Psychology Review, 26*, 47–60.

Gresham, F. M., Reschly, D., & Carey, M. P. (1987). Teachers as "tests": Classification accuracy and concurrent validation in the identification of learning disabled children. *School Psychology Review, 16*, 543–553.

Guskey, T. R. (1994). What you assess may not be what you get. *Educational Leadership, 51*, 51–54.

Harter, S. (1985). *Manual for the self-perception profile for children*. Denver: University of Denver.

Herman, J. L. (1998). The state of performance assessments. *School Administrator, 55*, 17–21.

Hoge, R. D. (1983). Psychometric properties of teacher judgment measures of pupil aptitudes, classroom behavior, and achievement levels. *Journal of Special Education, 17*, 401–429.

Hoge, R. D., & Coladarci, T. (1989). Teacher-based judgments of academic achievement: A review of the literature. *Review of Educational Research, 59*, 297–313.

Jitendra, A. K., & Kame'enui, E. J. (1993). Dynamic assessment as a compensatory assessment approach: A description and analysis. *Remedial and Special Education,* *14,* 6–18.

Kamphaus, R. W. (1991). Authentic assessment and content validity. *School Psychology* *Quarterly, 6,* 300–304.

Kaufman, A. S., & Kaufman, N. L. (1985). *Kaufman Test of Educational Achieve-* *ment—Brief Form.* Circle Pines, MN: American Guidance Service.

Kenny, D. T., & Chekaluk, E. (1993). Early reading performance: A comparison of teacher-based and test-based assessments. *Journal of Learning Disabilities, 26,* 277–286.

Kiresuk, T. J., Smith, A., & Cardillo, J. E. (1994). *Goal attainment scaling: Applications,* *theory, and measurement.* Hillsdale, NJ: Erlbaum.

Kratochwill, T. R., & Shapiro, E. S. (2000). Conceptual foundations of behavioral as- sessment in schools. In E. S. Shapiro & T. R. Kratochwill (Eds.), *Behavioral assess-* *ment in schools: Theory, research, and clinical foundations* (2nd ed., pp. 3–18). New York: Guilford Press.

Luce, S. R., & Hoge, R. D. (1978). Relations among teacher rankings, pupil-teacher in- teractions, and academic achievement: A test of the teacher expectancy hypothesis. *American Educational Resource Journal, 15,* 489–500.

McNair, K. (1978). Capturing inflight decisions: Thoughts while teaching. *Educational* *Research Quarterly, 3,* 26–42.

Merrell, K. W. (1999). *Behavioral, social, and emotional assessment of children and ado-* *lescents.* Mahwah, NJ: Erlbaum.

National Institute of Child Health and Human Development. (2000). *Report of the Na-* *tional Reading Panel. Teaching children to read: An evidence-based assessment of* *the scientific research literature on reading and its implications for reading instruc-* *tion* (NIH Publication No. 00-4769). Washington, DC: U.S. Government Printing Office.

Oliver, J. E., & Arnold, R. D. (1978). Comparing a standardized test, an informal inven- tory, and teacher judgment on third grade reading. *Reading Improvement, 15,* 56– 59.

Olson, A. E. (1995). *Evaluation of an alternative approach to teaching and assessing* *spelling performance.* Master's thesis, University of Wisconsin–Madison.

Radcliff, N. J. (2001). Using authentic assessment to document the emerging literacy skills of young children. *Childhood Education, 78,* 66–69.

Salvia, J., & Ysseldyke, J. E. (2004). *Assessment* (9th ed.). New York: Houghton Mifflin.

Sammons, K. B., Kobett, B., Heiss, J., & Fennell, F. S. (1992). Linking instruction and assessment in the mathematics classroom. *Arithmetic Teacher,* February, 11–15.

Sattler, J. M. (2001). *Assessment of children: Cognitive applications* (4th ed.). San Diego: Sattler.

Schurr, S. (1998). Teaching, enlightening: A guide to student assessment. *Schools in the* *Middle, 6,* 22–27.

Shapiro, E. S. (1996). *Academic skills problems* (2nd ed.). New York: Guilford Press.

Shapiro, E. S., & Elliott, S. N. (1999). Curriculum-based assessment and other performance-based assessment strategies. In C. R. Reynolds & T. B. Gutkin (Eds.), *The Handbook of School Psychology* (3rd ed., pp. 383–408). New York: Wiley.

Shapiro, E. S., & Kratochwill, T. R. (2000). Introduction: Conducting a multidimen- sional behavioral assessment. In E. S. Shapiro & T. R. Kratochwill (Eds.), *Con-* *ducting school-based assessments of child and adolescent behavior* (pp. 1–20). New York: Guilford Press.

Sharpley, C. F., & Edgar, E. (1986). Teachers' ratings vs. standardized tests: An empirical investigation of agreement between two indices of achievement. *Psychology in the* *Schools, 23,* 106–111.

Shinn, M. R. (1989). *Curriculum-based measurement: Assessing special children.* New York: Guilford Press.

Shinn, M. R., Collins, V. L., & Gallagher, S. (1998). Curriculum-based measurement and its use in a problem-solving model with students from minority backgrounds. In M. R. Shinn (Ed.), *Advanced applications of curriculum-based measurement* (pp. 143–174). New York: Guilford Press.

Stiggins, R. J. (1997). *Student-centered classroom assessment* (2nd ed.). Upper Saddle River, NJ: Merrill.

Ysseldyke, J. E., & Christenson, S. L. (1987). Evaluating students' instructional environments. *Remedial and Special Education, 8,* 17–24.

Wright, D., & Wiese, M. J. (1988). Assessment practices in special education: Adequacy practices in special education: Adequacy and appropriateness. *Educational Psychologist, 9,* 123–136.

SUGGESTED READINGS

DiPerna, J. C., & Elliott, S. N. (2000). *Academic Competence Evaluation Scales.* San Antonio: Psychological Corporation.

The manual for the Academic Competence Evaluation Scales (ACES) provides an exhaustive overview of the purpose and uses of the ACES within a problem-solving model of academic assessment. Detailed information is provided regarding the completion, scoring, and interpretation of each ACES scale as well a prescriptive overview of how to link assessment data to intervention. Information pertaining to the development of the scales as well as the psychometric properties of the scales is also detailed.

Fuchs, L. S., & Fuchs, D. (2000). Analogue assessment of academic skills: Curriculum-based measurement and performance assessment. In E. S. Shapiro & T. R. Kratochwill (Eds.), *Behavioral assessment in schools: Theory, research, and clinical foundations* (2nd ed., pp. 168–201). New York: Guilford Press.

This chapter provides an extensive overview of curriculum-based measurement and performance assessment. Both methods of assessment are presented within a problem-solving model of academic assessment. Examples of incorporating performance assessments within the context of conducting a curriculum-based measurement are detailed.

CHAPTER 5

♦ ♦ ♦

Population-Based Strategies for Identifying Schoolwide Problems

♦

BETH DOLL
MARY KELLY HAACK

Over the past 25 years, research in developmental psychopathology has revolutionized professional understanding of children's mental illness and their psychological well-being. In 1987, for the first time, the release of the revised third edition of the *Diagnostic and Statistical Manual of Mental Disorders* (DSM-III-R) provided developmentally sensitive criteria for traditional mental illnesses such as depression, the anxiety disorders, and conduct disorders (American Psychiatric Association, 1987). The availability of these criteria prompted a wealth of epidemiological studies on the incidence of mental illness in children and adolescents (Doll, 1996). The results are summarized in Table 5.1, and they were startling. Whereas pre-1980 estimates of childhood mental illness suggested that between 5 and 7% of school-age children met the criteria for one or more psychiatric disorders, the epidemiological studies consistently identified between 16 and 22% of their community samples as meeting the criteria. The pattern of disorders also shifted. The pre-1980 sources emphasized the prevalence of conduct disorders, attention-deficit disorders, and other externalizing disorders,

TABLE 5.1. Incidence of DSM-III-R Psychiatric Disorders among Children and Adolescents

	Incidence rates expressed in percentages	
Disorder	Elementary	Secondary
All major disorders	16.5–21.9%	16.4–20.3%
Anxiety disorders	17.6–21.0%	21.0%
Attention-deficit/hyperactivity disorder	2.3–6.7%	5.4%
Conduct disorders	3.3–5.1%	14%
Depression	.1–1.4%	1.8–5.7%

Adapted from Doll (1996). Copyright 1996 by the American Psychological Association. Adapted by permission.

while the epidemiological studies demonstrated that internalizing disorders such as depression and anxiety disorders were equally prevalent in school-age children.

More recently, researchers' attention has shifted to describing children's developmental trajectories into mental illness, and results are demonstrating that socioecological features of children's lives can be as important as individual child characteristics in predicting the incidence and severity of mental illness (Coie et al., 1993; Doll & Lyon, 1998). In particular, children's exposure to poverty, family violence, parental mental illness, or community violence significantly increases their chances of developing a debilitating mental illness, while their access to caring adults, high-quality parenting, and effective community support services can protect some children from severe mental illness (Coie et al., 1993; Doll & Lyon, 1998).

These altered understandings hold profound implications for how schools should address students' social, emotional, and behavioral problems. When the epidemiological studies identified large numbers of "hidden" disorders, they challenged the traditional refer–assess–treat continuum that had defined school-based mental health service delivery. Clearly, the adults who were referring children for mental health treatment were overlooking large numbers of children with internalizing disorders. Even children with externalizing disorders were underidentified, raising urgent questions about whether these "hidden" children had a legitimate claim to mental health services, and how their claim might differ from that of previously identified children. The functional impact of these psychiatric disorders on children's school success has not been adequately addressed in developmental psychopathology studies (Doll, 1996), but some research on severe emotional disturbances suggests that it is associated with low academic grades and increased truancy and school dropout (McInerney, Kane, & Pelavin, 1992). More important, the educational relevance of psychological health and wellness is amply documented in developmental research (Doll, Zucker, & Brehm, 2004).

The recognition of widespread child mental health needs has led to a number of important questions for practitioners. How must a community's child mental health identification procedures change so that these hidden children can be identified and served? Just as importantly, clinicians have been accustomed to using one-child-at-a-time assessment procedures to fully describe children's therapeutic needs. The child mental health system struggled to conduct these assessments with 5–7% of the population and could not possibly extend these to three times as many child clients. What kinds of assessments could support quality solutions for all children's problems? The emphasis on family and community factors as causal agents for children's mental illness raised important questions about the nature of, and responsibility for, services to support healthy socioemotional development in children. Causal factors such as poverty, parental health, or community violence lay outside the traditional mental health and school authority in most communities, suggesting that services of police departments, social welfare agencies, community health departments, families, religious groups, schools, and neighborhoods were as essential to child mental health as were those of the child mental health professionals.

Finally, developmental risk and resilience research has emphasized the importance of identifying children who are at high risk for developmental disruptions and concentrating protective resources on these children (Pianta & Walsh, 1996). A major contribution of the risk research was in specifying the chronic stressors that place children at risk for very limited academic and social success. The most prominent of these stressors include poverty, low parent education, marital discord or family conflict, ineffective parenting, child maltreatment, poor physical health of the child or parents, and parental mental illness or incapacity (Coie et al., 1993; Doll & Lyon, 1998). Many of these risk factors tend to concentrate in high-risk communities, a phenomenon that Pianta and Walsh (1996) refer to as "niches" of elevated risk. The implication is that social problem-solving services ought also be concentrated in these same communities. While the risk factors in this first list are difficult to modify, there are additional chronic life stressors identified by developmental risk researchers that are alterable. Included among these are low self-esteem, academic failure, peer alienation or isolation, and poor academic work habits (Coie et al., 1993).

Risk factors that have been identified as predictive of future life failures are high-priority problems that ought to be a focus of schools' problem-solving efforts. Other factors identified as predictive of future life success could become the mechanisms underlying solutions to some major social or academic problems. Examples of such protective factors include close peer friendships, high self-efficacy, high engagement in productive activities, access to warm relationships, and guidance from adults or access to responsive schools. Thus, taken in its entirety, the developmental risk and resilience literature provides a road map for planning responsive behavioral support services that address the academic and social problems of a school's students.

This chapter will build upon the risk and resilience literature to describe population-based assessment as an alternative framework for identifying the social, emotional, and behavioral problems that need to be addressed within a school. Rather than the refer–assess–treat model, population-based assessment strategies screen the full child population of a community or school and identify those children with a demonstrable need for socioemotional support. The framework borrows heavily from epidemiological research methods that have established standards for selecting community samples, screening for all instances of a disorder, confirming diagnoses to professional standards, identifying variables related to instances of the disorder, and using data to identify predictive and causal relations that point to useful intervention strategies. Similarly, this chapter's framework will reflect the influence of public health models of mental health services that emphasize wellness in addition to illness and that address psychological problems or wellness at a population level. Population-based interventions modify community factors to reduce the problems' rates or severity or alter community behaviors, attitudes, or access to resources so as to promote psychological wellness.

POPULATION-BASED MEASURES
OF CHILDREN'S MENTAL HEALTH

To be used in population-based assessments, measures must have attributes that make them uniquely suitable for accurately screening large numbers of children for mental health needs. First, population-based measures must be brief to administer so that the assessment of large numbers of children is neither time-intensive nor prohibitively expensive. For example, it would not be reasonable to expect that teachers could complete the 118-item Teacher Report Form (TRF; Achenbach & Rescorla, 2001) on every student in a class and still be reporting impressions that were accurate and insightful. Second, population-based measures must be efficient to code and simple to analyze so that the burden of interpreting them is not onerous. Hand scoring a brief 20-item checklist from every child in a 500-student elementary school could easily become an 80-hour task. Like traditional measures, population-based assessment strategies must have strong psychometric properties, including strong internal consistency and good test–retest reliability over brief intervals of time. The best measures also are capable of repeated administrations without practice effects distorting the results, and are sensitive to intervention effects, so that they can verify when changes in policy or practice diminish the prevalence or severity of a disorder. Finally, the screening procedures that incorporate population-based measures must be highly accurate in identifying all instances of disorder, with few or no "false-positive" and "false-negative" identifications of children.

Most but not all population-based assessments use multistage procedures in which the entire child population of a community is first screened to identify any evidence of the targeted problem. Measures used in this initial screening stage must minimize the number of false-negative identifications so that all children with legitimate need for services will be included in subsequent stages. The incidence of false-positive identifications in Stage 1 is less problematic, since the worst that will happen is that some children will be unnecessarily included in a second stage of assessment. In subsequent stages, more time-intensive measures are administered to fewer children and yield more certain identifications. At a minimum, the final result of the assessment will be a list of children with a demonstrated need for problem-solving services, but the most useful procedures also yield descriptive information about the identified group, including information about the prevalence of specific behaviors or risk factors. Population-based assessment procedures differ in the number of stages that define the procedures, the problems that are being identified, and the proportion of children identified as needing services. Most are designed to be repeated yearly, as part of annual planning for service delivery.

In this chapter, we will describe three prominent examples of population-based assessments that select out students with pressing problems that affect their academic or social success. The first example, the Systematic Screening for Behavior Disorders (SSBD), is a procedure for identifying elementary school students with marked behavior problems. The Early Screening Project (ESP) is a downward extension of the SSBD designed for use with preschool and kindergarten classrooms. The second example is Reynolds's (1991, 2002) procedure for identifying high school students who meet the diagnostic criteria for major clinical depression or who are at high risk for suicide. Third, we will describe sociometric procedures for identifying students with few friends or very low social acceptance. The chapter will close with a broader discussion of the implications of these three examples for planning schoolwide solutions to social, emotional, and behavioral problems.

SYSTEMATIC SCREENING FOR BEHAVIOR DISORDERS

The SSBD (Walker & Severson, 1992) is a procedure for identifying all children with behavior disorders in an elementary school. It uses a "multiple gating" design with three stages of assessment, each progressively more precise in identifying the children with the most significant problem behaviors. Stages 1 and 2 occur during a 60-minute school faculty meeting. In Stage 1, after a brief presentation alerting them to the distinctive behaviors of internalizing and externalizing students, teachers identify six students from their class: three who most demonstrate externalizing behaviors and three who most demonstrate internalizing behaviors. While referral-based identifications frequently underestimate the number of students with internalizing disorders (Doll & Lyon, 1998), carefully conducted training can prepare teachers to accurately nominate students with both internalizing and externalizing disorders (Walker et al., 1990). In Stage 2, teachers complete the SSBD's Critical Events Index and the Cumulative Frequency Index to describe the nature and frequency of critical behaviors that characterize each of the six students. Completion of the two indices' 45 items requires approximately 5 minutes per student. Those students who meet or exceed normative criteria on either index are systematically observed in both the classroom and the playground, and their observed behaviors are compared to those of at least two nonranked peers from their own class. Students are referred to the school's child study team for behavior planning when the observations confirm that they engage in excessive amounts of negative behavior, are unusually isolated, or are disengaged in classroom learning activities.

The SSBD is a time-efficient screening procedure. Stages 1 and 2 require approximately 1 hour for all teachers in a school to rank and rate their students, and Stage 3 requires 1 hour per student for a school psychologist, counselor, or resource teacher to observe students in classrooms and at recess (Walker & Severson, 1994). For a school consisting of 20 classrooms, administration of the SSBD Stage 1 and 2 ratings would take approximately 60 minutes of each teacher's time, and an additional 100 hours of observation time would be required to complete Stage 3.

Almost all of the research examining the technical adequacy of the SSBD and its measures has been conducted by Walker, Severson, and their colleagues (Walker & Severson, 1994; Walker et al., 1988; Walker et al., 1990). Results show that the procedures are moderately successful in identifying a school's students who have behavior disorders. The manual describes trial testing in which 90% of a school's students were correctly identified as internalizing, externalizing, or nonranked (Walker & Severson, 1992). Of the remaining 10%, 1% had externalizing problems but were identified as internalizing, 5% had problems but were not identified (false negatives), and 4% did not have problems but were identified (false positives). In a second study, 85% of a school's students were correctly classified (Walker et al., 1990). Of the remaining 15%, 7% were appropriately identified as having behavior problems even though the problems were mischaracterized as internalizing or externalizing, 6% were false negatives, and 2% were false positives. This accuracy is similar to that of the Teacher's Report Form (Achenbach & Rescorla, 2001), which correctly classified 85% of children referred for mental health services, with 7% false negatives and 8% false positives.

Since the SSBD uses its own measures, its integrity relies on the adequacy of its two indices and two observation procedures. The SSBD Critical Events Index is a 33-item checklist of child behaviors that are infrequent but are highly indicative of disorder when present. Examples include being physically aggressive with others or being cruel to animals. Teachers' ratings describe these behaviors as present or absent for each student. The SSBD Cumulative Frequency Index is a Likert scale describing the frequency of 12 adaptive behaviors (i.e., follows rules and initiates positive social interactions with peers) and 11 maladaptive behaviors (i.e., challenges teacher-imposed limits and manipulates other children and/or the situation to get his or her own way). The internal consistency of the SSBD scales generally falls above .80 and their test–retest reliability across 1-month intervals has been consistently found to fall at or above .80 (Walker & Severson, 1992, 1994; Walker et al., 1988; Walker et al., 1990). The scales' validity has been demonstrated in a series of studies showing significant correlations with other measures of behavioral adjustment (Walker & Severson, 1992; Walker et al., 1988)

The SSBD's Stage 3 observations provide specific data about the nature, severity, and frequency of behavior problems within and across students. The protocol incorporates four 15-minute observations of each identified student and two typical peers chosen at random from the same class—two observations during independent classroom seatwork and two observations during recess playtime. A training video included in the SSBD kit prepares observers to use an interval recording method, recording the amount of time each student is engaged in academic tasks and the type of social activities the student engages in during playground time (Walker et al., 1988). Adherence to these training procedures yields high interobserver reliability, with higher coefficients for observations of academic engaged time (.86 to 1.00) than for playground social engagement (.65 to 1.00). Again, the observations yield results that correlate with other measures of behavioral adjustment (Walker et al., 1988). School psychologists and general and special education teachers have recommended the SSBD as an effective tool in identifying children with externalizing and internalizing behavior problems (Walker & Severson, 1994).

EARLY SCREENING PROJECT

The Early Screening Project (ESP) is a downward extension of the SSBD for use with preschool and kindergarten children. While retaining the three-stage screening procedure, measures at each stage are adjusted to be developmentally appropriate for younger children (Feil & Becker, 1993; Feil & Severson, 1995; Feil, Walker, & Severson, 1995; Walker, Severson, & Feil, 1995). Specifically, in Stage 1, teachers nominate fewer externalizing and internalizing students, because preschool classes are usually smaller, averaging 15 students per class. In Stage 2, items on the ESP Critical Events Index and the ESP Cumulative Frequency Index were adjusted by omitting academic behaviors, problem behaviors that were developmentally normal in younger children, and problem behaviors that rarely occurred in younger children. Teachers also complete a third Stage 2 checklist for each child: the Aggressive Behavior Scale for externalizing children and the Social Interaction Scale for internalizing students. An optional parent questionnaire was added to Stage 2, and includes three four-item scales assessing peer play, interactions with caregivers, and playing with materials and self-care. Like the SSBD, Stages 1 and 2 are completed during a 60-minute school faculty meeting. Students who meet or exceed the normative criteria on Stage 2 checklists are only observed in social activities during Stage 3; classroom academic behaviors are not observed due to the limited academic expectations of young children. Specifically, two 10-minute observations are conducted of the children's antisocial behaviors (e.g., fighting or arguing and disobeying established rules), nonsocial behaviors (e.g., tantruming and solitary play), and prosocial behaviors (e.g., parallel play and following established rules). An optional parent questionnaire was added to Stage 3 and includes three four-item scales assessing peer play, interactions with caregivers, playing with materials, and self-care.

There is less research on the accuracy of the ESP selections. In one study, accuracy was examined by comparing the preschoolers it selected against those that teachers identified as possibly having serious behavior problems. Results showed that between 94 and 100% of young children identified as not having a behavior disorder were accurately categorized, and between 62% and 100% of young children selected as having a behavior disorder were correctly identified (Walker et al., 1995).

The reliability of the ESP's five scales has been examined by the authors and found to be somewhat less than that of the SSBD (Feil et al., 1995). Interrater reliability comparing ratings by teachers and assistant teachers fell between .48 and .93, depending upon the scale. These reliabilities are comparable to other measures of preschool behavior problems, such as the Preschool Behavior Questionnaire (Behar & Stringfield, 1974) and Conners Teachers Rating Scale (1989). Test–retest reliabilities across a 6-month interval were at or above .70. This is to be expected, given the variable behaviors at this age. Finally, significant correlations were demonstrated between the ESP scales and other measures of behavioral disturbance in preschool children (Feil et al., 1995).

Recommendation

An important outcome of the SSBD and ESP screening procedures is a list of students whose behavioral disturbances are severe enough to require careful behavioral assessment and planning. In addition, the procedures provide information about the normative behavior in the school's classrooms and on the playground and observational data describing typical and atypical behavior for each targeted student. Empirical studies demonstrate that these lists provide reliable and valid estimates of those students who are most in need of behavioral support. A school's behavioral support staff could use the lists to prioritize their services, precisely describe the behavioral resources needed in the school, and plan for a yearlong program of service delivery. Moreover, when data suggest that certain problem behavior patterns are especially prominent or problematic, classwide, or schoolwide behavior plans could be designed as a way to enhance the impact and increase the efficiency of behavioral support services. Just as importantly, the SSBD or ESP data could serve as a baseline against which to measure progress in individual or group behavior support plans. The ESP provides school districts with the option to begin this targeted behavioral support service at very young ages, when the potential impact on child outcomes is most pronounced.

The cost of the SSBD in staff time is not inconsequential, especially given the heavy time commitment necessary to conduct the behavioral observations. It is clear that a school would need to reorganize its staff time in order to conduct the SSBD screenings, and likely that a school would need to reallocate its behavioral support services in response to the SSBD results. Still, the screening procedure has the potential to identify significant behavior problems earlier in their trajectory, and could allow a school to be proactive in its behavioral interventions. Some schools will find this to be worth the SSBD's cost. The SSBD has been shown to require significantly less time and money than traditional referral and assessment procedures (Walker & Severson, 1994).

REYNOLDS'S SCREENING FOR DEPRESSION AND SUICIDE IN ADOLESCENTS

In a 20-year line of research, Reynolds (1991, 2002) developed a three-stage screening procedure to identify all clinically depressed adolescents in a high school. These procedures differ from the SSBD and ESP in their exclusive focus on internalizing psychiatric disorders and in their reliance on student self-report measures. However, both of these differences are appropriate to the secondary students that Reynolds's procedures target. Depression is strikingly prevalent among adolescents and is highly disruptive to student success, and self-report has been established as an accurate indicator of adolescent depression (Kessler & Walters, 1998; Reynolds, 1987, 1998). In Stage 1, the Reynolds Adolescent Depression Scale—2nd Edition (RADS2; Reynolds, 1987, 2002) is completed by all students during a large assembly. Students scoring above a clinical cutoff score return 2 weeks later to retake the RADS2. This second administration eliminates adolescents who were experiencing a transient depressed mood or for some other reason overendorsed depressive symptoms on the first RADS2. Those who score above the cutoff a second time are systematically interviewed by mental health professionals using the Hamilton Depression Rating Scale interview (Hamilton, 1967). If a diagnosis of major depression is confirmed by the interview, students are referred for mental health services using a combination of community, family, and school resources.

Investigations of the technical adequacy of this screening procedure were conducted principally by Reynolds and his colleagues. In Stage 1, approximately 12–16% of adolescents identify a "clinically relevant" level of depression on the RADS2 (Reynolds, 2002). Between 70 and 80% of the Stage 2 students are referred on to complete the depression interview. Ultimately, approximately half of the students identified as possibly depressed in Stage 1 have that diagnosis confirmed by the interview (Reynolds, 1994). This represents 7–12% of the total number of students who were originally screened. Using the Hamilton Depression Rating Scale as a criterion, results of one study showed that the two-stage screening procedure correctly identified 92% of clinically depressed adolescents as depressed and identified 90% of nondepressed adolescents as not depressed (Reynolds & Mazza, 1998).

Even allowing 5–10 minutes per protocol for scoring the RADS2, Stages 1 and 2 of the Reynolds screening procedure are quite time-efficient. However, Stage 3 represents a logistical challenge in administering 60-minute interviews to 10% of a high school's students. Reynolds accomplished this by recruiting volunteer mental health professionals from diverse agencies and schools to complete the required interviews. Subsequent to identification, students will need to be referred for appropriate treatment services. Studies with adult depression screenings have demonstrated that, subsequent to National Depression Screening Day, two-thirds of the adults recommended for treatment sought out services (Greenfield et al., 2000). It is not clear whether the high school students were similarly successful in securing treatment.

Reynolds developed scales specifically for use in this screening procedure. The RADS2 (Reynolds, 1989, 2002) is a 30-item self-report measure that assesses the occurrence, frequency, and duration of depressive symptoms using a four-point Likert response format ("almost never," "hardly ever," "sometimes," or "most of the time"). Results yield a total score and subscale scores for Dysphoric Mood, Anhedonia/Negative Affect, Negative

Self-Evaluation, and Somatic Complaints. The measure includes five critical items that assess dangerous symptoms. Adolescents are possible candidates for a diagnosis of major depressive disorder if they score above the clinical cutoff score or have a high score on four or more critical items (Reynolds & Mazza, 1998; Reynolds, 2002). Analysis of the RADS2 standardization sample demonstrated high internal consistency reliability, with coefficients of .93 for the total score and ranging from .80 to .87 for the subscales (Reynolds, 2002). The RADS2's test–retest reliability is similarly high, at .85 for the total score and ranging from .77 to .84 for the subscales across 6-week intervals (Reynolds, 2002). These results were similar to those of an earlier study demonstrating test–retest reliabilities for the RADS of .87 for 2- to 4-week intervals (Reynolds & Mazza, 1998). Construct validity was demonstrated through correlations with the Hamilton Depression Rating Scale (Reynolds, 1989, 2002; Reynolds & Mazza, 1989), other measures of depressive symptoms (Reynolds, 1989), and related measures of internalizing disorders (Reynolds, 2002).

Since suicidal ideation exists in adolescents who do not show clinical levels of depression, Reynolds has developed a similar but separate two-stage procedure to identify all suicidal students in a secondary school. In Stage 1, the Suicidal Ideation Questionnaire (SIQ; Reynolds, 1987) is administered to all students, and those who scored above the cutoff on this first administration are interviewed by mental health professionals using the Suicidal Behaviors Interview (SBI; Reynolds, 1991). Between 9 and 11% of adolescents score at or above the cutoff on the SIQ during the initial screening (Reynolds, 1991). More girls than boys are typically identified (Reynolds, 1989). The use of a conservative cutoff score of 30 for the SIQ screening yields no false negatives, but only half of the adolescents identified in Stage 1 are subsequently found to be at risk for suicide. The use of a less conservative cutoff score would lower the false positives, but also means that a few suicidal students might go undetected.

Reynolds (1989) developed the SIQ specifically for use in this screening procedure. It is a 30-item self-report measure that assesses the frequency of a continuum of suicidal thoughts ranging from general wishes that one is dead to specific plans describing how, when, and where an attempt will be made. The SIQ is suitable for senior high school students (grades 10–12), while a middle school version (the 15-item SIQ-JR) is provided for students in grades 7–9. Both forms use a 7-point Likert response format describing the frequency of suicidal thoughts during the past month.

Analysis of the standardization sample yielded internal consistency reliability coefficients at or above .90 for the SIQ-JR and the SIQ (Reynolds, 1989; Reynolds & Mazza, 1999). The two scales also demonstrate strong test–retest reliability greater than .70 across 4- to 5-week intervals (Reynolds, 1989; Reynolds & Mazza, 1999). Moreover, significant correlations have been demonstrated with the SIQ-JR and the Suicidal Behaviors Interview and with related instruments that measure psychological distress and hopelessness (Reynolds & Mazza, 1999). The SIQ-JR scores of adolescents who had attempted suicide in the past 12 months were significantly higher than scores of those who had not (Reynolds & Mazza, 1999).

The SBI (Reynolds, 1991) is a semistructured clinical interview that occurs in two parts. Part 1 incorporates four questions inquiring about generalized level of psychological distress, severity of daily hassles, level of social support, and recent negative life events that may intensify the risk for suicidal behavior. Part 2 consists of 14 questions about specific types of suicidal behavior and related risk factors. Responses are scored by the interviewer using prescribed scales, and cutoff scores are used to identify high risk of suicide. The SBI has strong internal consistency (alpha = .91), strong interrater reliability (r = .98), and correlates with adolescents' self-reports of suicidal behavior (Reynolds, 1991).

Recommendation

The outcomes of the Reynolds screening procedures are lists of all clinically depressed adolescents in a high school or of all students at high risk for suicide. Reynolds's research has demonstrated that these lists are reliable and valid, and will identify most (but not all) depressed or suicidal students in a building. Since these are students who were largely unidentified in traditional referral-based identification procedures, these lists could significantly reduce the morbidity associated with adolescence in many school communities. Left untreated, adolescent depression could diminish students' active participation in the school curricula and social activities. Like the SSBD/ESP, these are not cost-free evaluations. In addition to the heavy cost of the hourlong interviews, each identified student must be systematically linked to resources for therapy. Clearly, a communitywide commitment is required since schools cannot accommodate a therapy caseload of approximately 10% of the student body. School administrators may be reluctant to identify potentially lethal conditions like depression and suicide, worrying that the identification of adolescents in crisis could be construed as a responsibility for addressing the crisis. Still, when a communitywide collaboration can be established, Reynolds's screenings can identify depressed and suicidal students much earlier and reduce a major risk to adolescents in the school.

SOCIOMETRIC STRATEGIES FOR IDENTIFYING CHILDREN WITH SOCIALIZATION DIFFICULTIES

Disturbances in peer relations have not typically been considered a critical mental health problem. However, Achenbach's (2001) empirically derived diagnostic typology has identified "peer relationship disturbances" as a unique factor with important implications for developmental competence. Poor peer acceptance and having few or no friends are two important but distinct forms of peer disturbances (Parker & Asher, 1993; Rose & Asher, 1999). Both are related to recess problems, and particularly to problems with children being isolated or not allowed to play by classmates (Doll, Murphy, & Song, 2003). More importantly, peers' collective evaluations of classmates' social competence are powerful predictors of adult dysfunction including unemployment and underemployment, social dependence, or serious mental illness (Berndt, 1984; Dodge, 1989; Guralnick, 1986). Finally, social relations play a key role in insulating children against the onslaught of developmental risk and so have the potential to ameliorate risk and promote competence.

Peer relationship disturbances are best assessed using variations of sociometric procedures. Sociometric assessments were prominent in the 1950s as measures of classroom social networks, and then reemerged in the 1980s as a preferred strategy of researchers who were investigating children's social competence. Their widespread acceptance is due to sociometric measures' exceptionally strong psychometric properties. They have been repeatedly demonstrated to be stable over time and across situations (Berndt, 1984; Coie & Kupersmidt, 1983; Newcomb & Bukowski, 1984; Parker & Asher, 1989, 1993).

Variations on two sociometric procedures are used in both research and practice: sociometric nominations, in which classmates list their friends, or sociometric roster-ratings, in which children rate all of their classmates according to how much they liked to play with them (Asher & Hymel, 1986; Berndt, 1984; Parker & Asher, 1993). Sociometric nominations can be limited (i.e., list your three best friends) or unlimited (i.e., list your friends). However, limited nominations are problematic because they underidentify mutual friendships and can artificially lower the measure of peer acceptance reported for students (Parker & Asher, 1993). Sociometric ratings are generally preferred because they reflect a student's overall acceptance by every other student in the class (Parker & Asher, 1993) and appear to be more reliable than nominations (Asher & Hymel, 1986; Parker & Asher, 1989, 1993). The measures do not require sophisticated procedures or copyrighted forms and can be collected in less than 15 minutes per class. Analysis of the measures used to be unbearably time-consuming if done by hand, since this involves creating elaborate matrices of who chose whom for each sociometric question that is asked, and then computing the rank order and proportion of nominations received by each student. There are computer scoring protocols available as freeware and for purchase online that can reduce this task to one requiring only a few minutes. (As an example, see a free demo of Walsh's Classroom Sociometrics at *www.classroomsociometrics.com*.)

Both sociometric nominations and ratings are easily used to describe peer acceptance as well as to identify mutual friendship pairs in a school or classroom (Benenson, 1990; Parker & Asher, 1989). Using either sociometric rating or nomination procedures, peer acceptance is determined by ranking students according to the number of nominations that they receive or the magnitude of their peer ratings (Coie, Dodge, & Coppotelli, 1982; Parker & Asher, 1993), while mutual friendships are identified whenever nominations or high ratings of two students are reciprocal (Berndt, 1981; Berndt & Perry, 1986). In prior studies using unlimited-choice positive nomination procedures, approximately 4% of children were not chosen as friends by any classmate, while no mutual friendship choices were identified for 10% of the class (Asher, 1995). Important targets for intervention are children not chosen as friends by any classmate, rejected children who are rated as highly disliked by peers, and neglected children who are neither chosen as a friend nor disliked. Generally, fewer than 15% of a class will fall into the neglected or rejected subgroups.

Perhaps the most formidable barrier to the use of sociometric assessments is their unfavorable reputation. Sociometric assessment's requirement that children evaluate the likability of classmates is controversial in school districts (Bierman & McCauley, 1987; Crick & Ladd, 1989). Critics claim that peer nominations can cause children to view certain peers more negatively and violate school norms prohibiting derogatory comments about classmates (Bell-Dolan, Foster, & Sikora, 1989; Deno, Mirkin, Robinson, & Evans, 1980). Despite convincing evidence that peer evaluations do not alter ongoing peer interactions (Bell-Dolan et al., 1989; Hayvren & Hymel, 1984), administrators and parents frequently oppose the collection of sociometric assessments in schools (Cook & Iverson, 1993).

Recommendation

The outcome of sociometric assessment is lists of students with few or no friends, or with low peer acceptance. School staff can use these lists as an efficient and effective way to identify the students who are struggling to establish supportive friendships with their peers. Given the substantial evidence that peer relationship difficulties presage later, more serious, disturbances, these lists also can be prime tools in early prevention programs by picking out children who are at risk for later, more serious, disturbances. Still, sociometric procedures cannot be used when schools have policies prohibiting them, and are too time-expensive to use without analysis software to compile the ratings and peer matches. Given the key role that social competence plays in early identification and remediation of other socioemotional disturbances, some schools will value the information that sociometric assessment can provide.

EXAMPLE

A small religious school was struggling with unusually large numbers of playground fights, and these were especially disturbing to the very devout parents who sent their children to the school. Initially, the school staff attempted to select out the students that they believed were causing the conflicts, but the task was insurmountable. Instead, and with parent permission, the school psychologist administered sociometric nomination surveys to every class in the school, asking questions specific to the playground difficulties: Which students are often in fights on the playground? Which students often get picked on by other kids? Which students are good at keeping the peace? And which students take care of other kids on the playground? Results showed important grade-level differences. Lots of students were identified as "fighters" in the fifth grade, and very few were identified in the fourth grade. The recess problems of the second, third, and sixth grades appeared to be due to a few select students, and the teaching staff established some individualized behavior plans for those students. However, the recess problems of the fifth grade appeared to be widespread and nonspecific. In subsequent classroom meetings, the fifth-grade students discussed the problems that recess held for them: Students' feelings were hurt by the raucous arguments that ensued whenever they chose soccer teams. They disagreed about the rules to the soccer game, and were angry at each other's "cheating." They engaged in a lot of retaliation against each other for mishaps that happened on the field, and had long-standing grudges about misunderstandings from several months earlier. Their conflicts sometimes bled over into the other grades that were on the playground with them. In the fifth grade, the school psychologist and teaching staff initiated some intensive social problem-solving meetings in order to identify and resolve present peer disagreements and to prepare the students to use more effective disagreements in the future.

SUMMARY

Population-based assessments are a necessary first step in order for schools to respond planfully to their students' needs for problem-solving intervention. By screening the full student population of a school, the procedures identify children who would have slipped through the cracks in traditional referral-based services. In particular, most population-based procedures will identify more children with internalizing behaviors who are often overlooked. In most cases, students with significant needs for support will be identified much earlier than they would have been through referrals. Thus, population-based assessments allow schools to be proactive rather than reactive in responding to students' developmental risks.

By providing a shared set of information about the identified children, population-based assessments allow schools to create a profile of common socioemotional problems that need to be addressed and to prioritize services toward students with the most urgent needs. With this data-based description of the problem, schools gain the potential to respond systemically to high-frequency problems, using interventions that directly address the needs of groups of students. For example, Crone, Horner, and Hawken (2004) describe a schoolwide behavioral support system that could be used with students whose behavioral compliance is a continuing problem. In some cases, school staff may decide that there are ecological factors that facilitate problems of a particular sort in a building. For example, a middle school determined that large numbers of students were being expelled for behavioral conflicts that occurred at recess, and that the playground's emptiness contributed to the disruptions. They reduced expulsions significantly by adding more games to the noontime recess. In other instances, population-based assessments can provide important normative standards against which to judge any single student's behavior. In every case, the population-based procedures make it possible for schools to be more planful, thoughtful, specific, and comprehensive in their plans for addressing students' social and behavioral problems.

Population-based assessments are not inexpensive. In each case, they require considerable staff time "up front" in order to collect and analyze the schoolwide data. At a minimum, this will require that schools redirect some of the resources currently allocated to referral-based service delivery. While it is a premise of this chapter that the benefits of schoolwide assessments outweigh these costs, the ultimate benefits may not be readily available to key school decision makers until after the assessments are conducted.

Moreover, population-based assessments do not replace traditional problem-based assessments of individual students. In particular, the screening procedures described earlier have 90% accuracy rates, such that some students will not be identified for services when they should be. Further, even though data collected during screening and identification procedures can provide a head start toward a functional analysis of a student's particular problem, it rarely provides sufficient definitive information for a full behavior plan. The problem-based assessments described throughout this book will be important intermediate steps in creating effective behavior plans.

These examples should not limit the vision of what is possible using population-based measures. Notably, none of the measures described above has taken advantage of computer technology for the administration or analysis of schoolwide data; yet, doing so could substantially reduce the time and cost. Moreover, at each stage, the procedures generally relied on a single informant to make a decision. However, 38 years ago, Barclay

(1966) integrated teacher ratings and peer sociometric ratings by using a simple three-by-three grid and demonstrated that the majority of fourth-grade students who subsequently dropped out of school had very low peer ratings, very low teacher ratings, or both. Barclay (1992) went on to conduct a comprehensive series of correlational, cross-sectional, and longitudinal studies examining the combined power of peer sociometrics, teacher ratings, and self-reported descriptions of preferred activities in predicting school success. He used the then emerging computer technology to meld the three sources into a single model and published his tool as the Barclay Classroom Climate Inventory (BCCI; Barclay, 1972), which was later renamed the Barclay Classroom Assessment System (BCAS; Barclay, 1983). Results of the BCCI/BCAS identified students who experienced motivation and attitude difficulties 3 years later (Barclay, 1979), who dropped out of school 4 years later (Barclay, 1966; Davis, 1967) and whose achievement test scores declined 3 years later (Barclay, Covert, Scott, & Stilwell, 1975).

Barclay's innovative use of technology and measurement is evidence of the power with which population-based strategies could ultimately be applied. Technology could streamline the procedures by which screening questions are asked, classwide and schoolwide data are collated and analyzed, and data trends over time are identified and tracked. The increased efficiency and reduced cost of schoolwide data collection could remove many of the barriers to population-based assessments. Subsequently, it can become common practice to preface powerful problem-solving assessment strategies with empirically supported procedures for selecting out those students most in need of behavioral support. Ultimately, the promise of populationwide data is the possibilities it creates for thinking about populationwide intervention. The full potential of population-based assessments will not be realized until there are more evidence-based systemic interventions that allow schools to respond effectively and efficiently to the identified needs.

REFERENCES

Achenbach, T. (2001). Assessment of Psychopathology. In A. J. Sameroff, M. Lewis, & S. M. Miller, (Eds.), *Handbook of developmental psychopathology* (2nd ed., pp. 41–56). New York: Kluwer Academic/Plenum Publishers.

Achenbach, T. M., & Rescorla, L. A. (2001). *Manual for ASEBA School-Age Forms and Profiles*. Burlington: University of Vermont, Research Center for Children, Youth, and Families.

American Psychiatric Association. (1987). *Diagnostic and statistical manual of mental disorders* (3rd ed., rev.). Washington, DC: Author.

Asher, S. R. (1995, June). *Children and adolescents with peer relationship problems*. A workshop presented at the Annual Summer Institute in School Psychology: Internalizing Disorders in Children and Adolescents, Denver, CO.

Asher, S. R., & Hymel, S. (1986). Coaching in social skills for children who lack friends in school. *Social Work in Education, 8,* 203–218.

Barclay, J. R. (1966). Sociometric choices and teacher ratings as predictors of school dropout. *Journal of Social Psychology, 4,* 40–45.

Barclay, J. R. (1972). *The Barclay Classroom Climate Inventory: A research manual and studies.* Lexington, KY: Educational Skills Development.

Barclay, J. R. (1979). *A manual for the Barclay Learning Needs Assessment Inventory.* Lexington, KY: Educational Skills Development.

Barclay, J. R. (1983). *Barclay Classroom Assessment System manual.* Los Angeles: Western Psychological Services.

Barclay, J. R. (1992). Sociometry, temperament and school psychology. In T. R. Kratochwill, S. Elliott, & M. Gettinger (Eds.), *Advances in school psychology* (vol. 8, pp. 79–114.) Hillsdale, NJ: Erlbaum.

Barclay, J. R., Covert, R. M., Scott, T. W., & Stilwell, W. E. (1975). *Some effects of schooling: A three-year follow up of a Title III project.* Lexington, KY: Educational Skills Development.

Behar, L., & Stringfield, S. (1974). *Manual for the preschool behavior questionnaire.* Sunham, NC: Behar.

Bell-Dolan, D. J., Foster, S. L., & Sikora, D. M. (1989). Effects of sociometric testing on children's behavior and loneliness in school. *Developmental Psychology, 25,* 306–311.

Benenson, J. F. (1990). Gender differences in social networks. *Journal of Early Adolescence, 10,* 472–495.

Berndt, T. J. (1981). Effects of friendship on prosocial intentions and behavior. *Child Development, 52,* 636–643.

Berndt, T. J. (1984). Sociometric, socio-cognitive and behavioral measures for the study of friendship and popularity. In T. Field, J. L. Roopnarine, & M. Segal (Eds.), *Friendship in normal and handicapped children* (pp. 31–45). Norwood, NJ: Ablex.

Berndt, T. J., & Perry, T. B. (1986). Children's perceptions of friendships as supportive relationships. *Developmental Psychology, 22,* 640–648.

Bierman, K. L., & McCauley, E. (1987). Children's descriptions of their peer interactions: Useful information for clinical child assessment. *Journal of Clinical Child Psychology, 16,* 9–18.

Coie, J. D., Dodge, K. A., & Coppotelli, H. (1982). Dimensions and types of social status: A cross-age perspective. *Developmental Psychology, 18,* 557–571.

Coie, J. D., & Kupersmidt, J. (1983). A behavior analysis of emerging social status in boys' groups. *Child Development, 54,* 1400–1416.

Coie, J. D., Watt, N. F., West, S. G., Hawkins, J. D., Asarnow, J. R., Markan, H. J., Ramey, S. L., Shure, M., & Long, B. (1993). The science of prevention: A conceptual framework and some directions for a national research program. *American Psychologist, 48,* 1013–1022.

Conners, C. K. (1989). *Manual for the Conners rating scales.* North Tonawanda, NY: Multi-Health Systems.

Cook, G. R., & Iverson, A. M. (1993, April). *An investigation of parental non-consent in sociometric research.* Paper presented at the annual convention of the National Association of School Psychologists, Washington, DC.

Crick, N. R., & Ladd, G. W. (1989). Nominator attrition: Does it affect the accuracy of children's sociometric classifications? *Merrill-Palmer Quarterly, 35,* 197–207.

Crone, D. A., Horner, R. H., & Hawken, L. S. (2004). *Responding to problem behavior in schools: The Behavior Education Program.* New York: Guilford Press.

Davis, D. (1967). *The validity and reliability of a sociometric device.* Unpublished master's thesis, Idaho State University.

Deno, S. L., Mirkin, P. K., Robinson, S., & Evans, P. (1980). *Relationships among classroom observations of social adjustment and sociometric ratings scales* (Research Report No. 24). University of Minnesota: Institute for Research on Learning Disabilities.

Dodge, K. A. (1989). Problems in social relationships. In E. J. Mash & R. A. Barkley (Eds.), *Treatment of childhood disorders* (pp. 222–246). New York: Guilford Press.

Doll, B. (1996). Prevalence of psychiatric disorders in children and youth: An agenda for advocacy by school psychology. *School Psychology Quarterly, 11,* 20–46.

Doll, B., & Lyon, M. (1998). Risk and resilience: Implications for the practice of school psychology. *School Psychology Review, 27,* 348–363.

Doll, B., Murphy, P., & Song, S. (2003). The relationship between children's self-reported recess problems, and peer acceptance and friendships. *Journal of School Psychology, 41,* 113–130.

Doll, B., Zucker, S., & Brehm, K. (2004). *Resilient classrooms: Creating healthy environments for learning.* New York: Guilford Press.

Feil, E. G., & Becker, W. C. (1993). Investigation of a multiple-gated screening system for preschool behavior problems. *Behavioral Disorders, 19*(1), 44–53.

Feil, E. G., & Severson, H. (1995). Identification of critical factors in the assessment of preschool behavior problems. *Education and Treatment of Children, 18*(3), 261–271.

Feil, E. G., Walker, H. M., & Severson, H. H. (1995). The Early Screening Project for young children with behavior problems. *Journal of Emotional and Behavioral Disorders, 3*(4), 194–203.

Greenfield, S. F., Reizes, J. M., Muenz, L. R., Kopans, B., Kozloff, R. C., & Jacobs, D. G. (2000). Treatment for depression following the 1996 National Depression Screening Day. *American Journal of Psychiatry, 157,* 1867–1869.

Guralnick, M. (1986). The peer relations of young handicapped and non-handicapped children. In P. Strain, M. Guralnick, & H. M. Walker (Eds.), *Children's social behavior: Development, assessment and modification* (pp. 93–140). New York: Academic Press.

Hamilton, M. (1967). Development of a rating scale for primary depressive illness. *British Journal of Social and Clinical Psychology, 6,* 278–296.

Hayvren, M., & Hymel, S. (1984). Ethical issues in sociometric testing. The impact of sociometric measures on interactive behavior. *Developmental Psychology, 20,* 844–849.

Kessler, R. C., & Walters, E. E. (1998). Epidemiology of DSM-III-R Major Depression and Minor Depression among adolescents and young adults in the National Comorbidity Survey. *Depression and Anxiety, 7,* 3–14.

Kovacs, M. (1979). *Children's Depression Inventory.* Pittsburgh: University of Pittsburgh School of Medicine.

Krefetz, D. G., Steer, R. A., & Gulab, N. A. (2002). Convergent validity of the Beck Depression Inventory-II with the Reynolds Adolescent Depression Scale in psychiatric inpatients. *Journal of Personality Assessment, 78,* 451–460.

McInerney, M., Kane, M., & Pelavin, S. (1992). *Services to children with serious emotional disturbance.* Washington, DC: Pelavin Associates.

Newcomb, A. F., & Bukowski, W. M. (1984). A longitudinal study of the utility of social preference and social impact sociometric classification schemes. *Child Development, 55,* 1434–1447.

Parker, J. G., & Asher, S. R. (1989, April). *Peer relations and social adjustment: Are friendship and group acceptance distinct domains?* Paper presented at the biennial meeting of the Society for Research in Child Development, Kansas City, MO.

Parker, J. G., & Asher, S. R. (1993). Friendship and friendship quality in middle childhood: Links with peer group acceptance and feelings of loneliness and social dissatisfaction. *Developmental Psychology, 29*, 611–621.

Pianta, R. C., & Walsh, D. J. (1996). *High-risk children in schools: Constructing sustaining relationships.* New York: Routledge.

Reynolds, W. M. (1987). *Reynolds Adolescent Depression Scale.* Lutz, FL: Psychological Assessment Resources.

Reynolds, W. M. (1989). Suicidal ideation and depression in adolescents: Assessment and research. In P. Lovibond & P. Wilson (Eds.), *Clinical and abnormal psychology* (pp. 125–135). Amsterdam: Elsevier Science.

Reynolds, W. M. (1991). A school-based procedure for the identification of adolescents at risk for suicidal behaviors. *Family and Community Health, 14*, 64–75.

Reynolds, W. M. (1994). Assessment of depression in children and adolescents by self-report questionnaires. In W. M. Reynolds & H. E. Johnston (Eds.), *Handbook of depression in children and adolescents* (pp. 209–234). New York: Plenum.

Reynolds, W. M. (1998). Depresssion in children and adolescents. In T. H. Ollendick (Ed.), *Comprehensive clinical psychology: Vol. 4. Children and adolescents: Clinical formulations and treatment* (pp. 419–461). New York: Pergamon.

Reynolds, W. M. (2002). *Reynolds Adolescent Depression Scale—2nd Edition.* Lutz, FL: Psychological Assessment Resources.

Reynolds, W. M., & Mazza, J. J. (1998). Reliability and validity of the Reynolds Adolescent Depression Scale with young adolescents. *Journal of School Psychology, 36*, 295–312.

Reynolds, W. M., & Mazza, J. J. (1999). Assessment of suicidal ideation in inner-city children and young adolescents: Reliability and validity of the Suicidal Ideation Questionnaire—JR. *School Psychology Review, 28*, 17–30.

Rose, A. J., & Asher, S. R. (1999). Children's goals and strategies in response to conflicts within a friendship. *Developmental Psychology, 35*, 69–79.

Walker, H. M., & Severson, H. H. (1992). Systematic Screening for Behavior Disorders (SSBD): User's guide and administration manual. Longmont, CO: Sopris West.

Walker, H. M., & Severson, H. (1994). Replication of the systematic screening for behavior disorders (SSBD) procedure for the identification of at-risk children. *Journal of Emotional and Behavioral Disorders, 2*, 66–77.

Walker, H. M., Severson, H. H., & Feil, E. G. (1995). *Early Screening Project.(ESP): A proven child find process* (user manual). Longmont, CO: Sopris West.

Walker, H. M., Severson, H., Stiller, B., Williams, G., Haring, N., Shinn, M., & Todis, B. (1988). Systematic screening of pupils in the elementary age range at risk for behavior disorders: Development and trial testing of a multiple gating model. *Remedial and Special Education, 9*(3), 8–14.

Walker, H. M., Severson, H., Todis, B., Block-Pedego, A. E., Williams, G., Haring, N. G., & Barckley, M. (1990). Systematic screening for behavior disorders (SSBD): Further validation, replication, and normative data. *Remedial and Special Education, 11*(2), 32–46.

SUGGESTED READINGS

Pianta, R., & Walsh, D. J. (1996). *High-risk children in schools: Constructing sustaining relationships.* New York: Routledge.

This small volume provides a succinct and telling summary of the impact of developmental risk on children's schooling, and describes policies and practices that promote mentally healthier schools.

Walker, H. M., Severson, H. H., Nicholson, F., Kehle, T., et al. (1999). Replication of the systematic screening of behavior disorders procedures for the identification of at-risk children. *Journal of Emotional and Behavioral Disorders, 2,* 66–77.

This is an example of the research that supports the efficacy of the SSBD for identification of children, and discusses its implication for school practice.

Crone, D. A., Horner, R. H., & Hawken, L. S. (2004). *Responding to problem behavior in schools: The Behavior Education Program.* New York: Guilford Press.

This monograph describes an innovative schoolwide response program that is be built upon schoolwide discipline data.

CHAPTER 6

♦ ♦ ♦

Physiological Factors in Students' School Success

♦

GEORGE W. BROWN
CAROLYN V. BROWN

There are some obvious and basic physiological capabilities that influence a student's school success. These include mobility, hearing, speech capability, vision, and functional vital organs (heart, lungs, kidneys, and intestines). For most students, it is taken for granted that they have the physiological capacity to engage in school activities. Recognizing the role of basic physiological capability is an important, yet sometimes overlooked, aspect of school-based assessment activities. Less obvious, and therefore more easily overlooked, are health risk factors such as poor nutrition, family stresses, learning and behavior disabilities, emotional disorders, and environmental compromises. Accurate assessment with development of a treatment plan for students with physiological limitations is more likely when the child, family, school, and health care professionals work collaboratively. Such team efforts must be committed to short- and long-term involvement when appropriate.

Students with physiological and/or emotional problems face many challenges that are likely to influence their school performance. Even with appropriate team support, such problems may reduce a student's chances for school and life success. For students with physiological problems, early assessment and intervention reduces the extent to which such difficulties interfere with school success. A well-established model for early identification and treatment of health concerns involves three levels of care: primary, secondary, and tertiary (Fairbanks & Wiese, 1998). This model is a cornerstone of public health policy and includes steps to identify all children with physiological difficulties as early as possible. Primary prevention involves intervention and support for those who are *at risk* of a physiological condition. Secondary intervention includes treatment of the *first-stage symptoms* of a condition with the goal of reducing later symptoms and greater problems. Tertiary intervention includes comprehensive treatment for *chronic and advanced conditions*. Utilization of the primary and secondary prevention stages of public health intervention are more than just a humane ideal. These activities can promote cost-effective educational and health outcomes for students. Primary and secondary prevention efforts fit well with Deno's (1985, 1989) problem-solving model for school assessment in that they seek to identify and address gaps in student wellness problems before such problems become so great that they interfere with student school success.

In order to make sense of how problem solving and prevention-oriented activities can enhance student school success, the health conditions most prevalent in school-age children will be discussed. Five of the most common physiological problems seen in school-age children are (Nader, 1993):

1. Obesity and prediabetes symptoms
2. Attention-deficit/hyperactivity disorder (ADHD)
3. Emotional and behavior disorders
4. Respiratory complications
5. Chronic and congenital conditions

These five most common problems will be described within the context of the underlying causes and physiological effects that pose challenges to students. A case scenario will be provided that depicts a problem-solving-based approach for addressing physiological conditions affecting student school success.

PHYSIOLOGICAL CONDITIONS COMMON IN SCHOOL-AGE CHILDREN

Obesity and Prediabetes

Obesity causes multiple complications with direct impact on a student's school success (Rosenbaum, Leibel, & Hirsch, 1997). Obesity is defined as body mass index (BMI) of 27 or greater. In addition to the physical complications, obesity is socially unacceptable, especially among females, and promotes depression, social withdrawal, and poor school performance (National Institutes of Health Consensus Development Conference Statement, 1985). Severe obesity can cause sleep apnea (known as the Pickwickian syndrome). One of the most serious complications is high blood pressure with premature atherosclerosis from lipid damage to arteries (Belay, Belamarich, & Racine, 2004). More immediate physiologic effects for students are abnormal acceleration of physical growth and sexual development with early menarche and pubertal breast enlargement. The most dangerous physiological effect is on the endocrine system, with insulin resistance, elevated blood lipids, and eventually type 2 diabetes mellitus (American Diabetes Association, 2000).

Diabetes, both types 1 and 2, cause major swings in blood sugar levels from dangerously low (hypoglycemia) to life-threateningly high (diabetic ketoacidosis with hyperglycemia). Hypoglycemia alters brain function in several ways: altered neurotramission, energy failure for basic brain cell performance, and inteference with cell membrane depolarization. In rare cases, it can be fatal, especially among infants and toddlers, and more commonly can cause irreversible brain injury. Hyperglycemia alters brain function in multiple ways: abnormalities in cell fuel metabolism, disruption in brain blood flow, damage to brain blood vessels, and alteration of brain nutrient transport. In cases of severe diabetic ketoacidosis, excessive brain fluid (cerebral edema) may become irreversible and even fatal (Rovet, 2000).

Since the availability of insulin for the treatment of diabetes in the early 20th century, much more is understood at the cellular level. While most researchers initially considered diabetes to be primarily an inherited disorder, there is increasing evidence that obesity elevates the risk for diabetes among children and adults (Kaufman, 2002). The emerging worldwide epidemic of obesity is revealing two major environmental factors: fast food and television. For years, all childhood diabetes was considered to be inherited due to early loss of insulin production in the digestive organ, the pancreas. Adult diabetes was considered primarily environmental and secondary to chronic overweight. These conceptualizations led to the common medical diagnostic terms, type 1 diabetes in children and type 2 diabetes in adults. With the spreading epidemic of childhood obesity, type 2 diabetes is now being diagnosed in children. Obesity is now the most common physiological disorder among U.S. children (Health Resources and Services Administration, 2002). As a result of the dramatic increase in type 2 diabetes among children, a new diagnosis known as prediabetes has evolved (American Diabetes Association, 2000; Sinha et al., 2002). Prediabetes is defined as a fasting blood sugar level between 100 and 119 mg/dl, with diabetes mellitus observed when fasting blood sugar is above 120 mg/dl.

Data from students themselves reveal weight-related health concerns. In the U.S. 1999 Youth Risk Behavior Survey (Centers for Disease Control, 2000), 30% of high school students thought themselves overweight. This was a 10% increase since 1997. In 1999, nearly 40% of students were attempting weight loss, with females more than twice as likely as males to lose weight. The most common methods were use of moderate to vigorous physical and strengthening activities, but males used these more than females. Dieting and more drastic eating disorders are more common among females. The American Academy of Pediatrics (AAP) has conducted research in the area of television viewing habits of children and families with emphasis on advertisements for unhealthy high calorie and fast food use by children. Additionally, several national medical organizations, including the American Heart Association, American Public Health Association, American Medical Association, and American Diabetes Association and the U.S. Department of Health and Human Services, have joined the AAP to promote obesity awareness and healthy lifestyles among children. Importantly, a problem-solving and primary prevention approach to obesity and prediabetes involves identifying those students at risk for these conditions and helping them develop healthy eating and activity habits so that actual diabetes as well as other complications are prevented.

Attention-Deficit/Hyperactivity Disorder

Attention-deficit/hyperactivity disorder (ADHD) is the formal diagnostic term used to identify and describe individuals with chronic hyperactive and/or inattentive behaviors (American Psychiatric Association, 2000). ADHD has three subtypes: (1) hyperactive–impulsive, (2) inattentive, and (3) combined (those with both hyperactive and inattentive behaviors). Because there is no clinical laboratory test for ADHD, interviews and behavior rating scales with students, parents, and teachers, as well as classroom observations, constitute the best set of assessment and diagnosis procedures (DuPaul & Stoner, 2003). An essential characteristic necessary to support a diagnosis of ADHD is that the symptoms must be present in at least two settings (Blum, 2002). For example, students must show hyperactive and/or inattentive behaviors at school and home. Obvious discrepancies in interview, rating scale, and/or observational data suggest that other comorbid and/or family problems exist and ADHD may not be the correct diagnosis. For detailed descriptions of interview, observation, and rating scale methods, see Chapters 8, 9, and 10, respectively, of this volume.

Newer research techniques with isotope imaging and brain pharmacological studies are shedding light on the underlying pathophysiology of ADHD (Barkley, 1998). The major finding in the research has been identification of both anatomical and neurotransmitter differences in those with ADHD as compared to those without. Specifically, there are differences in the frontal cortex activation patterns of the brains of adults with ADHD. Additional research has suggested that these activation differences are related to deficits in two neurotransmitters, norepinephrine and dopamine.

Related studies have investigated the effectiveness stimulant medications for alleviating symptoms and correcting the neurotransmitter deficits. Experienced clinicians and researchers stress that medications alone are insufficient for reversing the student's diminishing chances of success from ADHD (DuPaul & Stoner, 2003). Some students have both ADHD and a learning disability. Many others, especially those with delayed school and clinical intervention until middle grades, have significant behavior problems. Family and school environments have major influences on a student's ADHD symptoms. Recent research has demonstrated the role of early and frequent television viewing as a significant increased risk for subsequent ADHD symptoms (Christakis, Zimmerman, DiGiuseppe, & McCarty, 2004). A combined treatment utilizing environmental features as well as medication appears to be the most effective way to help students with ADHD.

Estimates of the prevalence of ADHD vary from 5 to 10% of the school population (Barkley, 1998; DuPaul & Stoner, 2003). ADHD was once thought to be a condition exclusive to childhood. More recent epidemiologic studies have shown that ADHD symptoms continue into adulthood. Adults with ADHD have been effectively treated with combined family and clinical methods. There appears to be a consistently higher rate of ADHD in males, with four for every one female identified. Comorbid conditions, such as obsessive–compulsive disorder (OCD), oppositional defiant disorder (ODD), and posttraumatic stress disorder (PTSD) are common. These more complicated emotional and psychiatric disorders are discussed in detail in the next section. Genetic studies show a child's risk for ADHD as high as 25% if a first-degree relative has ADHD. This genetic component is confirmed by twin studies, with risks from 60 to 80% among identical twins compared to only 30% in fraternal twins (American Psychiatric Association, 2000). The effects of ADHD on a student's chances of school success can be enormous. A short list includes (1) school failure, (2) poor relationships with peers, (3) significant behavior problems, (4) sleep difficulties that can lead to school performance problems, (5) poor fine motor skills, (6) higher rates of accidental injuries, and (7) learning disabilities (Blum, 2002). This short list does not include additional psychiatric diagnoses.

Solving the problems of students with ADHD is usually less complicated with early diagnosis and intervention. When ADHD is identified early and effective treatment provided, the likelihood of related complications and comorbid disabilities is reduced. ADHD assessment is best done by teamwork, but team-based assessments may not always happen due to limited available educational and clinical resources. Thanks to educational efforts by the AAP and the National Association of School Psychologists (NASP), pediatricians and family practitioners have better access to continuing education on assessment and clinical management of ADHD. Students with ADHD benefit from ongoing communication among all members of the multidisciplinary team involved in both assessment and treatment. In cases of complex behavior and family dynamics, active participation and communication among the members of the team may make the difference between the student's long-term success or failure.

Emotional and Behavioral Problems

Emotional and behavioral problems among students include anxiety disorders, chronic depression, attachment problems, and severe aggressive behaviors. Dynamic changes in U.S. family structures over recent decades, including divorce, stepfamilies, public attention to issues like sexual abuse, substance abuse, and neglect, and economic pressures requiring both parents to work outside the home all contribute to the now common presentation of school behavior problems. Symptoms of behavioral problems are likewise wide-ranging, with multiple causes. Around 10% of all children will at some point go to the school nurse or other health facilities with a stomachache (American Academy of Pediatrics, 1993). Often their complaints are clues to existing behavioral and psychosocial difficulties. Behavior problems without physical complaints occur among 30–50% of all U.S. students. These are usually described by parents and teachers as disruptive and overactive behaviors that interfere with student learning. Some of the behavioral difficulties are subsequently identified as ADHD or as behaviors that mask underlying learning disabilities. Still, as many as 10% of students may have more significant emotional, behavioral mental health problems.

Ongoing research in neurophysiology and genetics is slowly revealing the marvelous capacities of human brain function. Importantly, this research has revealed that certain emotional and behavioral disorders result from significant genetic predispositions. We now understand family history to be vital for accurately identifying certain conditions such as bipolar disorder, OCD, PTSD, and risks for alcohol and other substance abuse disorders. Genetic studies show a greater than three times increase in risk for major depression among identical twins (Albee & Joffe, 2004; American Psychiatric Association, 2000). Neuroimaging studies, as in ADHD, suggest increased metabolic activity in the frontal lobes and basal ganglia in students with OCD. No exact causes for student emotional and behavioral disorders are understood except in PTSD, where specific stressful events are confirmed in a student's medical history.

The wide variety of emotional and behavioral disorders, and their myriad intertwined factors, can be grouped into six main categories: (1) ADHD, (2) vegetative, (3) habit, (4) anxiety, (5) mood, and (6) disruptive behavioral (American Psychiatric Association, 2000; Pickering, 2003). Vegetative disorders include pica (chronic ingestion of nonnutrient substances like plaster), daytime and nighttime wetting (enuresis), fecal soiling (encopresis), and sleep disorders. Habit disorders include repetitive tension-releasing activities such as nail biting, body rocking, hair pulling, tics, stuttering, and teeth grinding (bruxism). Grandmothers, experienced teachers, school nurses, and pediatricians often see and help parents handle these very common vegetative and habit problems before they become school learning impairments. In cases when such conditions interfere with school activities, integration of treatments into the school day may be necessary.

Anxiety disorders include phobias, avoidant behavior, OCD, ODD, and PTSD. PTSD is now better understood and more frequently diagnosed with expanding child neglect and sexual abuse awareness (Bernstein & Garfinkel, 1986). Mood disorders include the more serious and complex problems of major depression, dysthymic disorder, and bipolar disorder. Disruptive behavioral disorders comprise lying, impulsiveness, breath holding, defiance, and temper tantrums (Chun, 2002). These behaviors are appropriate in preschool and early elementary age children but become problematic if they occur too often or in older children. Estimates have suggested that about 50% of preschoolers in the United States are brought to the attention of physicians at some time because of disobedient and defiant behaviors. Often, such behaviors can be improved through changes in parenting style. If these behaviors continue into the early school grades, attention is needed to find underlying problems of a more serious nature such as ADHD, anxiety, or mood disorders.

If untreated, the physiological effects of these myriad disorders are pervasive. Vegetative disorders can lead to anemia, lead poisoning, nutritional deficiencies, skin rashes, urinary tract infections, and social ostracism at school. Habit disorders, such as tics and stuttering, that carry over into the early school years can have a negative influence on student success. Anxiety disorders such as phobias and avoidant behavior can be serious impediments to early school success because students with these disorders tend to miss out on so much instruction. Children with OCD, ODD, and PTSD will present significant challenges to families, teachers, psychologists, nurses, and physicians because the nature of these disruptive behaviors involves active resistance by the students to efforts to change their behaviors. Students with mood disorders such as major depression, dysthymic disorder, bipolar disorder, and PTSD need comprehensive evaluation and management to minimize the extent to which these conditions interfere with school success (Dalton, 1996; Silver, 1990).

Respiratory Problems

While infections such as the common cold and bronchitis by far outnumber all other childhood respiratory problems, appropriate family care with ongoing health education from school nurses, physicians, and public health professionals manages these with minimal risk of damaging student school success. The common chronic respiratory problem of asthma is another story. In medical terminology, "chronic" refers to conditions that are long-lasting or recurring. The physiologic definition of asthma consists of three components: reversible airway obstruction, airway inflammation (swelling), and airway excessive sensitivity (allergic) to stimuli (Hakonarson, 2002). Recent pharmacological research has produced preventive medications such as inhaled corticosteroids (Szelfler, 1998). These can be used for infants and hold promise of reversing the recent increased prevalence of asthma among school children. The old medical adage "All that wheezes is not allergic asthma" reinforces that there can be multiple causes of respiratory problems. Both medical and school personnel must be alert to inhaled foreign bodies in toddlers and conditions such as pneumonia (Shapiro, 1992). Nonetheless, allergic asthma is the most common chronic illness in children.

The most common cause for wheezing among school children is an inherited allergic condition with specific exposure to indoor tobacco smoke, dust mites, pollens, molds, and outdoor diesel motor fume exposures (e.g., school bus exhaust). Tobacco and diesel fume exposures are suspected underlying factors in increased numbers of children with asthma as well as increased asthma deaths during the 1980s and 1990s. While wheezing from asthma is as high as 30–60% in industrialized countries, most episodes of asthma follow viral infections in preschool children. Most of these asthma events subside before age 6. Asthma is more common among males up to 10 years of age; thereafter, the prevalence is equal between the sexes among older students and adults.

A consistently observed incidence of around 10% of the total population born with a genetic tendency to allergic disorders such as asthma, hay fever, and eczema has been documented for many decades (Shapiro, 1992). Children of asthmatic parents have a 20% risk of developing asthma if one parent has asthma and a 60% risk if both have asthma. This compares to a 6–7% risk if neither parent is affected with asthma. The most recent asthma research has pointed to the role of environment as being more important than genetics in the development of asthma. Evidence for the environmental contributions to asthma have been documented in the wide range of inherited severity, known as genetic penetrance. Individuals with only weak genetic asthma predisposition who are raised in relatively nonallergic and less lung-irritating air environments are less likely to develop clinical asthma (Richards, 1992). Public health research confirms the critical value of preventive education for students, parents, families, and the professionals who work with them. Despite the high rates of childhood wheezing in industrialized countries (30–60%), only 5–7% of all children go on to develop asthma.

Nonetheless, the physiological effects of chronic allergies, especially asthma, can cause frequent medical visits, including hospitalizations, and school absences (Richards, 1992). Additionally, lowered oxygen saturation levels to body organs cause fatigue, diminished attention, and may stunt physical growth. Asthma is associated with increased frequency of acute and chronic bacterial infections such as pneumonia, bronchitis, and sinusitis. Early detection and treatment of asthma symptoms can prevent negative school outcomes for students. School nurses, school psychological personnel, and school-based social services can play a significant preventive and early intervention role for such children and families. Many professional organizations promote early and ongoing family and public education about prevention of asthma.

Chronic and Congenital Problems

There are four basic types of chronic and congenital childhood health problems: (1) cancer, (2) congenital, (3) environmental, and (4) infectious.

Cancer

The most common childhood cancer type is acute lymphoblastic leukemia (Pui, 1997). It occurs in some 3,000 children annually, most under 4 years old (Waber & Mullenix, 2000). Effective treatment, which usually starts before kindergarten or first grade but continues for 3–5 years, achieves remission in 95% of cases, with long-term survival (over 5 years after completion of therapy) of 70% (Shankar, 2002). Specific toxicity to the central nervous system (brain) from anticancer drugs and radiation is well recognized. The short-term side effects of childhood cancer treatments include hair loss, severe immunosuppression, nausea, and energy loss.

The longer-term effects of leukemia therapies are of much greater concern to classroom teachers and those providing special education services. As leukemia treatments became more and more effective in the 1980s, an increasing number of survivors showed school difficulties far beyond the emotional stresses of such life-threatening illness and long school absences (Walker & Jacobs, 1985). These long-term side effects included lower-than-expected IQ scores and significant learning problems. As both chemotherapy and radiation treatments have been progressively defined, earlier treatment consequences like diminished IQ and pervasive learning problems have lessened. Still, subtle school difficulties like learning disabilities are still increased among childhood cancer survivors.

Congenital

The seven most frequent congenital childhood disorders are (1) dislocation of the hip, (2) club foot, (3) cleft lip, (4) cleft palate, (5) septal (dividing wall) defects of the heart, (6) pyloric stenosis (narrowing of the stomach outlet), and (7) neural tube defects of the lower spinal cord. Most of these have been successfully corrected by age 5 or 6 with effective medical, nursing, social, physical, and occupational therapy. Other less common childhood congenital disorders include common genetic syndromes such as Down, Turner, and Kleinfelter, as well as less well understood ones like fragile X and Rett syndromes. Families and their children with these problems have undergone extensive diagnostic and treatment procedures by the time they enter school. Children who need ongoing specialized instruction as a result of these conditions may be eligible both at the preschool and school-age levels for special education services (Walker & Jacobs, 1985). Rare but important to affected children and families is cystic fibrosis, which has more chronic effects in the teen years (American Academy of Pediatrics Committee on School Health, 1993).

Seizure disorders, also called convulsions or epileptic fits, are common chronic physiologic disorders that may or may not be genetic. Those children with seizures that affect nearly all of the muscles of arms, legs, torso, and face (known as major motor or generalized epilepsies) show an automosomal (not sex chromosomal) dominant genetic inheritance pattern (Brooks-Kayal, 2002). The degree of physiological inteference in school success varies greatly but is most influenced by the frequency of seizures. In other words, if an effective seizure medication (anticonvulsant) is found and used regularly, the number of seizures per month will be very low. If the seizure disorder is due to a recognized genetic or birth defect, effective treatment of the underlying cause is most important (Vining, 1998). For certain conditions, like neurofibromatosis or Sturge–Weber syndrome, there are limited effective treatments for the underlying cause. Impaired learning may be due more to the underlying brain malformation or metabolic disorder of brain cell function than to the seizures themselves. On the other hand, when seizures last for longer periods (i.e., more than 5–10 minutes), decreased supply of oxygen to brain cells may lead to impaired learning skills. A great majority of children with seizures fit into neither of these two higher-risk categories. Indeed, most children with seizures have normal cognitive and neuromuscular skills.

Infectious and Environmental

Fortunately infectious disorders, except for AIDS in some high-risk populations and geographical areas, are rare causes of physiological obstacles to student success in school. Prenatal environmental factors such as exposure to nicotine, alcohol, Dilantin (phenytoin), and other drugs commonly abused like cocaine and homemade methamphetamines cause chronic and often severe developmental delays and school success problems (Rasmussen, 2004). Postnatal environmental exposures to various slow poisons like lead and acute poison ingestions as well as physical injuries from choking, motor vehicle crashes, falls, drowning, and guns are major causes of permanent brain, motor, and skeletal disabilities. For comprehensive medical treatment of all these congenital and chronic problems, there are well-established pediatric center and subspecialty services that significantly decrease their long-term effects. Children with such conditions are best served when they can obtain early and ongoing treatment that includes supports for school and extracurricular activities.

PROBLEM-SOLVING ASSESSMENT AND TREATMENT

Before discussion of how best to conduct problem-solving-based assessment of the five major types of physiological conditions, a general framework appropriate to all of the conditions will be presented. A relatively new concept called "the medical home" is an emerging model for facilitating communication about a child's health treatment. The simple definition of the medical home is "the place where child patients and [their] families receive regular and reliable care for both acute illnesses and chronic medical problems" (Sia, 1992). Dr. Calvin Sia has specialized in developing community-based services for children and families with cancer, birth defects, learning disabilities, and child abuse and neglect problems. Other physicians have replicated this model in a variety of healthcare settings. The physician, nurse practitioner, or other healthcare provider gets to know the health, emotional, and social needs, strengths, and weaknesses of both the children and their families. These practitioners serve as centers of communication in all directions for the multitude of volunteer and professional services for families and children. The medical home model complements problem-solving assessment activities because it utilizes team-based decision making with continuous evaluation of treatment progress (Szilagyi, 2004).

This model can be used with a wide variety of childhood physical conditions, including the top five physiological problems discussed in this chapter. There are four guiding questions that can facilitate problem-solving approaches to physiological problems:

1. What are the student's strengths and weaknesses?
2. What are the behavioral objectives of treatment?
3. What are the optimum treatments or interventions?
4. What other resources are available for this child and family?

These questions complement the stages of Deno's (1989) problem-solving model of assessment and intervention.

Obesity and Prediabetes

While observation alone may identify most students with obesity, detection of evolving prediabetes in a given student involves several key steps. The basic early detection tools for obesity are regular physical examinations that include plotting height, weight, and body mass indexes on standard child growth charts. An individual student's trend toward increasing weight relative to height will allow calculation of the body mass index (BMI). BMI is calculated by dividing the child's weight in kilograms by the child's height in meters squared (BMI = kg/m^2; Centers for Disease Control, 2004). Growth charts have a graph for plotting BMI. Such measurements can be done in medical offices by practitioners or in school settings by school nurses. Once an increased body mass index is observed, nutritional and physical activity changes become imperative. Medical and pediatric literature continues to document the vital importance of family involvement for such changes to start (American Diabetes Association, 2000). Because obesity is two to three times higher in the children of families with obesity, parents and siblings should be involved with medical assessment and treatment planning. Some laboratory blood tests should be considered for the child and others in the family if there is a strong family history of diabetes, high cholesterol, or thyroid problems. Since no safe and effective medications for obesity are currently available, the combination of decreased calorie intake and increased physical exercise remain the cornerstones of obesity treatment (Weiss et al., 2004). Such treatment plans are more likely to be followed by obese children when all members of the family participate. Because such nutritional and physical activity prescriptions have lifelong preventive effects against diabetes, heart disease, arthritis, and common forms of cancer, they deserve vigorous and widespread application. An important component of the weight-loss plan is progress monitoring. Weekly weight data can be used to evaluate the effectiveness of the intervention and determine whether additional dietary and exercise changes are needed.

Diagnosis of diabetes in children usually follows symptoms of weight loss, fatigue, excessive thirst, and urination. Besides laboratory tests of blood sugar, the hemoglobin A1C level is measured. Once insulin treatment is started, regular medical visits and hemoglobin A1C assessments are mandatory. In some children with a pattern typical of type 2 diabetes, oral insulin may be used. Diabetic children and their families require regular teaching and support by either hospital-based diabetic or pediatric endocrinology clinics. Such clinics have pediatricians, nurses, diabetic educators, nutritionists, and physical therapists who can help the child and his or her family understand the lifelong implications of diabetes. School physical education, health, and athletic personnel are vital members of professional teams that work with obese, prediabetic, and diabetic children. Current standards of care call for control of blood sugar, with target levels of between 60 and 150 mg/dl. This is now relatively easy to achieve with accurate home glucose monitors, newer short- and long-acting insulins, and small computer-controlled glucose pumps. Early and continued diabetic education and medical supervision are key to good diabetic control. Prevention of prediabetes and obesity are more important goals because of their cost savings as well as avoiding later childhood diseases such as cardiovascular disease, hyperlipidemia, and hypertension (Belay et al., 2004). Given the lifelong risks associated with obesity, prediabetes, and diabetes, problem-solving and prevention-oriented health interventions are in students' long-term best interests.

Attention-Deficit/Hyperactivity Disorder

Whereas health professionals play lead roles in assessment and management of obesity and prediabetes, school psychologists, teachers, and educational administrators are the professional stars in the case of hyperactivity and attention difficulties. Recently, integration of educational, psychological, medical, and psychiatric models for the assessment and treatment of ADHD has been undertaken by the American Academy of Pediatrics, the American Academy of Child and Adolescent Psychiatry, and the National Association of School Psychologists (American Academy of Child and Adolescent Psychiatry, 2003; American Academy of Pediatrics, 2002). Assessment and treatment standards published by the AAP in 2002 include an emphasis on the important role of the multidisciplinary team in ADHD evaluations and treatment. Specifically, ADHD should not be diagnosed in school-age children unless there are data collected in school settings that validate other symptoms of ADHD.

ADHD evaluations usually begin after a parent or teacher identifies that a student is overly hyperactive or inattentive (Fergusson & Horwood, 1992). In many cases a co-occurring concern is that the student is not making satisfactory academic progress. For younger children, hyperactivity and behavior problems are the more common presenting problems. Thus, puzzled primary school teachers and frustrated parents are likely to seek school psychology and/or nurse-medical help. The assessment process should include the following key steps: (1) review of school records, (2) parent and teacher interviews, questionnaires, and rating scales, (3) direct observations of child behavior and school performance, and, for some, (4) formal psychological evaluation and physical and neurological examination (DuPaul & Stoner, 2003).

Either a school-based practitioner such as a nurse or school psychologist, or a medical professional, can initiate an ADHD evaluation as soon as parental consent is obtained. Usually, the ADHD evaluation will begin with a record review and interviews of the parent(s)/guardian(s), teacher(s), and student. Next, the parent(s) and teacher(s) will be asked to complete ADHD rating scales; if the student is old enough, he or she also may complete a self-report rating scale. Data must be obtained from the school setting, and either the school psychologist or teacher should complete observation(s) of the student's behaviors. Once these data are collected, the problem-solving team should meet to determine whether the data support a diagnosis of ADHD. In some cases, it may be important to schedule a physical examination of the child prior to diagnosis in order to evaluate and rule out other causes of the behaviors (Silver, 1990). If review of the rating scales, classroom observations, and the examination are consistent with a history of prolonged ADHD behavior both at home and school, such a diagnosis is warranted (American Psychiatric Association, 2000). If such a diagnosis is made, a treatment plan that includes school and extracurricular settings is needed.

The treatment plan should address several key questions:

1. What are the student's strengths and weaknesses?
2. What are the behavioral objectives of treatment?
3. What are the optimum treatments or interventions?
4. What other resources are available for this child and family?

When classroom and/or community-based interventions, coordinated with the family, show that neither behavioral nor academic improvements have occurred, other resources, such as referral for medication assessment, may be sought (Brown, 1998). Although assessment of medication effectiveness is more accurate when started blind to school personnel, the potential side effects of the medications as well as professional courtesy dictate that school personnel be notified when a child is placed on medication. The recent availability of effective long-acting stimulant medications given by parents at home can alleviate the need for students to take doses during the school day. For some students, more frequent dosages may be needed, so school nurses need to be involved in the treatment planning. Some families are not comfortable with the use of medication to treat ADHD (Solanto, Arnsten, & Castellanos, 2001). In such cases other interventions, such as environmental and behavioral adjustments, should be tried first. If medication is used as part of the treatment plan, it is vital that family and child return for follow-up visits with the medical practitioner to make necessary changes in dosages or medications in order to achieve optimal benefits.

For older secondary school children, both academic underachievement and behavior problems are more common presentations. Comorbid problems also are more common in this age group, and seeking other resources is often necessary. Further medical evaluations may include neurological and psychiatric consultations (Davilo, 1991). If subsequent diagnosis of comorbid problems like PTSD, OCD, or ODD occurs, then emotional counseling and/or other medications may be added. Because all medications have potential deleterious effects, close cooperation between prescribing physicians and school nurse and teacher personnel is important (Brown, 1998).

Emotional and Behavioral Problems

The large majority of emotional and behavioral obstacles to successful student learning occur during the preschool years. Vegetative disorders such as eating of non-nutrient materials like plaster, lack of urine or bowel control, and sleep difficulties are normal in toddlers and are seen more rarely in children over 5 years of age. Bed wetting and occasional daytime accidents are far more common in males and generally managed with medical guidance and occasional medications without need for school staff involvement (Chun, 2002). Habit disorders such as nail biting, hair pulling, and stuttering are more common in the early elementary grades. If these habits persist despite medical and family interventions, they may significantly impair school achievement. When accompanied with poor social development and increasing behavioral issues, school psychological referrals are appropriate (American Academy of Pediatrics Committee on School Health, 1993). Stuttering can be treated with speech therapy. Nail biting and hair pulling often require behavioral interventions.

Anxiety disorders like school phobias and avoidant behavior are common in kindergarten and first-grade students. The most important goal in cases of school refusal is to get the student into school as quickly as possible (Bernstein & Garfinkel, 1986). Cordial and consistent communications with parents are essential for evaluation and treatment of persistent anxiety problems. The four key assessment questions need to be answered. As the evaluation reveals answers about student strengths/weaknesses, behavioral objectives, optimum interventions, and available extra resources, a team conference with parents and appropriate professional persons should develop an individualized intervention plan. Such plans may incorporate counseling, needed therapy, medical interventions, and family supports with the educational and behavioral interventions by the school staff. Because many families and school districts have little or no medical or mental health insurance coverage or services, creative use of local nonprofit services is one way to help children have access to needed services (Sia, 1992; Sziglayi, 2004). Because significant family problems like domestic violence and substance abuse are associated with student anxiety problems, counseling services in shelter and alcohol and other drug abuse programs often offer alternative resources (Albee & Joffe, 2004; Udwin, 1993).

Methods for successful intervention for more complex anxiety disorders such as OCD, ODD, and PTSD should follow the same family-oriented and multidisciplinary team approaches. A significant number of students experiencing academic failures from these problems will have comorbidity with ADHD (Udwin, 1993). For all of these problems, comprehensive school, psychological, and family social service evaluations may be needed. In students with more severe symptoms and school failure, early pediatric and child psychiatric evaluation is imperative. Some of these students will have started either or both medication and counseling therapy, without improvement.

For students with PTSD, special consideration for social service evaluation of the child's family is also imperative. Current or previous domestic violence, family alcohol and other substance abuse, and even child abuse are quite common in the medical histories of children suffering with PTSD. As child protective and women's shelter services have expanded over the last 15 years, PTSD has become more frequently diagnosed. Many child and adult mental illness conditions like conduct and personality disorders have been shown to be related to specific events of psychological trauma. Life-threatening situations, especially when an infant or young child is repeatedly exposed to violence, predispose children to PTSD (Brown & Brown, 2000). These life-threatening situations may or may not be unintentional, but their severity and the quality of immediate family or social support influence risks for developing PTSD. Children living within family or other homes with substance abuse and infants and small children who experienced chronic neglect with little or no adult–infant bonding are among the most commonly found with PTSD.

A number of standardized, norm-referenced instruments for assessment of anxiety and depression are available, including the Achenbach scales, Behavior Assessment Scale for Children (2nd Ed.), and the National Institutes of Mental Health Global Rating Scale. For specific disorders, the Yale–Brown Obsessive–Compulsive Scale, Children's Depression Inventory, Beck Scale for Suicide Ideation, and Depression Self-Rating Scale may be useful (for a complete discussion of rating scales, see Chapter 10 of this volume). While standardized questionnaires may be helpful, experienced child psychiatrists and school psychologists rely more on individual and family interviews. There are no biological measures (i.e., blood tests) specific for anxiety and depression. Still, careful family histories are most valuable because of ample evidence of genetic influence. Use of continued and cooperative work with the parents and families, as well as team meetings such as case conferences with school, social service, and mental health professionals, are vital. Many children with mood and affective disorders will need to use specific medications for prolonged periods under the supervision of psychiatrists and other physicians (Brown, 1998).

Respiratory Problems

Assessment and intervention for childhood respiratory problems are typically conducted outside of school by parents, families, and health professionals. A huge majority of these are managed very well, with limited school complications. There are rare severe and chronic respiratory problems such as cystic fibrosis and tuberculosis, which are considered in the next section. The most common and potentially serious and life-threatening respiratory problem that reduces student school success is asthma. There are several ways school personnel, teachers, nurses, and physical education and athletic staff play key roles in optimal management of childhood asthma (Richards, 1992). Teachers are often the first to observe how uncontrolled asthma adversely affects students through chronic school absences, especially during the elementary grades and during the winter cold and flu seasons. In more subtle situations, teachers and physical education personnel will observe inability to continue running and bouts of prolonged coughing.

Because the mainstay of medical treatment for asthma is regular use of inhaled medicines that overcome the reversible airway obstruction (which is the major cause of the noisy wheezing respirations during an attack of asthma), school nurses should be aware of which students have parental permission for their use while at school. The most effective measurement of effective asthma control is the peak flow meter. School nurses can take these measurements on a regular basis, just as office nurses do when asthmatic children have regular doctor visits (Hakonarson, 2002). School personnel may be the first to observe deteriorating asthma control. Contact with the child's parents and physician can start the process of reevaluation and modification of home and school management. On some occasions, school personnel may be the first to observe suspicious symptoms that lead to the initial medical diagnosis.

A thorough family and past medical history is essential for asthma diagnosis. In childhood asthma, most patients have developed a typical pattern of recurrent acute wheezing episodes treated with both inhaled corticosteroids and bronchodilators before school entry. Laboratory blood tests, chest X-rays, nasal smears, and—in severely affected patients—allergy skin tests can lead to accurate diagnosis and appropriate medical treatment planning. The most critical variable for management of childhood asthma is helping parents and families reduce environmental exposure to the agents to which the child has become hypersensitive (allergic). House dust mites, molds, animal danders, flowering plants with airborne pollens, smoking, and viral upper respiratory infections (URIs) are by far the most common. Partially effective environmental controls, such as bedroom dust reduction, household mold removal, avoidance of high dander pet exposure, and no smoking have been shown to be highly effective. Because microbiologists have not yet developed effective vaccines for URIs, these continue to be the most common triggers of asthma in preschool children.

When the diagnosis of asthma is made, optimally at an early age, education, treatment, and family support are best provided in the child's regular medical home. While bronchodilator medications such as Albuterol are essential for reversing the bronchospasms in acute asthma attacks, the use of small doses of inhaled corticosteroids with home nebulizer equipment is the most important medication. This importance is due to the "prevention" effects of safe, low-dose inhaled corticosteroids (Szelfler, 1998). Physicians have relied upon high-dose oral (by mouth) and intravenous (by needle infusion into veins) corticosteroids (e.g., prednisone) for decades. This miraculous medicine has saved countless lives, but when used several times a year, especially in high doses, it causes significant side effects. Recent pharmacological research has made low-dose corticosteroids available in tiny droplets, when inhaled into the airway, that block the receptor sites where immune hypersensitivity produces the lung allergic process. This receptor site blocking prevents the process of inflammation during acute attacks and reduces the child's sensitivity to inhaled allergins. Thus, when exposure to the same allergin occurs again, the receptor sites do not react as much and there is even less inflammation. Studies now show that regular use of these new inhaled corticosteriods actually reduces the frequency and number of future asthma attacks (Brent & McGeady, 2000).

Bronchodilators like Albuterol are available in many forms. The metered dose inhaler (MDI) is the most common, and many school children use them. A major emphasis in child and family education for asthma management is early recognition of wheezing and prompt use of Albuterol. Concomitant use of inhaled corticosteriods is stressed. Most school-age asthma patients use both Albuterol MDIs for relief of bronchospasms and corticosteroid MDIs for reducing and preventing future inflammation. Specific and individual instructions about how each of these is to be used at school should be in writing and kept in the school nurse's office (Richards, 1992). For older students with asthma, a new inhaled system combines both a bronchodilator and a corticosteroid for regular use only twice a day. Again, research findings support using this combination of both rescue and prevention for many weeks or a few months—especially during the most allergic times of the year for the individual child. For students of all ages, avoidance of first- and second-hand smoking is true primary prevention. The benefits go far beyond individual students and their families with asthma. Newborn babies who have been exposed to prenatal and neonatal second-hand smoke are at a much higher risk for low birth weights and a variety of chronic health problems such as newborn respiratory distress and birth defects. Recent studies have shown links between second-hand smoke exposure and newborns with cleft lip and palate defects (Rasmussen, 2004).

Chronic and Congenital Problems

A brief listing of the more common chronic and congenital childhood disorders was given earlier. Because childhood leukemia and seizure disorders are more common and therefore more likely to be encountered by school personnel, they will be featured in this discussion of methods of problem solving to prevent and reduce school failure. As noted earlier, the most common of all childhood cancers, comprising over 75% of all childhood leukemia, is acute lymphoblastic leukemia (ALL). While the peak age of onset is at 4 years of age, the duration of needed treatment commonly extends into kindergarten through second grade. ALL progresses rapidly, thus early intensive and combined therapy with anticancer drugs and radiation is called "remission induction." This usually requires about 1 month. The second phase, called "intensification," involves drugs that attack leukemic infiltration into the brain as well as keep white cell proliferation under control; this phase usually takes several months. The third phase is called "maintenance therapy" and uses drugs (chemotherapy) injected into the cerebrospinal fluid to keep brain infiltration controlled and lasts about 2 years. Thus, a child diagnosed with ALL at age 4 will be near the end of the third, maintenance therapy, phase at age 6–7 years (Pui, 1997).

Improved accuracy in the initial diagnosis of specific types of leukemic cells now allows placing children into standard-risk and high-risk categories. Such risking can make a significant difference in rates of central nervous system (brain) toxicity and impaired learning (Waber & Mullenix, 2000). Medical care givers in the child's medical home are primarily responsible for early case finding and referral to children's cancer care centers (Sia, 1992). Because these specialized centers now place indwelling vein access ports (variously called "buttons" or "chemotherapy ports") at the time of initial treatment, many of the "standard risk" children return to their hometowns for ongoing chemotherapy treatments and maintenance blood tests. Once the treatment has reached the stage of regularly scheduled chemotherapy, most children with ALL are back in their regular schools and ready to resume academic growth.

Among several special needs of ALL survivors, and especially those back in school during their maintenance therapy, protection from infections is paramount. Chickenpox (varicella) is especially dangerous; thus, school faculty and nurse protocols must be followed to avoid exposing children with ALL. If exposure occurs, varicella zoster immune globulin must be given within 72 hours. Other more dangerous infections are influenza, epidemic diarrhea, and community-acquired pneumonia (commonly called viral pneumonia). Care must be taken to assure that children with ALL are not given routine vaccinations during chemotherapy treatment. Likewise, no live attenuated viral vaccines (measles, mumps, rubella, and varicella) should be given to any household member of the child while on ALL chemotherapy (Pui, 1997).

Accurate diagnosis and effective management of seizure disorders in childhood rests primarily with the person providing regular medical care, the child, and his or her family. Typical seizure evaluation procedures include a review of the history of seizure patterns, careful family and past medical history to uncover possible causes for the seizures, complete physical and neurological examinations, blood and urine laboratory tests, electroencephalogram (EEG), and, if suggested by the history, computed tomography scan (CT), or magnetic resonance imaging (MRI) of the brain (Vining, 1998). Because nearly two-thirds of children with seizures have no underlying cause such as a brain tumor, infection, or brain congenital malformation, these imaging studies are not usually needed. The EEG remains the mainstay of diagnosis of childhood seizures. These are interpreted by neurologists and can provide a good indication of the most likely favorable antiepileptic (AED) medication and some hints on prognosis for successful management. The family practitioner, pediatrician, or nurse practitioner in the child's medical home consults with the neurologist about starting and monitering AED medications. Generally, most children with seizures respond well to a core set of "first-line" AEDs. Most AEDs have potential side effects that require regular blood laboratory tests. If poor control of the child's seizures continues, either increases in the dose or changes to another AED will be undertaken. In some children with atypical seizures, such medication changes may require several months until the optimal AED and dosage is found (Brown, 1998). The essential goal of AED treatment of childhood seizures is to have no or only occasional seizures so that the child can engage in the usual school, social, and home activities. Access to timely medical care appears to be an important aspect of seizure prevention and treatment. Prompt evaluation and treatment of a child's first seizure has been linked with the best prognosis and often means children need AED medications for only a few years, to then be seizure-free for a lifetime. This is effective secondary prevention. For some children with seizures, the underlying causes and genetic predisposition result in a much longer, sometimes lifelong, need for AED medication.

Teachers, school psychologists, and nurses have a critical role in team management for children with seizure disorders. Teachers are often the first to begin to recognize certain signs of seizure activity. For example, absence seizures (previously known as "petit-mal" seizures) are characterized by blank staring for seconds or minutes at a time. Such staring is a major feature of absence seizures and teachers may be among the first to observe such behavior in a school-age child. Assisted by the school nurse, an early referral to the child's medical home assures good secondary prevention practice. All school personnel have a key role in monitoring the effectiveness of AED medications and being on the lookout for potential side effects. School staff also help by coordinating team conferences and helping to formulate and implement treatment. Such activities are key to reducing further deterioration of cognitive and motor skills, so key to successful student success in school.

CASE SCENARIO

Richard Smith had difficulty even in the first grade. Although Richard liked school and his parents were devoted to his success, he was the shortest in his class, he had a funny accent, and he was constantly moving, except when one of the class teaching aides sat close to him and helped him focus on the teacher, the blackboard, or the books and papers directly in front of him. This plan managed to get him through the end of December in his first year of public school. The small town in which Richard's family lived had a limited school budget, and state political changes brought about drastic cuts in education funding. In November of Richard's first-grade year, the teacher aide funding was cut, and all the aides learned they had no jobs after the new year.

Due to deteriorating outcomes in school, Richard was referred by his parents for a pediatric developmental evaluation. His mother accompanied him to the appointment. The history and examination unfolded as follows. Richard was adopted from Russia at age 3. He delighted his parents with his learning of English. While he was tiny by comparison with other toddlers, he ate heartily and his mild anemia was easily corrected with iron-rich foods. Because Richard had no siblings, he became quite used to excelling in his contacts with adults. His quick intellect endeared him to their conversations, and a few neighbors who spoke Russian especially enjoyed bilingual exchanges, so he could help them practice their less-used native tongue. His adoptive mother recalled the two trips she made to the Russian orphanage in arranging his foreign adoption. She was at first horrified at the stark surroundings of the mental hospital-like setting and somber moods of the few attendants. As she related this important data to the pediatrician, tears welled up and she asked for a brief pause.

The essential information was simply not there. Mrs. Smith had carefully brought in all of the medical information obtained at the orphanage. These records contained sparse data: his birth weight of 2.6 kilograms, the stark statement that he was left at the orphanage during his first week because his single mother had a drinking problem, a record of all the immunizations given at the orphanage, and a physical examination report written in Russian. The rather vague term "infantile marasmus" suggested that Richard was a "small for gestational age newborn" and evidenced "failure to thrive" as a toddler. Mrs. Smith knew nothing more about Richard's medical history, although she tried mightily to learn while in Russia. She is rather sure the father and his family had no involvement with Richard's care from the start of pregnancy.

During the fall, the teachers at Richard's school repeatedly told Mrs. Smith that he had ADHD. There were no psychological services directly available at the school, and his parents could not afford a private evaluation. Mrs. Smith brought along a stack of papers on ADHD, fetal alcohol syndrome (FAS), learning disabilities, and childhood mental disorders. All of these were obtained through the use of Google on their home Internet connection. These websites were all from either educational or parent advocacy organizations. None was medical. After reviewing the information she obtained on the Internet, Mrs. Smith concluded that Richard's problems were neither medical nor learning-related. She based this conclusion primarily on how well Richard did while a teacher's aide was available. In addition, Mrs. Smith made it quite clear that her husband would never accept use of medication for Richard. "We have seen such great improvement in our home, and we know full well he is smart!" she exclaimed. When queried about information from school, she showed scores from the teacher's Conners ADHD rating scales, which revealed high levels of both hyperactivity and attention difficulties.

Physical examination revealed Richard's weight to be 17.5 kg (38 pounds/10th percentile). His height was 111.5 cm (44 inches/25th percentile) and his head circumference was 51 cm (20.5 inches/50th percentile). Vision testing by the Snellen chart, hearing testing by audiometry, and blood pressure were normal. Richard sat quietly and was very cooperative for about 10 minutes, then he began to fidget and squirm. Careful examination for small nose, narrow space between eye lids, flattened filthrum (the small indentation of skin between nose and upper lip) and narrow upper lip revealed none of these features. Examination of his eyes, ears, nose, throat, mouth, and neck revealed no signs of infection or congenital defects. Lung, heart, abdomen, genitalia, extremities, and skin examination were all normal. A careful neurological examination of his affect, mental alertness, cranial nerves, and sensory and motor systems was likewise all normal. Richard was asked to perform motor coordination, right or left handiness, and detailed sensory writing and drawing tests. None of these showed the "soft" signs that may be present with ADHD. An office test for anemia by use of the hemoglobinometer showed no anemia.

During the postexamination review with Mrs. Smith, the doctor explained that a diagnosis of ADHD cannot be made by any specific physical or laboratory test. Much time was spent explaining the mechanism of action of stimulant medications for ADHD. Much emphasis was placed on their use only as an addition to good nutrition, nurturing, parenting, and extra learning support at school for children with ADHD. The doctor began to explain how a trial of such medication might be appropriate. Mrs.

Smith blurted out, "But doctor, I have brought you a videotape made at school with my camcorder. Is there some way you can view it here?" The doctor offered to take it home that evening and return it the next day, but she replied, "I was afraid you would not have a player here, so I brought my camcorder. Can you plug it in and view it now?" The doctor agreed.

The videotape showed Richard sitting quietly with the other first graders and attending well until the teacher's aide had to get up and physically remove another student who kept interrupting and would not calm down. Richard's head slumped, and he began to suck on his fist. Within about 1 minute he crawled away and hid under a nearby table. A discussion with Mrs. Smith about this behavior revealed similar responses at home if Mr. Smith scolded their pet dog loudly or if TV programs showed adults in verbal or physical conflict. He seemed especially more sensitive to the loud voices of any female.

The doctor stopped the video and offered a different formulation of Richard's school problems. Richard's physical examination, report cards of academic efforts, the Conners ADHD scales, and the evidence of withdrawal behavior from loud women's voices suggested that he suffered from PTSD. Importantly, other possible explanations for his behaviors were ruled out. There was no evidence of mental retardation, fetal alcohol syndrome, other congenital or birth defects, seizure disorder, autistic mannerisms, or any other neurological problem. The doctor provided Mrs. Smith with information about behavioral counseling for suspected PTSD. It was emphasized that such counseling is most effective if the family attends together. Mrs. Smith was given the names of three local child and family counselors who provide PTSD treatment. In order to evaluate Richard's progress a follow-up appointment was made for Richard in 6 weeks.

This case scenario provided an example of how a child's presenting problems may appear to fit neatly into a well-known diagnosis (ADHD), yet have entirely different origins. In Richard's case a trial of stimulant medication might have been very inappropriate because it could have exacerbated his anxiety without alleviating his PTSD symptoms. This case sheds light on the critical importance of gathering data from all relevant sources. In Richard's case, the classroom observation revealed essential information not otherwise available. This case shows the importance of school–home–physician communication for accurate assessment and treatment of a student's school difficulties.

SUMMARY

A number of physiological conditions can influence student success in school. School personnel play a pivotal role in linking medical and educational supports for children through their awareness of the top five medical conditions likely to influence school performance. The extent to which obesity, ADHD, emotional and behavior difficulties, respiratory problems, and chronic or congenital disorders will interfere with school success is related to how well school and health care professionals communicate with one another about students' needs. Application of a prevention-oriented problem-solving-based model of assessment and intervention is likely to help mitigate the negative effects of health problems on school success. Frequent, open, and solution-focused communication among parents, teachers, doctors, psychologists, and others is essential when children experience medical problems.

REFERENCES

Albee, G. W., & Joffe, J. M. (2004). Mental illness is not "an illness like any other." *Journal of Primary Prevention, 24,* 419–436.

American Academy of Child and Adolescent Psychiatry. (2003). *Guidelines: Attention-deficit/hyperactivity disorder.* Baltimore: Author.

American Academy of Pediatrics. (2002). *Caring for children with ADHD: A resource toolkit for clinicians.* Elk Grove Village, IL: Author.

American Academy of Pediatrics Committee on School Health. (Ed.). (1993). *School health: Policy and practice.* Elk Grove Village, IL: American Academy of Pediatrics.

American Diabetes Association. (2000). Type 2 diabetes in children and adolescents. *Diabetes Management, 23,* 381–389.

American Psychiatric Association. (2000). *Diagnostic and statistical manual of mental disorders* (4th ed., text rev.). Washington DC: Author.

Barkley, R. A. (1998). *Attention-deficit hyperactivity disorder: A handbook for diagnosis and treatment* (2nd ed.). New York: Guilford Press.

Belay, B., Belamarich, P., & Racine, A. D. (2004). Pediatric precursors of adult atherosclerosis. *Pediatrics in Review, 25,* 4–16.

Bernstein, G. A., & Garfinkel, B. (1986). School phobia: The overlap of affective and anxiety disorders. *Journal American Academy of Child and Adolescent Psychiatry, 25,* 235.

Blum, N. J. (2002). Attention-deficit/hyperactivity disorder. In M. W. Schwartz, L. M. Bell, Jr., P. M. Bingham, E. K. Chung, M. I. Cohen, D. F. Friedman, & A. E. Mulberg (Eds.), *The 5-minute pediatric consult* (3rd ed., pp. 160–161). Philadelphia: Lippincott Williams & Wilkins.

Brent, R. L., & McGeady, S. J. (2000). Efficacy and safety of inhaled corticosteroids. *Pediatrics in Review, 21,* 393–394.

Brooks-Kayal, A. R. (2002). Seizures—febrile and major motor. In M. W. Schwartz, L. M. Bell, Jr., P. M. Bingham, E. K. Chung, M. I. Cohen, D. F. Friedman, & A. E. Mulberg (Eds.), *The 5 minute pediatric consult* (3rd ed., pp. 736–739). Philadelphia: Lippincott Williams & Wilkins.

Brown, G. W., & Brown, C. V. (2000, September). *We are all the same people: We still do not recognize this.* Paper on statewide collaboration for domestic violence and child sexual/physical abuse management presented at the 13th International Congress on Prevention of Child Abuse and Neglect, Durban, South Africa.

Brown, R. T., & Sawyer, M. G. (1998). *Medications for school-age children: Effects on learning and behavior.* New York: Guilford Press.

Centers for Disease Control. (2000). *Youth behavior risk survey, 1999.* Retrieved July 31, 2004, from *www.cdc.gov/HealthyYouth/yrbs/data/index.htm*

Christakis, D. A., Zimmerman, F. J., DiGiuseppe, D. L., & McCarty, C. A. (2004). Early television exposure and subsequent attentional problems in children. *Pediatrics, 113*, 708–713.

Chun, T. H. (2002) Psychiatric or behavioral problems. In M. W. Schwartz, L. M. Bell, Jr., P. M. Bingham, E. K. Chung, M. I. Cohen, D. F. Friedman, & A. E. Mulberg (Eds.), *The 5 minute pediatric consult* (pp. 66–67). Philadelphia: Lippincott Williams & Wilkins.

Dalton, R. (1996). Anxiety disorders. In R. E. Behrman, R. M. Kliegman, & H. B. Jenson (Eds.), *Nelson textbook of pediatrics* (15th ed., pp. 122–136). Philadelphia: Saunders.

Davilo, R. R. (1991, September 16). *Clarification of policy to address the needs of children with attention deficit disorders within general and/or special education.* Unpublished letter to chief state school officers, Washington, DC: U.S. Department of Education.

Deno, S. L. (1985). Curriculum-based measurement: The emerging alternative. *Exceptional Children, 52*, 219–232.

Deno, S. L. (1989). Curriculum-based measurement and special education services: A fundamental and direct relationship. In M. R. Shinn (Ed.), *Curriculum-based measurement: Assessing special children* (pp. 1–17). New York: Guilford Press.

DuPaul, G. J., & Stoner, G. (2003). *ADHD in the schools: Assessment and intervention strategies* (2nd ed.). New York: Guilford Press.

Fairbanks, J., & Wiese, W. H. (1998). *The public health primer.* Thousand Oaks, CA: Sage.

Fergusson, D. M., & Horwood, L. J. (1992). Attention deficit and reading achievement. *Journal of Child Psychology and Psychiatry, 33*, 375–385.

Hakonarson, H. (2002) Asthma. In M. W. Schwartz, L. M. Bell, Jr., P. M. Bingham, E. K. Chung, M. I. Cohen, D. F. Friedman, & A. E. Mulberg (Eds.), *The 5 minute pediatric consult* (3rd ed., pp. 148–152). Philadelphia: Lippincott Williams & Wilkins.

Kaufman, F. R. (2002). Type 2 diabetes mellitus in children and youth: A new epidemic. *Journal of Pediatric Endocrinology and Metabolism, 15*, 737–744.

Nader, P. R. (1993). Special education: Historical and legislative underpinnings. In American Academy of Pediatrics Committee on School Health (Eds.), *School health: Policy and practice* (pp. 68–71). Elk Grove Village, IL: American Academy of Pediatrics.

National Institutes of Health Consensus Development Conference Statement. (1985). Health implications of obesity. *Annals of Internal Medicine, 103*, 1073–1077.

Pickering, L. K. (Ed.). (2003). *Report of the Committee on Infectious Diseases.* Elk Grove Village, IL: American Academy of Pediatrics.

Pui, C. H. (1997). Acute lymphoblastic leukemia. *Pediatric Clinics of North America, 44*, 831–846.

Rasmussen, S. (2004, June 1). Secondhand smoke linked to increase in fetal cleft risk. *Obstetrics—Gynecology News.*

Richards, W. (1992). Asthma, allergies, and school. *Pediatric Annals, 21*, 575–585.

Rosenbaum M., Leibel, R. L., & Hirsch, J. (1997). Obesity. *New England Journal of Medicine, 337*, 396–407.

Rovet, J. F. (2000). Diabetes. In K. O. Yeates, M. D. Ris, & H. G. Taylor (Eds.), *Pediatric neuropsychology: Research, theory, and practice* (pp. 336–341). New York: Guilford Press.

Shankar, S. M. (2002). Acute lymphoblastic leukemia. In M. W. Schwartz, L. M. Bell, Jr., P. M. Bingham, E. K. Chung, M. I. Cohen, D. F. Friedman, & A. E. Mulberg (Eds.), *The 5 minute pediatric consult* (3rd ed., pp. 100–101). Philadelphia: Lippincott Williams & Wilkins.

Shapiro, G. G. (1992). Childhood asthma: Update. *Pediatric Review, 13*, 403–412.

Sia, C. C. J. (1992). The medical home: Pediatric practice and child advocacy in the 1990s. *Pediatrics, 90,* 419–423.

Silver, L. B. (1990). Attention deficit-hyperactivity disorder: Is it a learning disability of a related disorder? *Journal of Learning Disabilities, 23,* 393–397.

Sinha, R., Fisch, G., Teague, B., Tamborlane, W. V., Banyas, B., Allen, K., Savoye, M., Rieger, V., Taksali, S., Barbetta, G., Sherwin, R. S., & Caprio, S. (2002). Prevalence of impaired glucose tolerance among children and adolescents with marked obesity. *New England Journal of Medicine, 346,* 802–810.

Solanto, M. V., Arnsten, A. F. T., & Castellanos, F. X. (2001). *Stimulant drugs and ADHD: Basic and clinical neuroscience.* Oxford, UK: Oxford University Press.

Szelfler, S. J. (1998). Early intervention for childhood asthma: Inhaled corticosteroids as the preferred medication. *Journal of Allergy and Clinical Immunology, 102,* 719–721.

Szilagyi, P. G. (2004). Improved access and quality of care after enrollment in SCHIP. *Pediatrics, 113,* 395–404.

Udwin, O. (1993). Annotation: Children's reactions to traumatic events. *Journal of Child Psychology and Psychiatry, 34,* 115.

Vining, E. P. (1998). Gaining a perspective on childhood seizures. *New England Journal of Medicine, 338,* 1916–1918.

Waber, D. P., & Mullenix, P. J. (2000). Acute lymphoblastic leukemia. In K. O. Yeates, M. D. Ris, & H. G. Taylor (Eds.), *Pediatric neuropsychology: Research, theory, and practice* (pp. 300–306). New York: Guilford Press.

Walker, D. K., & Jacobs, F. H. (1985). *Issues in the care of children with chronic illnesses.* San Francisco: Jossey-Bass.

Weiss, R., Dziura, J., Burgert, T. S., Tamborlane, W. V., Taksali, S. E., Yeckel, C. W., Allen, K., Lopes. M., Savoye. M., Morrison. J., Sherwin, R. S., & Caprio, S. (2004). Obesity and the metabolic syndrome in children and adolescents. *New England Journal of Medicine, 350,* 2362–2374.

SUGGESTED READINGS

American Academy of Pediatrics Committee on School Health. (Ed.). (1993). *School health: Policy and practice.* Elk Grove Village, IL: American Academy of Pediatrics.

This volume offers a concise summary of conditions and treatments that affect children's school functioning.

Walker, D. K., & Jacobs, F. H. (1985). *Issues in the care of children with chronic illnesses.* San Francisco: Jossey-Bass.

Although older, this book is one of very few that discusses the overall implications of chronic medical conditions on school functioning.

PART III

◆ ◆ ◆

Assessing School-Related Problems and Situations

◆

CHAPTER 7

♦ ♦ ♦

Functional Behavioral Assessment
The Cornerstone of Effective Problem Solving

♦

MARK W. STEEGE
RACHEL BROWN-CHIDSEY

Students who display behaviors that interfere with the acquisition or performance of academic and social behaviors present enormous challenges to professionals within educational settings. For example, behaviors such as aggression, verbal and nonverbal opposition, property destruction, threats of violence or harm, and bullying clearly violate school rules, social boundaries, and standards of acceptable behavior. Likewise, opposition to instruction, self-injury, stereotypy, and inappropriate social behaviors interfere with a student's educational progress. Historically, when students who exhibited such behaviors were referred for school psychological services, a descriptive or diagnostic approach was utilized. Generally, the outcome of the assessment resulted in the identification of a "disability," a determination of eligibility for services, and some form of special education placement. In all too many cases, descriptive/diagnostic assessments and subsequent special education placement became the expected outcome of the special education referral process and became the norm that defined school psychology practice (Reschly, Tilly, & Grimes, 1999). Indeed, Shinn (2002) reported that if schools are well practiced in any assessment activity, it is testing for purposes of special education placement.

In recent years the limitations of the assessment–placement service delivery model have been extensively reviewed, resulting in an increased recognition of the need for an assessment process that goes beyond mere descriptions of interfering behaviors and diagnostic determinations to a deeper understanding of the functions of these behaviors (Watson & Steege, 2003). This new assessment model is based on a theoretical framework and a firm foundation of empirical evidence showing that interventions based on the functions of behavior are more effective than those based solely on *diagnostic descriptions*. This model of assessing problem behaviors for the purpose of designing effective interventions is referred to as *functional behavioral assessment (FBA)*.

Paralleling the development and refinement of FBA methodologies has been the emergence of a problem-solving model of assessment, including Deno's (1989) model. Consistent with FBA, Deno's problem-solving model emphasizes the importance of going beyond a diagnostic model of service delivery to a process that includes an assessment–intervention–evaluation continuum. The purpose of this chapter is to describe and illustrate how FBA procedures contribute to the effectiveness of the problem-solving model.

WHAT IS FUNCTIONAL BEHAVIORAL ASSESSMENT?

Simply put, FBA is a process for understanding why interfering behaviors occur. FBA is both (1) a theoretical framework for understanding human behavior and (2) a set of assessment procedures. To understand FBA, one first needs to recognize that behavior does not occur in a vacuum. Rather, all behaviors occur as a result of interactions among an array of environmental variables and individual differences. By identifying the relationships between the unique characteristics of the student and the contextual variables that trigger and reinforce behavior, we begin truly to understand human behavior. FBA is a systematic process that results in the identification and description of those variables. Using these assessment results, school-based teams are able to work in concert with the student and his or her teachers, parents, and others to develop person-centered interventions that result in socially meaningful behavior change (Watson & Steege, 2003).

On a pragmatic level, the FBA process considers the "goodness of fit" among the student, environment, current behavioral supports, curriculum, instructional methodologies, and social relationships. For example, with a student identified with a severe emotional disability, the evaluator could examine the student's response to the immediate classroom environment, the appropriateness of current behavior, student-specific variables, curriculum features, and social variables. A combination of interviews, observations, rating scales, and curriculum-based assessments would constitute a comprehensive FBA with this student.

ORIGINS OF FUNCTIONAL BEHAVIORAL ASSESSMENT

FBA methodology is based on principles of applied behavior analysis. Although popularized with the Individuals with Disabilities Education Act Amendments of 1997 (IDEA, 1997), models for objectively analyzing problem behaviors were first developed in the 1960s. For example, in 1968 Bijou, Peterson, and Ault were among the first researchers to examine the contextual variables that trigger and reinforce problem behaviors. Their ABC (i.e., antecedent–behavior–consequence) method for understanding the function(s) of behavior continues to be used by practitioners. Subsequent researchers expanded the ABC model by including organism variables within the analysis of behavior. They supported the concept of *interactionism*, wherein behavior is best viewed as a function of both immediate environmental and organism variables (Nelson & Hayes, 1981). They described a model in which the Response (i.e., the problem behavior) was viewed as the result of an interaction among the following variables: Stimuli (e.g., noise, classroom setting, presentation of math worksheets, etc.), Organism (e.g., individual differences the student brings to the current environmental situation such as past learning, genetic factors, medical issues, physiological states, academic performance, etc.), and Consequences (e.g., environmental events that occur following a response that influence its frequency). Table 7.1 illustrates the S-O-R-C model.

Much of the early research on FBA focused on the assessment of severe behaviors that interfered with personal health and safety. For example, in 1977, Carr published a seminal article that examined the motivation for self-injurious behaviors (SIB). Carr reviewed numerous studies on SIB and concluded that SIB was found to be motivated by (1) socially mediated pos-

TABLE 7.1. S-O-R-C Model of Behavior

Stimulus	Organism	Response	Consequence
The teacher verbally directs a student to complete a math worksheet with 20 long-division problems	The student has a history of difficulties with language comprehension, difficulties in completing math worksheets, and "math anxiety"	The student displays opposition (e.g., a verbal statement "This is stupid. I won't do it, you jerk!")	The student is directed to leave the classroom and report to the in-school suspension classroom for the remainder of the school day

itive reinforcement, (2) socially mediated negative reinforcement, (3) sensory stimulation produced by the behavior, and (4) biologic or genetic disorders. In 1982, Iwata and colleagues published the first study demonstrating an empirical method for determining the function of problem behaviors that is now known as functional analysis. Iwata et al. (1982/1994) assessed the self-injurious behaviors of nine persons with developmental disabilities according to the hypotheses proposed by Carr (1977). Iwata and colleagues (1982/1994) found that the motivation for SIB varied across individuals. Specifically, for four of the individuals, SIB appeared to be motivated by automatic reinforcement (i.e., sensory consequences), with two others the SIB was motivated by negative reinforcement (i.e., escape from task demands), with one participant the SIB was motivated by positive reinforcement (i.e., social attention), and with three participants SIB appeared to be motivated by multiple functions.

During the past 20-plus years, the fields of applied behavior analysis, school psychology, and special education have seen a multitude of published studies, book chapters, and books devoted to the subject of functional behavioral assessment (Shapiro & Kratochwill, 1988, 2000). This body of literature has clearly demonstrated that (1) assessments of interfering behaviors need to be conducted on an individualized basis, (2) individual topographies of interfering behaviors may be maintained by multiple forms of reinforcement, and (3) interventions based on the function(s) of behavior are more effective and/or more efficient than interventions based on subjective opinion or diagnostic criteria (Watson & Steege, 2003). Indeed, the literature is replete with examples of the application of FBA methodologies across a wide range of variables, including handicapping conditions (e.g., autism, behavioral impairment, emotional disability, learning disability, mental retardation, typically developing students, etc.), populations (e.g., early childhood, K–12, adults), behaviors (e.g., aggression, opposition, reading errors, self-injury, stereotypy, written language, etc.), and settings (e.g., community settings, homes, hospitals, schools, etc.).

FUNCTIONAL BEHAVIORAL ASSESSMENT PROCEDURES

Conceptual models describing the use of FBA procedures have often relied on a multistage model of assessment. For example, Steege and Northup (1998) described a three-stage process involving (1) interviews and record reviews, (2) descriptive observations, and finally (3) functional analyses of behavior. In practice, the use of FBA procedures is not always so sequential. In our experience FBA is a *dynamic* process in which the evaluator uses a variety of assessment procedures throughout the assessment process. There are two major types of FBA: *indirect* and *direct*. Both types of FBA procedures may be used at any phase of the FBA process.

Indirect FBA methods are characterized by the assessment of behavior based on information provided by teachers, parents, staff, and in some cases the referred person. Examples of indirect FBA procedures include record review, unstructured interviews, semistructured interviews, recording forms, behavior rating scales, adaptive behavior scales, social skills assessments, and self-report measures. Table 7.2 includes examples of several published indirect FBA procedures. One example is the FAIR-T, developed by Edwards (2002). The FAIR-T is a teacher-completed record form designed to address problem behaviors that enables educators to identify interfering behaviors and to report and describe information about setting events, antecedents, consequences, and previously implemented interventions.

Due to their relative efficiency and cost-effectiveness, conducting an FBA using only indirect FBA procedures may be tempting. However, filling out a one-page form that is entitled "Functional Behavioral Assessment" or simply conducting brief and informal interviews may not constitute a valid FBA. Indeed, such practice often results in inaccurate results, faulty hypotheses, and ineffective interventions (Watson & Steege, 2003). In most cases the indirect FBA is the first step in conducting a comprehensive functional behavioral assessment. If the results of the indirect FBA are consistent

TABLE 7.2. Indirect FBA Methods

Method	Examples
Unstructured interviews	*Clinical and Forensic Interviewing of Children and Families* (Sattler, 1998)
Semistructured interview	*Manual for the Semistructured Clinical Interview for Children and Adolescents* (McConoughy & Achenbach, 2001)
Structured interview	*Diagnostic Interview Scale for Children* (Shaffer, Fisher, Lucas, Dulcan, & Schwab-Stone, 2000)
Recording form	*Interval Recording Procedure* (Watson & Steege, 2003)
Behavior rating scales	*Behavior Assessment Scale for Children*, 2nd Ed. (Reynolds & Kamphaus, 2004) *Child Behavior Checklist* (Achenbach, 2001) *Teacher Report Form* (Achenbach, 2001)
Adaptive behavior scales	*Scales of Independent Behavior—Revised* (Bruininks, Woodcock, Weatherman, & Hill, 1998) *Checklist of Adaptive Living Skills* (Bruininks & Moreau, 1995)
Social skills assessment	*Social Skills Rating System* (Gresham & Elliott, 1991)
Self-report measures	*Behavior Assessment Scale for Children*, 2nd Ed. *Student Form* (Reynolds & Kamphaus, 2004) *Conners' Rating Scales—Revised* (Conners, 2003) *Youth Self-Report* (Achenbach, 2001)

across informants and the practitioner is able to form solid hypotheses regarding behavioral function, then additional assessments may not be indicated. If, on the other hand, the practitioner is *not confident* about the results of assessment and the hypotheses are tentative at best, then additional assessments are necessary. In these cases, direct assessment procedures are indicated.

Direct descriptive FBA procedures involve the observing and real-time recording of interfering behaviors and *associated* antecedents and consequences. Unlike indirect assessment methods, where information is based on informant-report, with direct descriptive FBA procedures data are based on systematic observations of the individual within natural settings (e.g., classrooms, cafeteria, playground, home, etc.). Direct types of recording procedures range from anecdotal recording (i.e., observing and writing a narrative description of behaviors and relevant variables) and the use of prescribed recording procedures. Direct descriptive FBA procedures may involve a process in which the school psychology practitioner (or other evaluator) observes and records target behaviors as well as antecedent and consequence variables. In those cases in which direct observation by the evaluator is not possible, an observation form such as the Functional Behavior Observation Form (FBAOF; Watson & Steege, 2003) may be used by teachers, parents, or staff to record interfering behaviors and contextual variables. Table 7.3 includes examples of several direct descriptive FBA procedures.

One example is the FBAOF (Watson & Steege, 2003), which involves directly observing and recording interfering behaviors and associated contextual variables. The FBAOF is particularly useful in recording low-frequency behavioral episodes. An instrument that is geared toward teachers is the Interval Recording Procedure (IRP; Watson & Steege, 2003), which involves a process of (1) identifying and describing interfering

TABLE 7.3. Direct Descriptive FBA Methods

Method	Source
Antecedent–Behavior–Consequence (ABC)	O'Neill et al. (1997)
Behavioral Observation of Students in Schools (BOSS)	Shapiro (1996)
Conditional Probability Record	Watson and Steege (2003)
Functional Behavioral Assessment Observation Form	Watson and Steege (2003)
Functional Assessment Observation Form	O'Neill et al. (1997)
Interval Recording Procedure	Watson and Steege (2003)
Scatterplot Analysis	Touchette, MacDonald, and Langer (1985)
Task Difficulty Antecedent Analysis Form	Watson and Steege (2003)

and appropriate behaviors, (2) identifying recording procedures that are matched to the dimensions of each interfering behavior, (3) identifying predetermined intervals to record behavior (e.g., 5, 10, 15, 30 minutes), (4) designing a behavior recording form, and (5) recording behaviors and related contextual variables (e.g., setting events, immediate antecedents, relevant staff persons) at specified intervals throughout the school day. The IRP allows for an examination of the relationship of interfering variables with factors such as time of day, setting events, other interfering behaviors, appropriate behaviors, and teaching staff. In addition, the IRP serves as a running record of the rate of occurrence of each target behavior.

Direct descriptive FBA procedures have two major purposes. First, they are used to document the occurrence of interfering behaviors and associated triggers, antecedents, and consequences. Second, they measure the magnitude (e.g., frequency, duration, intensity) of interfering behaviors. While these procedures are valuable in identifying associated contextual variables, a true functional relationship between these variables and interfering behaviors will not have (yet) been demonstrated. Just as with the familiar saying of "correlation does not mean causation," within FBA we say "association does not mean function." In order to validate hypotheses regarding functional relationships between the interfering behavior and contextual variables, the necessary step is to conduct a *functional analysis*.

Functional analysis refers to an assessment model in which environmental events are systematically manipulated and examined within single-case experimental designs (McComas & Mace, 2000). Within this model, a functional relationship is said to exist when the change in one variable results in the change of a specific behavior. While a complete description of functional analysis procedures is beyond the scope of this chapter, the following sections briefly define these procedures. Relative to the assessment of problem behaviors, functional analysis procedures involve an experimental analysis of the cause–effect relationships between interfering behavior and specific predetermined antecedents and consequences. A structural analysis is a process for testing hypotheses about variables that appear to trigger interfering behaviors and involves arranging antecedent conditions and recording subsequent interfering behaviors (O'Neil et al., 1997). A consequence analysis is conducted in order to confirm hypotheses about variables that appear to reinforce interfering behaviors and involves arranging situations and providing specific consequences contingent on the occurrence of interfering behaviors (e.g., Steege et al., 1989, O'Neil et al., 1997). Both brief (Steege & Northup, 1998) and extended (e.g., Iwata et al., 1982/1994) models for conducting functional analyses have been described. Both procedures involve the observation of behavior and the direct manipulation of antecedent and/or consequence variables for the purpose of empirically determining the motivating function(s) of behavior. The brief functional analysis model incorporates the same general procedures as the extended analysis, except the number and duration of assessment sessions is limited (Watson & Steege, 2003).

While a functional analysis is the "gold standard" process of assessing interfering behaviors, there are many situations that preclude its use. For example, functional analysis methods may be contraindicated in cases in which (1) the interfering behavior is dangerous to the individual (e.g., severe self-injury) or to others (e.g., aggression), (2) the interfering behavior is of such a low rate that observation is unlikely (e.g., high-intensity but low-rate property destruction), (3) direct observation causes the individual to change his or her behavior, (4) the situation is at a point of crisis and immediate intervention is required, and/or (5) staff members trained to complete either a brief or extended functional analysis of problem behavior are not readily available. Thus, many school-based practitioners may find that indirect and direct descriptive procedures are applicable to the vast majority of referrals in which an FBA is indicated.

Functional Behavioral Assessment and the Problem-Solving Model

During its formative years, FBA was described as a prescriptive assessment method that resulted in the design of individually tailored interventions (e.g., Steege et al., 1989). Used in this way, FBA procedures are conducted *prior* to the design and subsequent implementation of interventions. This is a two-stage model in which the FBA (stage 1) is viewed as the prelude to intervention (stage 2). In many ways this model mirrors the two-stage diagnostic–placement process that has been dominant within school psychology and special education practice. Most school-based personnel know the drill (1) obtain the referral, (2) conduct the assessment, (3) write the report, (4) share the report at an interdisciplinary team meeting, and (5) move on to the next case. In contrast, when infused within the problem-solving model, FBA procedures do not end with the onset of intervention. Rather, within a problem-solving model, FBA is an *ongoing* process that occurs *prior to*, *during*, and *following* the implementation of interventions. Table 7.4 illustrates the infusion of FBA within the problem-solving process.

Functional Behavioral Assessment Methods Used within the Problem Identification Stage

During the *problem identification* stage, FBA procedures such as interviews, rating scales, and anecdotal observations are typically used to identify those behaviors that interfere with the student's academic and/or social behaviors (e.g., aggression, self-injury, tantrum, verbal opposition, etc.). The problem identification stage is completed when the team has ade-

TABLE 7.4. FBA Procedures According to Problem-Solving Stages

Problem-solving stage	FBA procedure(s)	Outcome(s)
Problem identification	Indirect FBA (e.g., interviews, rating scales)	Identify the behaviors that interfere with the student's acquisition or performance of skills. Identify the replacement behaviors.
Problem definition	Indirect FBA	Define the behavior in concrete terms.
	Direct descriptive FBA (e.g., observations and recording of behaviors and relevant contextual variables)	Identify relevant antecedent, organism, and consequence variables. Measure the magnitude of the behavior. Identify functions of behavior.
Exploring solutions	Reviewing FBA results	Base interventions on the results of the FBA. Implement assessment-based interventions using single-case design methodology to measure initial individual response to intervention.
Monitoring solutions	Direct descriptive FBA (i.e., ongoing data collection)	Use single-case design methodology to evaluate the effectiveness of interventions over time.
Problem solution	Analysis of data. Data-based decision making	Compare measures of behavior during intervention to baseline levels to determine effectiveness of intervention. Modify intervention based on analysis of data. Employ ongoing FBA to evaluate possible shifts in function of behavior.

quately identified behaviors that interfere with the student's acquisition or performance of academic and social behaviors. During the *problem definition* stage the three aspects of those behaviors are clarified. First, the identified behaviors are described in concrete terms. Second, the behaviors are assessed relative to antecedent, individual, and consequence variables. Third, the magnitude of each behavior is measured and compared to the behaviors of the student's peers as well as what the teachers and other school personnel expect.

During this stage, clear and unambiguous definitions are used to describe each behavior. Behaviors are defined in sufficient detail to provide for their accurate measurement. For example, physical aggression could be defined as "the student uses his hand (with an open hand or closed fist) to slap or hit teachers or classmates," or verbal opposition could be defined as "the student verbally refuses to comply with teacher requests or directives, to complete assignments, or to follow classroom rules." Within this stage, indirect and direct descriptive FBA procedures are used to identify and describe the contextual variables that are associated with each interfering behavior. For example, the Antecedent Variable Assessment Form (Watson & Steege, 2003) could be used during a semistructured interview with a classroom teacher to identify antecedent variables that appear to trigger the onset of interfering behaviors. Also, the Functional Behavior Assessment Observation Form (Watson & Steege, 2003) could be used in the assessment of interfering behaviors over a period of 2 weeks to record the occurrence of interfering behaviors and related setting events, antecedents, consequences, and staff interactions.

Finally, specific direct descriptive FBA procedures could be used to document objectively the current levels of occurrence of interfering behaviors (e.g., number of occurrences of aggression per hour, cumulative duration of tantrum behavior per school day, etc.). This process could range from the use of very basic behavior rating charts to a more comprehensive procedure such as the Interval Recording Procedure (Watson & Steege, 2003), which is used to record multiple interfering behaviors and related contextual variables throughout the school day. The problem definition stage is complete when the team has adequately described interfering behaviors in concrete terms, identified and described relevant antecedent, individual, and consequence variables, measured the magnitude of interfering behaviors, and developed hypotheses regarding the function(s) of interfering behaviors.

The *exploring solutions* stage of the problem-solving model is characterized by the use of a collaborative problem-solving process for the purpose of designing individually tailored interventions. Historically, this stage often was characterized by a process in which interventions were selected based only on subjective criteria (Watson & Steege, 2003). For example, interventions based solely on the topography of the behavior, the preferences of team members for specific strategies, the history of success of the intervention with other students, rigid institutional rules, or personal philosophy have been generally ineffective because they failed to recognize the function(s) of the student's behavior(s). While noble, often creative, and occasionally effective processes, all too often interventions based on subjective opinion have unfortunately resulted in behavioral instability.

A better model for the exploring solutions stage includes having team members first review and discuss the results of the FBA. In doing so, team members typically find that interventions become self-evident. For example, in discussing environmental antecedents (i.e., triggers of interfering behavior), strategies for modifying the environment to reduce the probability of interfering behavior are operationalized. Moreover, in discussing individual variables, teams often discover that each interfering behavior is associated with one or more skill deficits. These skills, if taught and reinforced, could replace the interfering behavior. Generally, interventions based on the results of the FBA will include antecedent modifications, individual interventions, and/or replacement behavior.

Antecedent Modification

This set of procedures involves modifying the antecedents that "trigger" interfering behavior, thereby reducing the probability of the occurrence of problem behaviors. For example, if the problem typically occurs with peers when the student is passing between classes in the halls, three possible antecedent modifications could be (1) providing an escort when the student passes between classes, or (2) requiring the student to pass from one class to the next at the very end of class periods, thus eliminating contact with peers, or (3) modifying the student's class schedule to decrease time in the halls and contact with known peers, among others.

Interventions Directed at Individual (Organism) Variables

These procedures involve directly treating those variables that contribute to the occurrence of interfering behaviors. For example, if a student's behavior is related to fatigue due to irregular sleep, then assessment and treatment of the sleep disorder is indicated. This could include medical intervention, a change of sleeping routines/habits, or a combination of the two.

Replacement Behavior

This type of intervention involves teaching functionally equivalent behaviors as the replacement for the interfering behaviors. This procedure first involves identifying the function of interfering behavior, reframing the interfering behavior as a skill or performance deficit, and teaching/reinforcing the replacement behavior. Increasing a replacement behavior that is functionally equivalent with the interfering behavior results in the increase of the former and a decrease in the latter. In short, the behaviors co-vary: as one behavior increases the other decreases. For example, if problem behaviors are motivated by negative reinforcement (i.e., avoidance and cessation of difficult tasks), the student could be taught to request a brief break following the completion of assignments. Over time, the behavior of requesting a break would replace the problem behavior because both behaviors resulted in the same outcome (i.e., a brief break from task). Or, for a behavior motivated by social attention, teaching and reinforcing appropriate social skills serves to increase social behavior and to reduce socially motivated inappropriate behaviors.

FBA procedures are used within the *monitoring solutions* stage of problem solving for two purposes: (1) to continue to monitor the relationships among interfering behaviors and contextual variables and (2) to document the effectiveness of interventions. It is important to monitor the relationships between interfering behaviors and contextual variables because in some cases the function of behavior may shift over time, resulting in the need for revisions in behavioral support plans. Consider the case of a student who displayed interfering behavior (e.g., swearing) within the classroom setting. The results of the original FBA showed that swearing behaviors were motivated by positive reinforcement (i.e., social attention from classmates). A time-out from reinforcement procedure was used, as a consequence, each time that the interfering behavior occurred. After a few weeks, the classroom teacher reported that swearing behavior was "out of control" and was occurring with increased frequency. A subsequent FBA documented that, indeed, swearing behaviors were occurring much more frequently than during the initial assessment and, furthermore, the function of swearing had shifted from social attention to one of negative reinforcement (i.e., escape or avoidance of difficult academic assignments). An ongoing FBA process allows practitioners to monitor closely the function(s) of behaviors and to pinpoint the need for modifications in behavioral support plans.

As discussed previously, within the problem solving model, FBA procedures are used both before and during the implementation of the intervention. Once the team has designed function-based interventions, FBA procedures are used to confirm baseline levels of performance and are used in an ongoing fashion to measure target behaviors over time. This provides team members with objective documentation of the effectiveness of the intervention. When evaluating the efficacy of an intervention, the team is concerned with determining whether or not the intervention resulted in meaningful behavior change. For example, the team would want to know whether a direct cause–effect relationship between the independent variable (i.e., intervention) and target behaviors (e.g., increase in appropriate behavior, decrease in interfering behavior) has been experimentally demonstrated. As outlined in Steege, Brown-Chidsey, and Mace (2002) the "best-practices" approach to demonstrating such functional relationships is with the use of single-case experimental design methodology. These methods are useful in that they provide objective determination of student progress and allow the team to make data-based decisions regarding intervention modifications. By using single-case experimental design methods, the team is able to demonstrate that the intervention was responsible for the measured change in behavior and rule out the possibility that confounding variables caused the behavior to change (Steege et al., 2002). Single-case experimental design methodology includes procedures for accurately recording behaviors as well as specific designs that allow for control of confounding variables (i.e., threats to internal validity). Designs such as the case study, withdrawal, alternating treatments, changing criterion, and multiple base-lines are described and illustrated by Steege et al. (2002). In-depth discussion of methods for evaluating the effectiveness of interventions is found in Chapter 16 of this volume.

The final stage of the problem-solving model, *problem solution*, is characterized by a data-based decision-making process in which interventions are critically examined and, when necessary, modified to meet the emerging needs of the student. Ongoing FBA procedures and the objective measurement of student outcomes in relation to intervention strategies serve as the basis for data-based decision making. Team review of direct descriptive FBA data and analysis of graphed data should occur on a regular basis. During the initial phases of intervention, daily reviews of data may be necessary. As the intervention continues, weekly and then monthly review may be sufficient. Identification of one or two key team members with the assigned role of data management and analysis is often critical to the success of this final stage.

EXAMPLE OF FUNCTIONAL BEHAVIORAL ASSESSMENT

Student: Margaret Wilson   *School*: Lincoln Elementary
Date of birth: July 4, 1994   *Date of report*: May 24, 2004
Grade: 4   *School psychologist*: Sally Andrews, NCSP

Referral Question/Statement of the Problem

The FBA was requested by team members at Margaret's school because of Margaret's ongoing display of the following behaviors: bolting, self-injury, tantrums, and physical stereotypy. The purpose of the FBA was to:

- Identify and describe behaviors that interfere with Margaret's academic and social behaviors within the school setting.
- Identify and describe the antecedent, individual, and consequence variables that contribute to the occurrence of interfering behaviors.
- Identify hypothesized function(s) of interfering behaviors.
- Report the magnitude of these behaviors.
- Identify interventions that could be used within a positive behavioral support plan.

Background Information

Margaret has received special education services since the age of 3 years under the eligibility category of autism. Margaret was diagnosed with autism at the age of 2 years, 8 months. She has attended the Moose Valley Child Development Center (MVCDC) since age 3. Margaret attends the MVCDC full-time, 6 hours per day throughout the year, including the summer session. Additional information about Margaret's educational history can be obtained from prior evaluation reports.

Procedures

Indirect Functional Behavioral Assessment

- Record review
- Interviews with MVCDC teachers

Direct Descriptive Functional Behavioral Assessment

- Observations at Margaret's school
- Interval recording procedure

Results

The results of the FBA are included in the FBA Documentation Form (see Figure 7.1). The functions hypothesized to contribute to Margaret's behaviors are social attention, task avoidance, and self-arousal/stimulation. In order to reduce the frequency of the interfering behaviors and help Margaret participate more fully in her educational program, the following potential solutions are suggested.

Possible Solutions for the Team to Consider

1. Ongoing FBA of interfering behaviors is supported. The use of the interval recording procedure is recommended.

2. Behavioral consultation using a collaborative problem-solving process in the design, implementation, and evaluation of positive behavior support interventions is recommended. In designing the positive behavior support plan, the team is encouraged to consider each of the environmental antecedents that appear to trigger interfering behavior, the individual variables that contribute to the occurrence of these behaviors, and the consequences that appear to reinforce these behaviors. The team is encouraged to consider the following:

   a. *Antecedent modification*: This involves modifying the variables that appear to trigger interfering behaviors. For example, the FBA revealed that Margaret engages in bolting behaviors at transition times. In order to facilitate stabilization of Margaret's behavior, minimal daily transitions in Margaret's program should be planned.

b. *Addressing individual variables*: This involves addressing each of those individual variables that contributes to interfering behaviors. For example, bolting occurs during recess. Margaret evidences marked delays in independent play and cooperative play skills. The use of a picture activity schedule paired with 1:1 social coaching procedures will teach Margaret independent play skills and reduce socially motivated bolting.

c. *Differential reinforcement of incompatible behavior (DRI)*: This includes social, token, and activity reinforcement of behaviors that are functionally equivalent to and incompatible with interfering behaviors.

d. *Differential reinforcement of other behavior (DRO)*: This involves social, token, and activity reinforcement at prespecified intervals contingent on the nonoccurrence of interfering behaviors.

e. *Functional communication training (FCT)*: Team members may consider teaching functional communication skills as a replacement for interfering behaviors. For example, teaching Margaret to sign "all done" or to exchange a "break" symbol is likely to reduce the occurrence of escape/avoidance-motivated interfering behaviors.

f. *Social stories*: Social stories address appropriate behaviors within the context of transitions and recess.

g. *Picture/word schedule*: Margaret could use a visual schedule (e.g., task analysis with pictures and words of the steps of transitions) paired with visual feedback contingent on appropriate behaviors.

h. *Social coaching*: This could include individualized coaching and reinforcement of social behaviors during recess.

i. *Interspersed instruction* (i.e., a combination of strategies to increase participation in tasks and activities) might include presenting Margaret with mastery-level tasks prior to instructional-level tasks and interspersing high-probability (preferred) activities within the context of low-probability (nonpreferred) tasks.

j. When interfering behaviors occur, a combination of planned ignoring of interfering behaviors, redirection to appropriate behaviors, and reinforcement of appropriate social and academic skills is suggested.

k. Teaching Margaret independent recreation skills as a replacement for stereotypy that occurs during "down times" is suggested. For example, Margaret could be taught to press a microswitch that activates preferred music, videos, or tapes.

l. Staff training in the implementation of positive behavior support interventions and data recording procedures is supported.

Student: Margaret Wilson
Date of birth: July 4, 1994
Grade: 5

School: Lincoln Elementary
Date of report: May 24, 2004
School psychologist: Sally Andrews, NCSP

Interfering behavior	Operational definition	Antecedents	Individual variables	Consequences	Functions(s)	March 2004	April 2004	May 2004 (through May 20)
Bolting	Running from teacher or educational technician	Transitions (e.g., hallway and during recess)	Delays in social and functional communication skills	Social reaction (e.g., chase her, verbal comment, eye contact)	Positive reinforcement (social attention)	Frequency recording: 25 occurrences per day	27.0 occurrences per day	34.0 occurrences per day
Self-injury	Hitting self with open hand or fist	Individual instruction; verbal prompts	Delays in social, academic, and functional communication skills	Avoidance or cessation of task, activity, or teacher directions	Negative reinforcement (avoidance of or escape from tasks/activities)	Frequency recording: 48.5 occurrences per day	62.0 occurrences per day	33.3 occurrences per day

| Tantrum | Swiping items from table, throwing objects; kicking walls, furniture, doors; crying or screaming. Each incident is separated by 30 seconds or more of no tantrum behavior. | Individual instruction; teacher directions | Delays in social, academic, and functional communication skills | Avoidance or cessation of task, activity, or teacher directions | Negative reinforcement (avoidance of or escape from tasks/activities) | Duration recording: 27.5 minutes per day | 37.2 minutes per day | 48.4 minutes per day |
| Physical stereotypy | Repetitive movements (e.g., shaking head/weaving, tapping objects with fingers) | No specific antecedent; behavior occurs across all settings | Delays in self-regulation | Sensory consequences | Automatic reinforcement (arousal induction) | Performance-based recording: 8.3% per day | 7.3 % | 8.7% |

FIGURE 7.1. Functional Behavioral Assessment Documentation Form.

EXAMPLE OF A POSITIVE BEHAVIOR SUPPORT PLAN

Student: Margaret Wilson   *School*: Lincoln Elementary
Date of birth: July 4, 1994   *Plan implemented*: September 8, 2004
Grade: 5   *Case manager*: Sally Andrews, NCSP

Goals of the Positive Behavior Support Plan

The overall goals of the PBS plan are to increase functional skills and to decrease interfering behaviors. It is expected that by modifying the antecedents that "trigger" interfering behaviors, teaching Margaret functional skills, and reinforcing her active participation in tasks/activities, her functional skills/active participation will increase and interfering behaviors will be reduced and eventually eliminated. The results of the FBA indicated that escape and tantrum behaviors are members of the same response class. These behaviors typically occur at transition times or when new instructional materials are used. Specific steps designed to reduce her escape and tantrum behaviors are outlined in Figure 7.2.

Supports for Staff

Positive Behavior Support Team

This is a team composed of the special education teacher, special education consultant, school psychologist, speech/language pathologist, and mainstream teacher. The team will use a collaborative problem-solving process to develop, implement, and evaluate the positive PBS plan.

Staff Training

All staff assigned to working with Margaret will be trained to implement each of the PBS plan interventions. Staff will also receive instruction in the recording of each of the target behaviors. Staff training will include the following: (1) written descriptions of each intervention procedure and data recording procedures, (2) modeling and discussion of each component of the PBS, and (3) ongoing performance feedback and consultation from members of the PBS team.

Evaluation of the Effectiveness of the Positive Behavior Support Plan

The effectiveness of the PBS plan will be evaluated using single-case experimental design methodology. Using the aforementioned data recording procedures, target behaviors will be recorded prior to (i.e., baseline) and dur-

Student: Margaret Wilson
Date of birth: July 4, 1994
Grade: 5

School: Lincoln Elementary
Date of report: May 24, 2004
School psychologist: Sally Andrews, NCSP

Interfering behavior	Definition	Function	Antecedent modifications	Replacement behaviors	Reinforcement procedures	Reactive procedures	Data recording
Bolting	Running from teacher/ educational technician	Positive reinforcement (social attention)	Modify daily schedule to reduce transitions in the hallway. Use the "working walk" method during transitions and recess. Social coaching/ systematic instruction of social skills during transitions and recess. Picture activity schedule to promote cooperative play skills during recess.	Increase active participation (AP) in tasks and activities. Increase reciprocal social interaction skills. Increase independent and cooperative play skills. Increase generalization of academic and social skills.	DRI: social and token reinforcement contingent on behaviors that are incompatible with bolting behaviors. DRA: social and token reinforcement of appropriate academic, social, and play skills	When bolting occurs, implement: 1. Redirection to the picture schedule procedure 2. Redirection to the picture/ symbol classroom rules	Performance-based recording of AP. Frequency-based recording of bolting behaviors

(continued)

FIGURE 7.2. Summary of Margaret's positive behavior support plan activities.

FIGURE 7.2. (continued)

Interfering behavior	Definition	Function	Antecedent modifications	Replacement behaviors	Reinforcement procedures	Reactive procedures	Data recording
Self-injury	Hitting self with open hand or fist	Negative reinforcement (escape/ avoidance of tasks/ activities)	Minimize use of verbal prompts Picture activity schedule Interspersed Instruction model Token Board	Increase AP in tasks and activities	DRI: social and token reinforcement contingent on behaviors that are incompatible with self-injury DRA: social and token reinforcement of appropriate behaviors	When self-injurious behaviors occur, implement: 1. Planned ignoring of self-injurious behaviors 2. Redirection to the picture schedule procedure 3. Redirection to the picture/ symbol classroom rules	Performance-based recording of AP Frequency recording of self-injury

Tantrum	Swiping items from table, throwing objects; kicking walls, furniture, doors; crying or screaming. Each incident is separated by 30 seconds or more of no tantrum behavior.	Negative reinforcement (escape/ avoidance of tasks/ activities)	Minimize use of verbal prompts Picture activity schedule Interspersed Instruction Model Token Board	Increase AP in tasks and activities	DRI: social and token reinforcement contingent on behaviors that are incompatible with tantrums DRA: social and token reinforcement of appropriate behaviors	When tantrum behaviors occur, implement: 1. Planned ignoring of tantrum behaviors 2. Redirection to the picture schedule procedure 3. Redirection to the picture/ symbol class- room rules	Performance- based recording of AP Duration recording of tantrum
Physical stereotypy	Repetitive movements (e.g., shaking head/ weaving, tapping objects with fingers)	Automatic reinforcement (arousal induction)	Keep Margaret engaged in tasks and activities Reduce "down time"	Active participation in all tasks and activities Teach independent play and leisure skills	DRI: social and token reinforcement contingent on behaviors that are incompatible with stereotypy DRA: social and token reinforcement of appropriate behaviors	When stereotypy occurs, implement: 1. Redirection to the picture schedule procedure 2. Redirection to the picture/ symbol classroom rules	Performance- based recording of AP and stereotypy

ing the implementation of the PBS plan. The school psychologist will be responsible for analyzing collected data, including graphing of data on a regular basis.

SUMMARY

Functional behavioral assessment refers to a broad range of assessment procedures that serve to identify the function of specific behaviors. Indirect and direct descriptive FBA procedures are used to (1) identify interfering behaviors, (2) describe behaviors in concrete terms, (3) identify associated environmental antecedents and consequences, (4) identify related individual variables, (5) measure the magnitude of behavior, and (6) identify hypotheses regarding the function(s) of behavior(s). A separate stage involving functional analysis procedures may be used experimentally to test these hypotheses and objectively determine which variables are controlling the occurrence of interfering behaviors.

FBA methodologies are perfectly suited to problem-solving-based assessment because they can operationally define the steps necessary at each stage of the problem-solving model. FBA methodologies provide practitioners the tools to identify and define problems, explore solutions, monitor the effectiveness of interventions, and refine the supports that promote student success. FBA procedures also are very well suited to team-based problem-solving methods because they involve key stakeholders at each stage of the FBA process, from initial assessment through problem solution.

REFERENCES

Achenbach, T. M. (2001). *Achenbach System of Empirically Based Assessment*. Burlington, VT: Research Center for Children, Youth, and Families, Inc.

Bijou, S. W., Peterson, R. F., & Ault, M. H. (1968(. A method to integrate descriptive and experimental field studies at the level of data and empirical concepts. *Journal of Applied Behavior Analysis, 1*, 175–191.

Bruininks, R. H., Woodcock, R. W., Weatherman, R. E., & Hill, B. K. (1984). *Scales of Independent Behavior—Revised*. Itasca, IL: Riverside Publishing.

Bruininks, R. H., & Moreau, L. (1995). *Checklist of adaptive living skills*. Itasca, IL: Riverside Publishing.

Carr, E. G. (1977). The motivation of self-injurious behavior: A review of some hypotheses. *Psychological Bulletin, 84*, 800–816.

Conners, C. K. (1997). *Conners Rating Scales—Revised*. Toronto: Multi-Health Systems.

Edwards. R. P. (2002). A tutorial for using the Functional Assessment Informant Record—Teachers (FAIR-T). *Proven Practice: Prevention and Remediation Solutions for Schools, 4*, 31–38.

Gresham, F. M., & Elliott, S. N. (1991). *Social skills rating system*. Circle Pines, MN: American Guidance Service.

Individuals with Disabilities Act Amendments, 20 U.S.C. § 1400 *et seq.*(1997).

Iwata, B., Dorsey, M. F., Slifer, K. J., Bauman, K. E., & Richman, G. S. (1982). Toward a functional analysis of self-injury. *Analysis and Intervention in Developmental Disabilities, 2,* 3–20. Reprinted in *Journal of Applied Behavior Analysis, 27,* 197–209 (1994).

McComas, J. J., & Mace, F. C. (2000). Theory and practice in conducting functional analysis. In E. S. Shapiro & T. R. Kratochwill (Eds.), *Behavioral assessment in schools: Theory, research, and clinical foundations* (2nd ed., pp. 78–103). New York: Guilford Press.

McConoughy, S. H., & Achenbach, T. M. (2001). Manual for the Semistructured Clinical Interview for Children and Adolescents (2nd ed.). Burlington: University of Vermont Research Center for Children, Youth, and Families.

Nelson, R. O., & Hayes, S. C. (1981). Nature of behavioral assessment. In M. Hersen & A. S. Bellack (Eds.), *Behavioral assessment: A practical approach* (2nd ed., pp. 3–37). New York: Pergamon.

O'Neill, R. E., Horner, R. H., Albin, R. W., Sprague, J. R., Storey, K., & Newton, J. S. (1997). *Functional assessment and program development for problem behavior: A practical handbook.* Pacific Grove, CA: Brooks/Cole.

Reschly, D. J., Tilly, W. D., & Grimes, J. P. (Eds.). (1999). *Special education in transition: Functional assessment and noncategorical programming.* Longmont, CO: Sopris West.

Reynolds, C., & Kamphaus, R. (2004). *Behavior Assessment Scale for Children* (2nd ed.). Circle Pines, MN: American Guidance Service.

Sattler, J. M. (1998). *Clinical and forensic interviewing of children and families.* San Diego: Sattler.

Shaffer, D., Fisher, P., Lucas, C. P., Dulcan, M. K., & Schwab-Stone, M. E. (2000). NIMH Diagnostic Interview Schedule for Children—Version IV (NIMH DISC-IV): Description, differences from previous versions, and reliability of some common diagnoses. *Journal of the American Academy of Child Adolescent Psychiatry, 39,* 28–38.

Shapiro, E. S. (1996). *Academic skills problems workbook.* New York: Guilford Press.

Shapiro, E. S., & Kratochwill, T. R. (Eds.). (1988). *Behavioral assessment in schools: Conceptual foundations and practical applications.* New York: Guilford Press.

Shapiro, E. S., & Kratochwill, T. R. (Eds.). (2000). *Behavioral assessment in schools: Theory, research, and clinical foundations* (2nd. ed.). New York: Guilford Press.

Shinn, M. R. (2002). Best practices in using curriculum-based measurement in a problem-solving model. In A. Thomas & J. Grimes (Eds.), *Beat practices in school psychology IV* (pp. 671–698). Bethesda, MD: National Association of School Psychologists.

Steege, M. W., Brown-Chidsey, R., & Mace, C. F. (2002). Best practices in evaluating interventions. In A. Thomas & J. Grimes (Eds.), *Best practices in school psychology IV* (pp. 517–534). Bethesda, MD: National Association of School Psychologists.

Steege, M. W., & Northup, J. (1998). Brief functional analysis of problem behavior: A practical approach for school psychologists. *Proven Practice: Prevention and Remediation Solutions for Schools, 1,* 4–11, 37–38.

Steege, M. W., Wacker, D. P., Berg, W. K., Cigrand, K. K., & Cooper, L. J. (1989). The use of behavioral assessment to prescribe and evaluate treatments for severely handicapped children. *Journal of Applied Behavior Analysis, 22,* 23–33.

Touchette, P. E., MacDonald, R. F., & Langer, S. N. (1985). A scatter plot for identifying stimulus control for problem behavior. *Journal of Applied Behavior Analysis, 18,* 343–351.

Watson, S., & Steege, M. W. (2003). *Conducting school-based functional behavioral assessments: A practitioner's guide.* New York: Guilford Press.

SUGGESTED READINGS

O'Neill, R. E., Horner, R. H., Albin, R. W., Sprague, J. R., Storey, K., & Newton, J. S. (1997). *Functional assessment and program development for problem behavior: A practical handbook*. Pacific Grove, CA: Brooks/Cole.

This book provides a good conceptual overview of FBA theory and methods, particularly for individuals with developmental disabilities.

Watson, T. S., & Steege, M. W. (2003). *Conducting school-based functional behavioral assessments: A practitioner's guide*. New York: Guilford Press.

This book provides a thorough description of how to conduct FBA in school settings. Using a number of case examples and formats, it offers detailed information about FBA practices. The book includes a number of reproducible forms and a "Frequently Asked Questions about FBA" section.

CHAPTER 8

♦ ♦ ♦

Using Interviews to Understand Different Perspectives in School-Related Problems

♦

PEG DAWSON

Interviews are the staging ground for assessment. Any problem-solving process begins with someone saying, "I have a problem." The response to that statement is for some other person, often a psychologist, to say, "Tell me about this problem." Thus the interview begins.

The interview is integral to the first two stages of Deno's (1989) problem-solving model. Indeed, it can be argued that interviews may be a useful procedure for all five stages. While other data collection mechanisms also will inform the process, the interview is essential in problem identification and problem definition. Based on interviews, judgments are made about whether additional assessment is necessary and what form that assessment may take. The quality of these interviews may have a profound impact not only on what course the assessment will take but also on the ability to translate assessment results into effective action designed to solve the problem.

This chapter will detail how interviews are used to identify and define school-related problems and how they contribute to the decision-making process designed to solve those problems. The essential skills required for effective interviewing will be described, the process that good interviews follow will be outlined, and a rationale for conducting interviews with the key people involved, including parents, teachers, and students, will be presented. Finally, a case study incorporating interviews in a problem-solving process will be provided.

BACKGROUND

Theoretical Models

Historically, both the format and use of interviews have been shaped by the theoretical model to which the clinician subscribes (Beaver & Busse, 2000). Those from a psychodynamic orientation, one of the earliest models used in the history of psychotherapeutic intervention, tend to use more open-ended questions and encourage more free-floating or stream-of-consciousness responses. Such an approach is based on the assumption that the causes of behavior problems are often unconscious and not available to the client for direct description. In part because the psychodynamic model assumed that the clinician was the "expert" and therefore established a hierarchical relationship between clinician and client that some considered unhelpful, Carl Rogers developed a more nondirective interviewing style during the 1950s (e.g., Rogers, 1951). This approach emphasized using interviews to develop a therapeutic relationship between clinician and client, based on the use of active listening, reflection of feelings, and unconditional positive regard.

More recently, to address shortcomings associated with this nondirective approach, practitioners with a behavioral orientation developed an interview methodology that emphasized problem definition, identification of environmental conditions that contributed to the problem, and intervention planning designed to reduce the problem (Gresham & Davis, 1988). While the use of interviews in the problem-solving process is most closely aligned with a behavioral model, elements of the other theoretical models can be incorporated with good effect.

Interview Structure and Format

Beaver and Busse (2000) describe three levels of structure (unstructured, structured, semistructured) and three interview formats commonly employed (omnibus, behavior-specific, problem-solving). Clinicians who use *unstructured interviews* do so in order to collect a wide range of information, including family, developmental, and medical history, as well as a history of the presenting problem and the factors that might be contributing to the problem. This format has the advantage of flexibility, since the clinician is free to pursue any issues that arise in the course of the interview that the clinician believes may be relevant to the presenting problem. The disadvantages include both the time-consuming nature of this approach as well as concerns about reliability and validity of the data obtained in the course of this kind of interview. Although comprehensive in nature, this interview format varies across practitioners, and so the same results may not be obtained in every case.

Structured interviews, in contrast, follow a standardized questioning procedure with clear guidelines for follow-up questions and for sequencing the interview questions. They have the advantages of reducing interviewer bias and increasing reliability and validity. The lack of flexibility associated with this approach is a distinct disadvantage, as is the fact that rapport is more difficult to establish using this more formal questioning approach. Additionally, most structured interview formats are designed for diagnosis rather than problem solving or intervention planning and hence are less applicable to a problem-solving approach. For a discussion of structured diagnostic interviews, see McConoughy (2000).

Semistructured interviews allow for greater flexibility than structured interviews while having greater reliability and validity than that offered by unstructured interviews. Semistructured interviews provide the clinician an organizing framework and specific questions but also allow for different lines of inquiry depending on the responses of the interviewee. Examples of semistructured interview formats include the Vineland Adaptive Behavior Scales (Sparrow, Balla, & Cicchetti, 1984) and the Schedule for Affective Disorders & Schizophrenia for School-Age Children (Ambrosini & Dixon, 1996). Although the Vineland can be used for intervention planning, most semistructured interviews are designed for diagnostic purposes and are therefore also less relevant when a problem-solving process is followed.

With respect to interview formats, *omnibus formats*, associated with more traditional clinical interviews, are used when the purpose of the interview is broad in scope. The advantage of this format is that it enables the clinician to obtain information on a wide range of issues and concerns that may shed light on what is causing or maintaining the behavior of concern. This approach often uncovers information that may be critical to understanding the variables having an impact on the problem behavior. For instance, parents may consult a psychologist because they are concerned that their 15-year-old son has an attention disorder. During the course of the initial interview, the clinician asks about sleep patterns, and the parents remark that their son is having trouble falling asleep at night and is therefore chronically sleep-deprived on days he has to rise early to get to school. If the interview had focused only on the immediate behaviors of concern (e.g., difficulty paying attention in class, failure to complete homework), the sleep deprivation might never have come to light.

Behavior-specific interviews focus on problem behaviors with the intent of accurately describing them in terms that are specific and measurable. The advantages of this kind of interview are that they are efficient and lead naturally to the intervention-planning phase. The disadvantage of this approach is that the problem definition may be incomplete, too narrow, or incorrect, and this can lead to inappropriate or ineffective interventions. Finally, *problem-solving interviews* focus not just on problem behaviors but on the conditions that are maintaining those behaviors, with the intent of developing appropriate interventions to solve the problem.

Gresham and Davis (1988) describe three kinds of interviews that should be employed when engaged in a problem-solving process: *problem identification, problem analysis,* and *problem evaluation.* The purpose of the first interview, problem identification, is to define the problem to be solved, obtain an objective description of the behaviors of concern, identify the environmental conditions associated with the problem behavior (including antecedent, sequential, and consequential events), and establish the data collection procedures that will be used to better understand the problem behavior. These collection procedures may include formal and informal assessment methods, curriculum-based measurement, classroom observations, and the completion of rating scales by parents, teachers, or students.

The second problem-solving interview, the problem analysis interview, is held after the data collection procedures are conducted. The purpose of this meeting is to use the data collected during the problem identification interview to validate the problem, analyze the conditions that influence the problem behavior, and design an intervention plan to alter the problem behaviors. Finally, the problem evaluation interview occurs after the intervention plan has been implemented. Its purpose is to determine if the intervention has been effective. Because these two interviews are associated with intervention design rather than assessment, the remainder of this chapter will focus on the problem identification interview. The focus in Chapters 15 and 16 on implementing and evaluating interventions will address how assessment data are used in interventions when using a problem-solving model.

Good interviewers understand the various formats and structure interviews and select an approach that is appropriate to the situation. While the use of interviews within the context of a problem-solving process will draw on a behavioral methodology more than any other, there are appropriate applications of other methodologies within this context. A further discussion of this will be incorporated into the following section.

INTERVIEW METHODS

This section describes in greater detail the actual interviewing process. It includes a description of the clinical skills that are prerequisites for conducting effective interviews, an outline of the steps involved in conducting interviews, and a discussion of the use of interviews with relevant audiences (teachers, parents, students).

Prerequisite Clinical Skills for Effective Interviews

Good interviewers, it almost goes without saying, possess good communication skills. The most important communication skill is the ability to listen effectively. Good interviewers listen far more than they talk. And when they talk, they are often clarifying, summarizing, or paraphrasing what they have just heard to be sure that their perceptions are accurate. Good listeners not only hear the words the client says but they notice *how* they speak—tone of voice, hesitations, words emphasized, inconsistencies. They pick up on what the speaker *doesn't say*. Did the speaker change the subject, stop in midsentence, only partially answer the question? Good listeners set aside their own biases and preconceived notions so that they can really *hear* what the client is saying.

Good interviewers not only communicate that they understand what the client has said, but they also communicate empathy. They translate facts into feelings (e.g., "That must make you really angry"), and when the client talks about feelings directly, good interviewers express understanding and sympathy for those feelings. This may be difficult when the interviewer doesn't agree with what the client is saying or how he or she has handled the problem situation, but unless the client feels heard and understood, he or she is unlikely to be receptive to a different point of view or a different solution. Good interviewers are also aware of their own reactions to and feelings about what the client is saying. This is both because it can be a source of insight into some hidden or unspoken motives on the part of the client but also because it is important for interviewers to be able to modulate their feelings (e.g., to avoid becoming defensive or accusatory).

Good communication skills are particularly important in situations where interviewers are interviewing more than one person at a time (e.g., several teachers or two or more parents/stepparents). In these situations, interviewers need to be able to read both the person speaking as well as the other members of the group being interviewed, and they need to be able to make good decisions about whether to solicit input or reactions from other participants. This is especially important when the body language of a participant suggests he or she doesn't agree with what another participant is saying.

In addition to good communication skills, good interviewers need good meeting management skills. They need to be able to estimate correctly how much time they will need to conduct the interview, and they need to be able to gauge whether the interview is proceeding at an appropriate pace in order to conduct the necessary business within the time allotted. They also have to be able to strike a balance between allowing for a free-ranging discussion and focusing on the problems of primary concern. If they are interviewing more than one person at a time, they need to make sure that all participants are heard and no participant dominates.

Finally, good interviewers need to be knowledgeable about both the problem-solving process and how interviews should be conducted to facilitate this process. This is because an interviewer needs to go into an interview with a clear idea of the purpose of the interview and the steps that should be followed to ensure that that purpose is achieved.

Steps in Conducting an Effective Problem-Solving Interview

Establish Rapport

The first stage in conducting an effective interview is to connect with interviewees on a personal level and make them feel comfortable (see Table 8.1). Attention to the physical setting in which the interview is conducted includes choosing a quiet room, free from distractions, and selecting furniture appropriate to the occasion (Sattler, 1998). Interruptions should be kept to a minimum. This means forwarding phone calls, turning off cell phones, and asking colleagues not to interrupt. Establishing rapport may

TABLE 8.1. Interview Steps

Step 1. Establish rapport.	Attend to physical setting; put client at ease; engage in informal conversation, but keep it brief.
Step 2. Begin with open-ended questions.	Examples: "Tell me about your concerns." "What led you to make this referral?" The answers to these questions will help identify the most critical problems to be addressed.
Step 3. Identify the most salient concerns.	Move from broad questions to more specific questions; ask client to prioritize problem behaviors or target behaviors.
Step 4. Develop precise descriptions.	Translate vague or general descriptors in concrete, observable behaviors.
Step 5. Generate hypotheses about causes of behaviors of concern.	Consider all conditions external to the child (i.e., antecedents, consequences, environmental factors) as well as internal to the child (e.g., skill deficits, medical condition, etc.).
Step 6. Develop an assessment plan.	Identify what behavior will be assessed, when, and how. Determine who will be responsible for the assessment component.
Step 7. Set a date to review assessment results.	State and federal laws mandating time lines may need to be considered; follow-up should be as timely as possible.

also involve engaging in informal conversation to help put interviewees at ease, but this should be fairly brief because time is always at a premium, and getting down to business fairly quickly sets the tone for the remainder of the interview.

Good interviewers also take into account the ethnocultural context when establishing rapport. Merrell (2003) has noted that certain demographic trends in the United States favor an increasingly diverse population, with much of that growth coming among the Asian American and Hispanic American communities. The more interviewers understand diverse cultural traditions, the more effective they will be. In particular, Merrell noted that interviewers should be sensitive to cultural differences in comfort with eye contact and physical proximity in situations in which strangers are holding conversations.

Begin with Open-Ended Questions

With both parents and teachers, an appropriate first question might be "So, tell me about your concerns" or "What led you to make this referral?" When the interviewer begins with open-ended questions such as these, several things happen. First of all, this approach continues the rapport-building phase by allowing clients to ease into a discussion of their concerns. In many cases, individuals who come to psychologists because they have a problem have uncertainties about engaging in the process at all. They fear that by admitting they have a problem they can't manage on their own, they will appear inadequate or incompetent to the interviewer. Most parents and teachers take their roles very seriously, and by coming to someone for help, they worry that they will be seen as "bad" or failing at an important life skill. By beginning with an open-ended question, clients can tiptoe carefully into what, to them, may seem like a minefield.

Another reason for beginning with an open-ended question is that the answer to this question gives the clinician important information about what clients view as the most critical problem. A parent might say, "I can't get my son to do his homework!" and this statement not only reveals an important problem to be addressed but it also tells the clinician something about the impact this problem has on the parent. Associated with this, the clinician has an opportunity to gauge the kind and degree of emotion the client feels about the problem. Based on the level of stress the client feels, the interviewer may choose to conduct the interview differently, such as making a decision to focus on short-term relief for the client first before focusing on more long-term problem solving.

A third reason for beginning with an open-ended question is that the answer may tell the clinician something about how clients frame the problem in their own minds. If a first-grade teacher says, "I'm concerned that Sarah is just not ready to handle first-grade work," then that suggests that the teacher has a maturationist philosophy about child development and education that may need to be addressed as the problem-solving process moves forward. Finally, as noted previously, by beginning with open-ended questions, the interviewer will be less apt to zero in on specific problem behaviors too soon. By exploring the broader context within which problem behaviors occur, the clinician is likely to pick up useful information that will facilitate intervention planning when that stage of the problem-solving process is reached.

In addition to asking questions about areas of concern, interviewers should also ask the client about the student's perceived strengths and interests. This is particularly important with parents. I have seen the whole tenor of an interview change when I move away from asking about the child's problem behaviors to asking questions as simple as "So, tell me, what does your daughter like to do for fun? How does she spend her spare time?" For teachers, the question can be "What do you see as this child's strengths?" Questions like this enable parents and teachers to set aside points of friction or disappointment and to see the child as someone with passions and talents. This information can be used by the clinician in later interviews with the child as well as supplying useful insights for intervention design.

Finally, this portion of the interview can be used to follow up on information that may be available to the clinician from other sources, such as developmental history forms, behavior rating scales completed prior to the interview, the child's cumulative folder, or impressions or data obtained from other informants. Following up on medical information is particularly important. If a parent notes on the developmental history form that the child sustained a head injury at the age of 2, learning more about the nature of that injury might be important in placing the child's problem behavior in a broader context.

Identify the Most Salient Concerns

At this stage in the interview process, the interviewer's task is to take all the information gleaned in the early phases of the interview and narrow it down to areas of specific concern. Whereas the previous line of questioning has been broad and open-ended, questions now become more probing, with a goal of having the client be as specific as possible in describing the areas of concern. If the client lists a number of problem behaviors, the interviewer may want to ask him or her to prioritize by selecting the behavior that is either the most disruptive or the easiest to change. Gresham and Davis (1988) also point out that by carefully selecting a target behavior (such as work completion) several problems can be addressed at once (e.g., daydreaming, off-task, or acting-out behaviors).

Develop Precise Descriptions of the Behaviors of Concern

Once the behaviors of primary concern have been identified, the interviewer helps the client develop precise definitions of those behaviors. This often involves translating vague terms into concrete, observable behaviors. Terms such as *disruptive, immature,* or *impulsive* lack specificity that, unless refined, may doom the problem-solving process during the beginning phase. By disruptive, does the teacher mean the student calls out, interrupts, refuses to participate, or knocks over desks? Does immature mean giggling at the wrong time, fidgeting during circle time, or that the student has large and messy handwriting?

It should be noted that this phase of the interview process also can be used to obtain a clearer understanding of academic skill deficits. When a teacher reports that a child is "behind in reading," what does this mean? Has the child failed to acquire a sight vocabulary, is he or she unable to sound out words, or does the child read words accurately but very slowly? Similarly, problems with math or written language need to be carefully delineated. Does the child break down in math because he or she doesn't have the math facts memorized, because the child doesn't understand the language of word problems or because he or she makes careless mistakes or doesn't follow procedures such as regrouping or performing multistep processes? In writing, does the child have difficulty generating ideas or content, does he or she have trouble writing complete sentences or organizing his or her thoughts, or does the child have difficulty with the mechanical aspects of writing such as spelling words correctly or following spelling/capitalization rules? Often, when interviewing teachers and parents, it becomes apparent they can't answer these questions. In the case of concerns about academic deficits, asking parents or teachers to bring work samples to the interview may be useful, since the child's work may help answer those questions.

Generate Hypotheses about What May Be Causing or Maintaining the Behavior of Concern

The next step is to use the interview information to create summary statements that capture the presenting concerns. To achieve this, the interviewer must delineate the environmental conditions in which the target behavior occurs. What happens just before, during, and just after the occurrence of the behavior? When and where is the behavior most likely to occur? Are there things that happen just prior to the behavior that are triggering its occurrence? Are there things that happen just following the behavior that might be acting to reinforce the behavior, thus increasing the likelihood that the behavior will occur in the future? Along with understanding the environmental conditions that might be contributing to the problem behavior, it is useful to have the interviewee estimate the severity of the behavior in terms of frequency, intensity, and duration. In the case of highly disruptive and dangerous behaviors, then, this portion of the interview becomes critically important and may require a more fine-grained analysis, such as is used with functional behavioral assessment (FBA) procedures (see Chapter 7 for a discussion of FBA).

In terms of generating hypotheses about the cause(s) and solution(s) to problems, a strict behavioral approach would involve having the interviewer focus on environmental conditions, especially antecedents and consequences surrounding the behaviors of concern. Special education laws, however, frame learning and behavior problems more from a medical model. Such a model focuses on understanding disorders as being within the child and leading to behaviors that prevent him or her from profiting from regular classroom instruction. As a result of the use of the medical model of disability, teachers often want to know if the child has a learning disability or an emotional disorder that might be causing the behavior of concern.

Parents, too, are often looking for a label to help them understand why their children behave the way they do. While parents are eager to find interventions that address specific behavioral problems, that alone is often insufficient. The behaviors of concern often persist over time and require ongoing, and often changing, treatment depending on how those behaviors manifest themselves. Diagnoses become a way of understanding a set of sometimes disparate and often persistent problems. Another reason parents often look for a diagnosis is because it helps them explain their children to friends and relatives. While labels can be constraining and run the risk of placing a child in a box by oversimplifying the problem, it is easier for parents to explain to a concerned friend or relative that their son or daughter has an attention disorder than to talk about antecedents, consequences, and reinforcement schedules and the impact of these on the child's behavior.

Beyond the fact that parents and teachers are often looking for a diagnosis, a case can be made for exploring the possibility that traits within the child help explain why that child is failing within the educational setting. Dyslexia, anxiety, depression, and attention-deficit disorder, to name just a few, are all conditions that can impact a child's ability to learn or the speed with which progress is made. Some of these conditions have implications for medical intervention as well. Using dyslexia as an example, parents find it helpful to understand the cognitive processes that affect their child's ability to learn to read (e.g., phonological processing, rapid word retrieval, auditory sequential memory, complex language processing). Even though diagnostic labels may be useful, detailed descriptions of students' behaviors are still needed because such information conveys how a given condition (e.g., learning disability) is manifest in a given child. Understanding how, and the extent to which, certain processes are impaired in a child can help teachers and special educators plan appropriate interventions for that child.

Interview Summary and Next Steps

A problem identification interview typically ends with the interviewer providing a brief summary and review of the information obtained. This summary serves the purpose of both reflecting back the information obtained to verify accuracy and setting the stage for the next phase in the problem-solving process. Any inaccuracies in the obtained information should be corrected and the schedule for next steps explained to the interview participants. The summary usually takes the form of hypotheses about the problem and assessment steps necessary to validate these hypotheses. Once hypotheses are generated regarding the factors that are causing or maintaining the problem behaviors, the next stage in the interview is to lay out a plan for data collection. For behavior problems, this will most likely involve designing procedures for establishing a baseline with respect to frequency, intensity, or duration of the target behavior. Decisions need to be made regarding what behavior will be measured, when it will be measured, how it will be measured, and who will be responsible for collecting the data. Gresham and Davis (1988) recommend that for school-related problems teachers should be responsible for collecting the baseline data whenever possible. Thus, procedures have to be practical and disrupt teaching routines as little as possible.

When the concerns relate to academic performance, then data collection procedures may involve administering either formal or informal academic measures. They may also involve collecting information about cognitive processes that might be contributing to the learning problem (e.g., memory, processing speed, language comprehension or expression). Whether the assessment procedures will be broad or narrow will, of course, depend on the severity of the problem and the hypotheses established during the previous interview stage. Historically, schools have tended to use lengthy and comprehensive assessment methods that may not be necessary to address the behaviors of concern and that may slow down the process and impede the development of effective interventions.

The National Association of School Psychologists (NASP, 2003) has promoted a multitiered model that begins by providing high-quality instructional and behavioral supports within general education, followed by a second-level program of "targeted intensive prevention or remediation services for students whose performance and rate of progress lag behind the norm for their grade and educational setting." Only at the third stage would there be a "comprehensive evaluation by a multi-disciplinary team to determine eligibility for special education and related services" (p. 2). It is the role of the interviewer to explain the nature of planned assessments and ensure agreement and understanding regarding the kind of assessments to be conducted. When the interviewer is also a psychologist, and therefore an assessment specialist, the interviewer can certainly offer an expert opinion regarding the assessment processes to be used. Nonetheless, it is always important for the client to be comfortable with the assessment plans. In all cases, parent/guardian written consent for assessment must be obtained before any activities can begin.

Set a Date to Review Assessment Results

The final step in the problem-solving interview is to set a time and date to review the assessment results. When this interview is used as part of the special education process, there are state and federal laws that mandate time limits. When the interview is used more informally, there are no mandated time constraints, but it is reasonable to complete the process in as timely a manner as possible in order to avoid delaying the implementation of interventions.

The Use of Interviews with Specific Target Populations

When interviews are used within a school setting to help solve a student's learning or behavior problem, it is rare that the child's teacher is not interviewed. Unfortunately, it is all too common that parents and the students themselves are not included in the interview process. The kinds of interviews one conducts and the kinds of questions one asks may vary depending on the target audience, especially where students are concerned, but as frequently as possible an assessment process should include interviews with the student, parent(s), and teacher(s). This section will provide interview guidelines for each.

Interviewing Teachers

The most salient point to keep in mind when interviewing teachers is that time is usually at a premium. The focus, in this case, should be less on establishing rapport, or spending a lot of time exploring broad issues, and more on zeroing in on the specific behaviors of concern. This does not mean that rapport building and asking open-ended questions should be ignored, but this portion of the interview may reasonably be truncated, especially when the interviewer already knows the teacher from prior contacts. Rapport building might include arranging to meet the teacher at a time and place convenient to him or her. Rapport will be easier to maintain if the psychologist conducts the interview using a colleague-to-colleague approach rather than coming at it from an expert perspective.

While beginning with an open-ended question is still recommended, the interviewer should be able to move quickly to the problem definition phase of the interview. Since teachers often have multiple concerns, the interviewer should help the interviewee prioritize those concerns. This can be done by having him or her prioritize the concerns or answer the question "If we could clear up one of these problems tomorrow, which one would you choose?" When interviewing teachers, clinicians should be particularly alert to unspoken feelings and motives and should be particularly sensitive to the level of stress the teacher is feeling. Placing the problem within the larger context of how the classroom is functioning as a whole may be important. For example, a particular problem may not seem that urgent to the person conducting the interview, but it may be that the student in question is one of several students exhibiting problem behavior and the teacher feels overwhelmed.

Establishing the purpose of the interview is particularly important when working with teachers. Teachers may be resistant to participating in a problem-solving interview because the refer–test–place model has been ingrained in them and they view a problem-solving approach as requiring them to shoulder the intervention burden on their own. Lentz and Wehmann (1995) recommend that in-service training be used to help teachers transition from this traditional approach to service delivery to a problem-solving model. They note that "failure to inform consumers of the nature of new methods, including the use of interviews that closely explore classroom environments, can result in teacher suspicions about psychologist motives and interfere with the accomplishment of interview objectives" (p. 641).

As noted previously, teachers often frame problems in terms of traits within the student (e.g., "immature," "lazy," etc.). In this case, it becomes particularly important for the interviewer to translate those vague terms into specific behaviors. "Lazy" is not a reasonable target for intervention; "fails to complete homework" or "makes numerous mistakes on class assignments," in contrast, do lend themselves to intervention. By specifying the target behaviors, the rationale for collecting baseline data becomes much more persuasive. If we know what percentage of homework assignments the student is completing now, then we can set a specific goal and determine whether the intervention we design enables us to meet that goal. Some teachers will embrace this way of looking at problems because they see it as empowering them to intervene; others will see it as simply causing more work for them. This again speaks to the need for in-service training in the problem-solving process when schools move to adopt this approach to managing students' learning and behavior problems.

Interviewing Parents

The writer Elizabeth Stone has been widely quoted as saying after the birth of her son in the early 1980s that the decision to have a child "is to decide forever after to have your heart go walking around outside your body." When clinicians interview parents, they would do well to keep this thought foremost in mind. Interviewing parents requires good listening skills and sensitivity. Attempting to understand children's learning or behavior problems without talking with parents not only misses critical information that only a parent may possess but also shortchanges intervention efforts. A student generally remains with a teacher for a single year, but parents live with their children until adulthood. Even if the home is not the primary environment in which the intervention will occur and even if it is not parents' behavior that is a target for change, it is parents who have the greatest capacity to advocate for their children and to ensure that the needs of their children will continue to be met from year to year.

Even when a child is referred by a teacher, it is best to begin an interview with parents with an open-ended question such as "What concerns do you have about your child?" A parent's perspective may be very different from a teacher's, and this kind of question is the best way to get at that. Parents might say, for instance, "*Our* concern is that our daughter has a teacher who doesn't understand her," suggesting that they see a personality conflict at the root of the problem. Parents may also have insight into aspects of the problem that teachers are not aware of. A math teacher might express concern about a child's disruptive behavior in his or her class, and when asked about this, parents may note that from working with their child on math homework they've noticed he or she doesn't grasp concepts—and furthermore, this is not a new problem but one they have seen in past years as well. Thus, parents are a rich source of a child's history. If the problems teachers are reporting are ones that weren't present in past years, then it suggests there is something about either the classroom environment or the academic demands placed on the child that the child has been unable to accommodate.

The parent interview also affords the clinician the opportunity to clear up misperceptions parents may have about learning and behavior problems. I've had parents say to me, "My daughter reverses her letters and reads some words backwards. She must have dyslexia," or "I know my son doesn't have attention problems—he can play video games for hours." The interview may offer a way to educate parents about the nature of learning or behavioral difficulties.

The interview also may provide a way to help parents move away from a medical model of student difficulty when this does not appear to be appropriate. If a school is implementing a multitiered intervention model, then helping parents understand the graduated nature of the intervention process will be critically important. Otherwise, parents may not be satisfied that the school is doing everything it can to meet their child's needs.

Interviewing parents during a special time, apart from a larger team meeting, is recommended. Parents are more likely to confide sensitive information to a single receptive clinician than they are to divulge this information in a larger, more impersonal, group. Furthermore, parents often feel intimidated coming into team meetings where many school employees are present. Many feel they walk into an "us-against-them" forum. By meeting alone with a school psychologist during the early phases of a problem-solving process, trust can be established and the parents are more likely to be reassured that the school psychologist is there to advocate for the best interests of their child, no matter what the outcome of the problem-solving process is.

It is rare that an intervention will not include a parent component, especially if the problem-solving process is reserved for more complicated and intractable school problems. Although there will be situations when parents are unavailable for interviews and ill equipped to participate in intervention planning, every effort should be made to contact them and involve them in the process. In situations in which the student lives with a guardian or other caregiver, those individuals should be interviewed. Sometimes, more than one person or couple may have information about a child that can help with the problem-solving process. This may mean arranging for interviews outside regular school hours or in locations other than the school.

Interviewing Students

For many reasons, students present more challenges in an interview than do parents or teachers. First of all, there are developmental factors to consider. Young children in particular often lack the verbal skills and insight to discuss their own behavioral or learning problems. To discuss learning problems knowledgeably, for instance, requires metacognitive skills (i.e., the ability to think about thinking or the learning process), and these skills tend not to develop until upper elementary school at the earliest. However, at the same time that children develop the cognitive capacity to talk about problems, they tend to become more sensitive and often more defensive about problem behaviors. By the middle school years, for instance, the need to conform to peers becomes an important developmental task; thus, these young teenagers are heavily invested in looking and acting no different from their classmates. And by high school, years of failure may make teenagers with learning or behavioral problems both fearful of further damage to their fragile self-esteem and distrusting of adults, whom they often view as the source of their problems. Nonetheless, students are often a source of very useful information, both in terms of understanding the dynamics of the problem situation and in terms of identifying potential solutions. Steps that can be taken to facilitate the interview with students include:

1. Spend time getting to know the child before tackling sensitive topics. Often the best way to begin an interview with a child is to talk with him or her about how he or she spends his or her spare time. If the child has a particular hobby or interest, ask questions about these interests in such a way that the student is able to assume an expert role. An example of this would be to ask a skateboard enthusiast how he or she does difficult maneuvers (e.g., "When you do a 180, how do you make the skateboard spin around with you, anyway?").

2. Hold off interviewing the child until after you have engaged in other assessment procedures. This not only gives the child a chance to get to know you better, but also it enables you to use his or her performance on tests, or responses to checklists, as an entrée into the interview. Ask students about their responses to specific items on anxiety or depression inventories in order to better understand the nature and extent of their worries or concerns. Similarly, asking about behaviors observed while performing cognitive or academic tests can help one understand learning problems. Making comments such as "I noticed you got really frustrated when you couldn't put that puzzle together," or "I saw that you were using your fingers when you were doing those math problems," may either give the interviewer important information or may begin the process of helping the child to understand his or her own behavior and learning problems better.

3. Use all the same active listening and empathy skills that are effective in communicating with adults. Children who feel you understand and accept how they are feeling are more likely to trust you to disclose important information to enable an interviewer to obtain a fuller understanding of the nature of the problem.

4. With older youngsters, consider using a structured or semistructured interview format. Going through a written set of questions in a matter-of-fact way is often less threatening to teenagers than asking them open-ended questions that put the burden on them to confess problems or worries. While there are published interview formats for children—for example, The Semistructured Clinical Interview for Children and Adolescents (McConoughy & Achenbach, 1994)—you may also consider developing your own checklist. See Sattler (1998) for a wide variety of semistructured interview formats for students, parents, and teachers.

Although it may not be appropriate or feasible to interview all students, in all cases where it could provide important information concerning the presenting problem, student interviews are recommended.

Unlike parents and teachers, minor students do not have the same legal rights concerning confidentiality and disclosure of information. Students may not initially understand the purpose of the interview. For these reasons, it is very important to preface student interview questions with an explanation about why the information is being sought and how it will be used. In order to prevent misunderstanding later, it is best to let all students know that if they reveal information during the interview that suggests they might hurt themselves or others, certain people will have to be notified and a safety plan will be developed.

CASE SCENARIO

David is a 15-year-old sophomore attending a midsized suburban high school. At the time the interviews were conducted, he had been receiving special education services for many years and had been identified as having a specific learning disability. His individualized education plan stated that he had problems processing complex language that affected classroom performance as well as written production, and poor organizational and time management skills. He was assigned to the resource room for one period daily for assistance with school work and homework (the school had block scheduling).

David was a B/C student in ninth grade, but his grades fell over the course of the fall of 10th grade so that, at the time the interviews were conducted, he was earning C's and D's on progress reports and was in danger of failing some classes. Both David's mother and his resource room teacher were concerned about the declining grades, and the school hired a consulting psychologist to assess the situation and make recommendations regarding steps that could be taken to enable David to become more successful.

The psychologist conducted several interviews, including an interview with the resource room teacher, with David's mother, a group interview with David's general education teachers, and finally an interview with David. Each of those interviewed had different perspectives and different opinions about what was causing David's declining grades.

David's resource room teacher expressed concern about David's resistance to working with her. She maintained a system of sending home weekly progress reports to David's mother regarding homework and test grades, but when she attempted to offer help to David in organizing his work or understanding assignments, he rebuffed her. She described David as a difficult student to work with, but she also expressed dismay at her own inability to be more effective in helping David.

David's mother was concerned that David's learning needs weren't being adequately addressed. She felt that his ability to understand instruction in the classroom was affected by his language processing problems, and she worried that the school was not doing enough to help him understand figurative and abstract language. She recognized that the situation was complicated by the fact that David tended to be a rigid thinker and often felt he understood material better than he did. "He's resistant to help because he thinks he already 'gets it,' " she stated in her interview.

David's classroom teachers were interviewed as a group. One teacher reported that David socialized with students in her class and this led him to be off-task. She felt he understood the material, but she was concerned about inconsistent homework completion. A second teacher also expressed concern about incomplete assignments, noting that the work that was done was of good quality. David's math teacher reported that he observed greater effort on David's part at the beginning of the year but that his performance had declined as the year progressed. He felt David had difficulty grasping the concepts but noted that David declined to go for extra help.

The final phase was the interview with David. He came to the psychologist's office for the interview and spent about 45 minutes with her. He acknowledged that his grades had declined, and when asked why that was, he attributed it primarily to poor test grades. In math, for instance, he reported that he thought he understood the material when it was presented in class, but when he went to do his homework or to study for a test, he found he really hadn't understood the concepts. He also acknowledged that he was not consistent in getting homework handed in. "Sometimes I forget to do it or I forget to hand it in. Sometimes I do half of it and then stop because I don't understand."

David was vocal in his dislike of the resource room. He felt that it did not offer real help with the homework and had a "bunch of stupid rules" that did not make sense to him and did not match how he learned (for example, strict requirements about how he organized his notebooks). He expressed a strong desire to get out of the resource room, adding that he would be willing to stay after school for extra help from his teachers when he had missing assignments or got low grades on tests. He was asked what his academic goals were, and he identified the grades he would like to earn in each of the academic subjects he was taking that marking period. The grades he wanted to earn ranged from B's to C's, depending on the subject.

David had had extensive testing in the past, and it was not felt that additional assessments needed to be conducted. Test grades, homework completion rates, and report card grades served as the baseline measures that indicated the current program was not successful. These same measures would be used to measure the success of interventions.

Based on all interview results, with a particular effort to incorporate David's input, the following intervention plan was developed:

1. Remove David from the resource room and have him work during that same time block with a tutor, using a coaching model (Dawson & Guare, 1998). Coaching sessions should include two primary elements: (a) making a study plan for the day, including reviewing assignments and mak-

ing sure David understands the assignment; and (b) practicing study techniques using real tests and assignments in order to identify strategies that are effective for David. Any free time at the end of the block would be used to begin following the study plan.

2. Put systems in place for homework not handed in and poor test grades. Using David's input, it was suggested that he stay after school to complete any missing homework assignments. When he earned test or quiz grades of 75 or less, David should stay after school to review the material with the teacher who gave the test and retake the test.

3. Close daily communication between David's coach and his classroom teachers was seen as essential to ensure that the coach knew about homework assignments and test grades since it was the coach's job to ensure that David stayed after school when he needed to.

The psychologist met with David's teachers and then later with David, the resource room teacher, and his mother to review the plan. Both David and his mother had some reservations about the plan but agreed that it met many of their concerns and were willing to go along with its implementation. The school assigned a coach who was thought to be compatible with David. Follow-up meetings were arranged to monitor the intervention.

SUMMARY

Interviews are a critical component of a problem-solving approach to assessment. They serve as a key data collection mechanism, and the success or failure of interventions often hinges on how interviews are conducted. While the problem definition phase of interviewing may be the most important element of the process, interviews are also key to ensuring that all people involved—parents, teachers, and students—feel that they are heard and contribute to the assessment process. Finally, by laying this groundwork, the likelihood is increased that the interventions designed will be acceptable to all and ultimately successful.

REFERENCES

Ambrosini, P., & Dixon, J. F. (1996). *Schedule for affective disorders & schizophrenia for school-age children (K-SADS-IVR)*. Philadelphia: Allegheny University of the Health Sciences.

Beaver, B. R., & Busse, T. T. (2000). Informant reports: Conceptual and research bases of interviews with parents and teachers. In E. S. Shapiro & T. R. Kratochwill (Eds.). *Behavioral assessment in schools: Theory, research, and clinical foundations* (2nd ed., pp. 257–287). New York: Guilford Press.

Dawson, M. M., & Guare, R. (1998). *Coaching the ADHD student*. Toronto: Multi-Health Systems, Inc.

Deno, S. (1989). Curriculum-based measurement and special education services: A fundamental and direct relationship. In M. Shinn (Ed.), *Curriculum-based measurement: Assessing special children* (pp. 1–17). New York: Guilford Press.

Gresham, F. M., & Davis, C. J. (1988). Behavioral interviews with teachers and parents. In E. S. Shapiro & T. R. Kratochwill (Eds.), *Behavioral assessment in schools: Conceptual foundations and practical applications* (pp. 455–493). New York: Guilford Press.

Lentz, F. E., & Wehmann, B. A. (1995). Best practices in interviewing. In A. Thomas & J. Grimes (Eds.), *Best practices in school psychology III* (pp. 637–649). Silver Spring, MD: National Association of School Psychologists.

McConoughy, S. H. (2000). Self-reports: Theory and practice in interviewing children. In E. S. Shapiro & T. R. Kratochwill (Eds.) *Behavioral assessment in schools: Theory, research, and clinical foundations* (2nd ed., pp. 323–352). New York: Guilford Press.

McConoughy, S. H., & Achenbach, T. M. (1994). *Manual for the Semistructured Clinical Interview for Children and Adolescents.* Burlington: University of Vermont, Department of Psychiatry.

Merrell, K. W. (2003). *Behavioral, social, and emotional assessment of children and adolescents* (2nd ed.). Mahwah, NJ: Erlbaum.

National Association of School Psychologists. (2003). *NASP recommendations for IDEA reauthorizing: Identification and eligibility determination for students with specific learning disabilities.* Retrieved from *www.nasponline.org*

Rogers, C. R. (1951). *Client-centered therapy.* Boston: Houghton-Mifflin.

Sattler, J. M. (1998). *Clinical and forensic interviewing of children and families.* San Diego: Sattler.

Sparrow, S. S., Balla, D. A., & Cichetti, D. V. (1984). *Vineland Adaptive Behavior Scales.* Circle Pines, MN: American Guidance Service.

SUGGESTED READING

Sattler, J. M. (1998). *Clinical and forensic interviewing of children and families.* San Diego: Sattler.

This is a very comprehensive volume on all types of interviews that might be useful when working with children. It includes many sample interview questions and considerations appropriate for different interview participants and settings.

CHAPTER 9

◆ ◆ ◆

Conducting Systematic
Direct Classroom Observations
to Define School-Related Problems

◆

EDWARD S. SHAPIRO
NATHAN H. CLEMENS

When students are having difficulties in school, it is almost always the teacher who notices the problem and asks for help from education professionals to solve the problem. Indeed, the starting point for all problem-solving assessment is to obtain information from the referral source about his or her perception of the problem. These data are acquired usually by interviewing the teacher or asking the teacher to complete a rating scale that includes judgment of the nature and severity of the problem area.

Although data obtained from teachers through interviews or rating scales can offer valid perceptions, teacher reports alone cannot be assumed to be entirely valid. If a teacher's report alone was assumed to be a valid indicator of a problem, then it would make sense to move directly from the teacher's report to intervention development. Such a link would be equivalent to going into a doctor's office with complaints about discomfort and having the doctor move directly to a surgical intervention. Clearly, the doctor needs to investigate in detail whether the physical complaints are consistent with an existing medical condition, and it is the diagnosis of the condition that leads to selecting the right intervention. When a teacher reports a child to be physically sick, the child is sent to the school nurse, a health care professional who confirms or disconfirms the teacher's suspicions that the child is ill. In schools, when a teacher refers a child for a school-related problem, the teacher's perceptions of the problem as reported through interviews or rating scales need confirmation by professionals designed to assess school-related problems. Systematic direct observation is the methodology used to provide such confirmation. Not collecting systematic direct observation for a referred school-related problem is tantamount to not taking a child's temperature when he or she complains of not feeling well. Indeed, systematic direct observation is the core method linked to multiple stages of the problem-solving process and needs to be used in every case to better understand the nature of the child's problem. This includes referrals for children who display problems of behavior such as inattentiveness, calling out in class, fighting, and showing aggression toward others; for children who display excessive withdrawal or have few friends; as well as for those with academic skills problems who do not complete their homework or do not accurately complete their reading, math, social studies, or science assignments.

The purpose of this chapter is to show how systematic direct observations can be linked to the problem-solving process in defining school-based problems. After a brief discussion of the importance and value of systematic direct observation in the problem-solving process, the methods of systematic direct observation are described briefly. The relationship of each type of observation method to the solving of specific types of school-related problems will be identified. Two brief case studies illustrating the use of systematic direct observation to define school-related problems will also be provided.

BACKGROUND

Over the past decade, the best practices involved in conducting school-based assessments for children referred for behavioral and academic problems have become increasingly well defined. Early studies that examined the assessment practices of school and child clinical psychologists noted that almost all assessments included the use of measures of intellectual functioning, academic achievement, and personality (e.g., Goh, Teslow, & Fuller, 1981; Hutton, Dubes, & Muir, 1992; Wade & Baker, 1977; Wilson & Reschly, 1996). As assessment practices were refined, the use of multimethod and multimodal assessment strategies became required strategies for completing effective evaluations. Labeled as Behavior Systems Assessment (BSA; Mash & Terdal, 1997) or Multidimensional Behavioral Assessment (MDBA; Shapiro & Kratochwill, 2000a, 2000b), it has been clearly recognized that one must assume an ecological perspective in evaluating childhood problems and assess across the various systems that impinge on a child's difficulties.

Methods used to conduct a BSA or an MDBA have long been identified within behavioral assessment. In an early conceptual model of conducting behavioral assessment, Cone (1978) indicated that methods of assessment are on a continuum of direct to indirect. The distinction between direct and indirect assessment is based upon the contiguity of the observed or reported behavior and its actual occurrence. When behavior is recorded at the time it occurs, one is using a direct form of assessment. For example, the use of systematic direct observation or self-monitoring is considered a form of direct assessment (Shapiro & Kratochwill, 2000a, 2000b). Assessment becomes indirect when the behavior being observed or recorded is not occurring at the same time as the assessment data are collected. For example, the use of informant or self-report rating scales is a good example of indirect assessment. Data obtained from both direct and indirect assessments are considered essential elements that work together to complete a BSA or MDBA (DuPaul, 2003; DuPaul & Stoner, 2003; Shapiro & Heick, 2004).

Use of rating scale and other indirect methods of assessment are often viewed as efficient, economical, and valuable in obtaining information from multiple perspectives (e.g., DuPaul, Power, McGoey, Ikeda, & Anastopoulos, 1998; Shapiro & Heick, 2004). However, the relationships between data obtained through direct observation and indirect methods such as rating scales are not usually strong. For example, Demaray and Elliott (1998) found that in the assessment of academic skills stronger relationships between the actual behavior and ratings occurred when more direct measures of the academic skill were used as the source of the ratings. Feinberg and Shapiro (2003) also found that a teacher's overall judgment of a student's performance of oral reading fluency was not always a strong predictor of how the student actually performed such a skill. Such outcomes are not surprising since the data obtained through indirect methods provides information on one's perception of the behavior problem and not data on the actual nature or levels of occurrence. Given the questionable level of relationship between direct and indirect methods, one cannot rely on rating scales and other indirect methods alone in completing effective child assessments.

Among the direct methods of assessment, systematic direct observation remains the hallmark of behavioral assessment methodology (Merrell, 2003; Skinner, Dittmer, & Howell, 2000). Through data collection, the assessor obtains an observable, verifiable record of events. The data serve multiple functions such as identifying agreed-upon targets for intervention, a baseline against which progress of interventions can be measured, and opportunities to set empirical goals against which both the change agent and the targeted individual can judge the outcomes of strategies to change behavior. In addition, when assessing children for the purpose of determining educational classification, there is a legal mandate through the Individuals with Disabilities Education Act of 2004 for observational data to be included as part of the diagnostic process.

Observational data can be collected using either quantitative/systematic methods or more informal qualitative/narrative methods. In a quantitative or systematic method of data collection, the behaviors to be observed are well defined before the observation begins, and data are collected in a formal way that provides quantitative syntheses of the outcomes of the data collection process. Typically, this involves counting the behavior in some way that captures the nature of what has occurred and how often. The data can provide an empirical record that offers confirmation or disconfirmation of teacher perceptions obtained through interviews or rating scales. Equally important, the data obtained through systematic data collection processes provide a replicable record of the child's behavior and can be used to judge whether changes occur in the desired direction once an intervention is implemented. The data also can be used effectively to help education professionals select the intervention they believe will be most effective for the referral problem. Empirically validated goals can be established to determine if the intervention has reached its expected level of success and to offer feedback that all other school professionals, parents, and the child him- or herself can use to gauge the success of the intervention.

When more qualitative methods for observation are used, observers usually provide a narrative description of the behavior and its context. Extensive methodologies for qualitative data collection processes have been defined in the literature (Kratochwill, 1985). Trained professionals write down the events that they have observed, along with their personal impressions based on those observations. The information is then examined for consistencies and inconsistencies to better understand the nature of the referral problem. Although such qualitative records are certainly valuable for achieving an initial understanding of the problems, this type of observational data collection does not offer an approach that can be easily replicated. The observations by their nature are expected to contain personal interpretation, as the data are being filtered through the perceptual lens of the individual collecting the data. Likewise, it is not possible to set empirically based long-term goals using such data collection methods, nor is it possible to determine clearly whether changes have occurred related to intervention implementation.

Systematic direct observation has a significant role in multiple stages of the problem-solving process. At *problem identification*, systematic observation is useful in offering a clear indication that a problem does or does not exist, including evidence of the severity of the problem. In particular, systematic direct observation recognizes that all school-related problems are context-specific. For example, consider a teacher who refers a third-grade student because the student does not pay attention in her math class. When systematic direct observation is conducted, it is found that the student is on-task and attentive about 75% of the time. However, the teacher's expectations are that students will be attentive during instruction 95% of the time, and, indeed, data collected across peers in the same classroom as the referred child find an average level of on-task behavior across these students to be 94%. Thus, for this teacher the referred student has a behavior problem that would not have been noticed easily unless systematic observation data were collected. At the same time, this student has a different teacher for reading, and when data are obtained in that teacher's classroom, the student has an on-task level of 70%. When asked about the student's attentiveness the reading teacher indicates that this student is one of the more attentive in her class. Indeed, data collected on peers in her classroom finds a classroom average on-task level of only 62%.

The example above also illustrates how systematic direct observation plays a role in the *problem definition* stage of the problem-solving process. One of the important decisions that must always be addressed is whether the referral problem is severe enough to justify the resources for intervention development. One mechanism for making this judgment is to examine the relationship of the severity of the student's problem to those of his or her peers. Because behavior is context-specific, it is most important that the comparison group be one's peers within the same context where the behavior problem is occurring. Although this student is on-task 75% of the time in math class, and such levels are less than that expected by the teacher, one would raise the question whether a 95% level of expected on-task behavior is a reasonable expectation for third-grade students. At the same time, intervention for this student may be justifiable, given that the student is clearly visible to the teacher as an attention problem, and given the high expectations for behavior in her classroom.

Another important use of systematic direct observation is in the *exploring and implementing solutions* stage of problem-solving assessment. Over the past decade, functional behavioral assessment has become a mainstay of many assessments for students referred for behavior problems (e.g., March & Horner, 2002; Scott, Nelson, & Zabela, 2003; see Chapter 7 in this volume). In a functional behavioral assessment, systematic direct observational data are collected to point education professionals toward hypothesized solutions that link the behavior occurrence to a specific function (e.g., Gresham, Watson, & Skinner, 2001; Watson & Steege, 2003). For example, a functional behavioral assessment of a student who becomes disruptive whenever independent math assignments are distributed needs to determine if the problem (disruptiveness) is a "can't do" or a "won't do" problem. If the problem is a skills problem ("can't do"), the designed solution would be very different than if it's a performance problem ("won't do"). In a skills problem, the focus of the intervention would be on teaching and instruction, whereas in a performance problem the intervention would focus on strategies to increase motivation. Indeed, several studies (Daly & Murdoch, 2000; Daly, Witt, Martens, & Dool, 1997) have shown that functional behavioral assessment can be equally applied to academic skill problems as well as behavior problems. Systematic direct observation is a critical part of making these functional behavioral determinations that will lead to the selection of the most successful interventions. Boyajian, DuPaul, Handler, Eckert, and McGoey (2001) have demonstrated that brief functional assessment can be a very powerful tool for practitioners in developing the most effective intervention strategies.

Finally, systematic direct observation has a role in the final stage of problem solving, *problem solution*. Using systematic direct observation, the education professional can set reasonable and empirical goals for determining the success of intervention strategies. Such goals offer concrete objectives for students, teachers, and parents in examining whether real gains are made. Indeed, goal setting itself using systematic direct observation to obtain the data often can be an effective intervention strategy for both behavior (e.g., Ruth, 1996) and academic skills problems (e.g., Fuchs, Fuchs, & Deno, 1985).

In conclusion, systematic direct observation can play an important role in multiple stages of the problem-solving process. Whether the goal is to identify and define the problem or to determine which intervention is likely to be successful, systematic direct observation offers the data upon which decisions can be made.

METHODS OF SYSTEMATIC DIRECT OBSERVATION

Choosing the best method of systematic direct observation is an important first step in the problem-solving process. There are multiple methods at the disposal of the practitioner, and choosing the method that best captures the referral problem of interest requires that the evaluator consider variables such as the topography of the behavior, the context in which the behavior occurs, and/or the logistics of conducting the observation. One method of data collection does not fit all. More importantly, the objective of the data collection is to capture accurately the behavior problem as it is described by the referral source. Selecting an appropriate method of observation will better enable the practitioner to capture the behavior precisely and specifically, as well as understand the context in which the behavior problem is occurring.

This section will describe the various methods of systematic direct observation and how each can help define specific school-related problems. As a guideline, Figure 9.1 provides a list of many of the typical school-related behavior problems and the methods that are deemed most

Observation method	Behaviors	Rationale
Event/frequency recording	Calling out, throwing objects, aggression, whining, cursing, teasing, tattling, arguing or talking back, lack of independence with tasks, failure to complete work, cheating, stealing, lying, noncompliance, vocal or other disruptions, self-stimulatory behavior, self-injurious behavior, skipping class, carrying weapons, drug use, smoking, tardiness, negative self-statements, dress code violations, vandalism, food refusal, property destruction, homework incomplete	How bothersome the behavior is to the teacher is reflected in how often it occurs. Behaviors that are of a more discrete nature or occur at low frequencies are best assessed by using event recording. If behavior occurs at high rate, consider a time-sampling procedure.
Duration recording	Out-of-seat behavior, noncompliance, fighting, crying, sleeping, insufficient time to complete tasks, tardiness, tantrums	Behavior length is of interest (can indicate intensity). Intervention goals might initially target reductions or increases in length.
Latency recording	Lack of time to comply with requests or instructions, tardiness, time to provide a response	Time between stimulus (i.e., teacher instruction) and occurrence of behavior is of interest. Intervention goals would target reduction or increase of latency.
Time Sampling	Academic engaged time, passive engaged time, off-task behavior, playing with objects, tapping feet or objects, rocking in chair, vocal or other disruptions, self-stimulatory behavior, self-injurious behavior, social isolation or withdrawal, sleeping, lack of independence with tasks, noncompliance, out-of-seat behavior	Used when behaviors are continuous, it is difficult to continuously monitor, behaviors are of high frequency, or when monitoring more than one behavior. Consider whole interval for behaviors in which continuous occurrence of the behavior is desired, partial interval when behaviors are of high or moderate rate, and momentary time sampling when behavior lengths can vary or it is difficult to continuously monitor.
Performance-based recording	Any of the foregoing behaviors when a less demanding method of data collection is desired	Used when you are unable to collect data at the time behavior occurs. Can provide efficient rating-type data collection of the perception of behavior occurrence.
Permanent product	Academic work, vandalism, graffiti, property destruction	Used when the behavior cannot be observed at the time it occurs; inspection of products can reflect intensity or frequency of behavior.

FIGURE 9.1. Use and examples of systematic direct observational methods.

appropriate for collecting systematic direct observational data. The figure is by no means exhaustive but can provide practitioners with guiding principles on the data collection process. Figure 9.2 provides a decision chart designed to help guide practitioners toward the most appropriate form of systematic direct observation matched to the type of behavior problem presented by the referral source.

Operational Definition of Behavior

Prior to conducting a systematic direct observation, regardless of the method being employed, the behavior of interest must be defined in a manner that allows it to be objectively observed. A good operational definition is one that describes what the behavior looks like in clear, concrete terms as well as the context in which the behavior most frequently occurs. The operational definition does not attempt to make assumptions regarding the function of the behavior; rather, it identifies the topography of the behavior—in essence, what the behavior *looks like*. In addition, the definition should provide clear discrimination between instances and noninstances of the behavior.

Developing an operational definition can be difficult for those who may be unfamiliar with or inexperienced with the process. Likewise, developing an accurate and precise operational definition through an interview with a teacher, based solely on his or her perspective and interpretation, poses obvious pitfalls. For example, a teacher may tell the assessment professional that a child "often appears to be lethargic and inattentive." To assess this problem accurately, operational definitions of the terms "lethargic and inattentive" need to be developed. By conducting more in-depth interviewing such as that defined by Bergan and Kratochwill (1990), one is able to begin the process of better understanding the nature of the problem. However, by conducting additional behavioral observation (especially more qualitative and narrative recording), a sound operational definition of the behavior can be developed (Skinner, Ditmer, & Howell, 2000). Thus, in this example the term *lethargic* could be defined by the lack of response to direct questions asked by the teacher and *inattentive* could be defined as, for example, staring out the window during independent work periods.

After the behavior(s) of interest have been objectively defined, a method of systematic direct observation can be used. The first step in deciding which observation method to employ is to identify the nature of the presenting problem: Is the behavior a problem because it occurs too often (or not often enough)? Is the behavior a problem because it occurs for too long a period of time (or not sufficiently long)? Is the behavior a problem because of how long it takes for the behavior to occur (or because the behavior is not delayed long enough)? Each of these problems requires a different form of systematic direct observation.

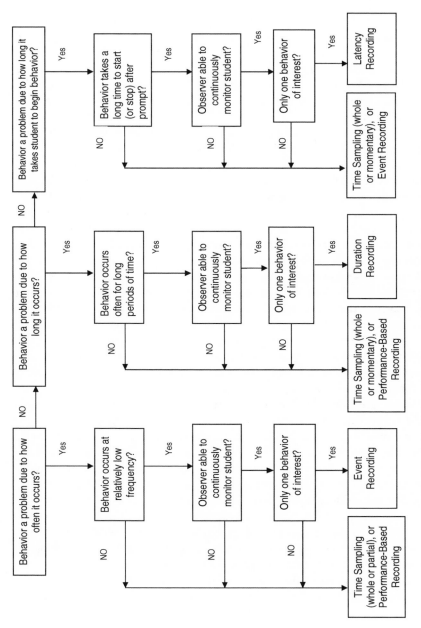

FIGURE 9.2. Decision chart for conducting systematic direct observations.

183

Event Recording

Behaviors that pose problems for teachers and other school personnel often do so because of the frequency at which they occur. Certain behaviors become "problem behaviors" simply because they occur either too often or too infrequently. Event (or frequency) recording is one method of systematic data collection that measures the number of occurrences of a behavior during a given observation period. When conducting event recording, the observer simply tallies the number of times the target behavior occurs, based upon the predetermined operational definition, thus providing the frequency of the behavior during the session.

Some behaviors are more amenable to event recording than others. Behaviors that have an observable beginning and end, such as calling out, completing work assignments, and throwing objects are best suited for event recording. Observers can determine directly when such behaviors have started and when they have stopped. Additionally, behaviors well suited for event recording are those that typically occur with a relatively short duration. Because the observer must record each occurrence of the behavior, this method of data collection may not result in accurately collected data if the behavior occurs at a very high frequency. Alternative methods described later in this chapter are better suited to efficiently capture higher-rate behaviors for which event recording could be conducted.

Although event recording can be used simply to confirm a teacher's report of the presence (or absence) of a reported behavior, simply reporting the number of times that a behavior occurs may not fully explain the nature of the problem. For example, if a teacher referred a student for calling out, an event recording of calling-out behavior may reveal that a student called out five times during the observation. Unless one knows the amount of time within which the observation was conducted, the data reflecting events would be meaningless. Thus, if the student was found to be calling out five times within a 30-minute observational period, his behavior may be deemed problematic and worthy of further intervention. On the other hand, if the student had called out five times across a 2-week period of observations made throughout the entire school day, the problem would not be viewed as significant and probably would not be considered substantial enough to warrant intervention. Recording the length of the observation allows a frequency or event count to be converted into a rate by dividing the number of occurrences of the behavior by the number of minutes observed. Thus, a behavior that occurs eight times in a 30-minute session occurs at a rate of 0.23 per minute, or in other words, occurs approximately once every four minutes. Rate data provide meaningful information because they allow frequency data to be compared across sessions that are of different lengths.

Frequency counts of a target behavior also can be converted into percentage data. For example, a frequency count of a behavior might be converted into a percentage of opportunities (Skinner, Skinner, Rhymer, & McDaniel, 2000). Suppose a problem behavior is a student's failure to carry out a teacher's instruction or requests. A systematic direct observation session might record 11 opportunities to follow a teacher's instruction, of which the student carried out 4 requests appropriately. By dividing the number of occurrences of the target behavior (in this case, following a teacher's direction) by the total number of opportunities and multiplying by 100, a percentage can be found. In this example, the student followed 36% of the teacher's instructions.

Duration Recording

Some behaviors are considered problematic not because of their frequency but because of how long the behavior continues once it starts. Measurement of the behavior's duration provides a metric of the behavior's intensity or problematic nature. For example, out-of-seat behavior is a behavior that has the potential to occur for long periods of time. In a 30-minute observation session, suppose a student gets up out of his chair only one time but is out of his seat for 18 minutes. In this instance, the particular occasion of the behavior was particularly problematic, as he was out of his seat for over half the class period, but a frequency count would only reflect one instance of the behavior. A frequency count alone would not necessarily capture the problematic nature of this behavior. Duration recording would reflect that the behavior was more of a problem.

Duration recording is appropriate for collecting data on behaviors that may have an extended duration, or behaviors in which a change in their duration signifies a change in the problem posed by the behavior. Examples of these types of behaviors include out-of-seat behavior, tantrums, noncompliant episodes, fighting, crying, and on-task behavior. Change in the duration of these behaviors would be of interest to the teacher and interventionist. For a student who displays tantrum behavior, a reduction in the duration of his or her tantrums would suggest a reduction in the intensity of the behavior and possibly a change in how problematic the behavior is for the teacher. Likewise, an increase in the duration of a student's time on-task would signify an improvement in his or her classroom behavior and would likely be viewed favorably by classroom personnel. Thus, duration recording is a method well suited to help define and monitor behaviors whose principal characteristic is that of the length during which they occur.

Duration recording is accomplished through the use of a timing device, usually a stopwatch. When conducting duration recording, the observer starts the stopwatch when the behavior begins and stops the watch when the behavior has ceased (again, a good operational definition of the target behavior will indicate when the behavior is considered to begin and when it is considered complete). Then, without resetting the stopwatch, the observer begins timing the behavior on the next occasion it is observed. This pattern continues until the observation session is completed. The observer then records the total time the observation occurred. To find the percentage of time the student engaged in the behavior during the observation session, the observer divides the number of minutes the behavior was observed by the number of minutes in the observation, then multiplies by 100.

Although the previously described method of duration recording is a simple way of determining the amount and percentage of time the student is engaged in the target behavior, the result is total duration and does not allow the observer to determine the average time of each occurrence of the behavior. Another form of duration recording can address this concern by recording the duration of each occurrence of the behavior after it has concluded, and resetting the stopwatch following each occurrence. This method provides the observer with the length of time each episode occurred, allowing one to calculate the average duration of each episode. In addition, this method provides a frequency count of the occurrence of the behavior. Although more sensitive information regarding the average duration and frequency of the behavior can be collected using this method, more logistical complications are introduced as the observer's attention may be repeatedly diverted from the target student to the stopwatch and data sheet. This can be especially problematic if a behavior occurs frequently.

While teachers or other school practitioners may be able to provide fairly accurate estimates of a behavior's duration when asked, duration recording can help validate these reports. Estimates of behavior length offered by teachers such as "it occurs for a while" or "most of the class period" may suggest how bothersome the behavior is to the teacher. However, duration recording provides a means to validate these estimated durations.

Latency Recording

Student behavior may be deemed problematic not necessarily based upon how often the behavior is exhibited or how long it occurs, but by how long it takes for a behavior to begin (or stop). In other words, latency, or the time it takes a student to display a behavior following a given stimulus, may be the presenting problem. Latency recording involves the measurement of the amount of time between the presentation of a stimulus and the onset of the target behavior. In many cases where latency is of interest, the target behavior is one that is desired. For example, the amount of time it takes a student to begin working following an instruction to do so from the teacher would be a behavior amenable to latency recording. In this case, a reduction in the time a student delays in responding appropriately to the instruction would be needed. Another example of a behavior amenable to latency recording might be a student's tardiness in changing classes. Here, the time it takes, or latency, from when the bell rings ending the period until the student arrives at his or her next classroom would be measured by latency recording. Latency may also apply to behaviors in which an increase in latency is desired. For example, a behavior such as calling out responses to questions before a teacher requires a response may be reflected in a measure of the time between when a question is asked and when a student calls out an answer.

The procedure for conducting latency recording is similar to that of duration recording. The observer starts a stopwatch when the stimulus is delivered (i.e., teacher delivers an instruction), and timing is stopped when the target or expected behavior is elicited by the student (i.e., student compliance to the request). If several opportunities to elicit the behavior occur during the observation session, the observer can obtain an average latency by not resetting the stopwatch to zero and then dividing the total time by the total number of opportunities.

As with the duration of a behavior, latency can be difficult to estimate and communicate accurately when one is removed from the context in which the behavior occurs. Thus, latency recording provides a method to both validate teacher reports and obtain more precise measurements.

Time-Sampling Procedures

The methods of data collection discussed thus far all involve the recording of essentially each occurrence of behavior that is observed. To be accurate with this type of recording, the observer may need to have a quick hand with the tally sheet or quick finger on the stopwatch, especially if the behavior occurs frequently. Furthermore, collecting data using event, duration, or latency recording prevents the observer from monitoring and recording other behaviors that may be co-occurring. In some instances, such as behaviors of a high frequency, the nature of the behaviors is such that accurate recording is simply not possible. Likewise, when behaviors are of very high frequency and occur in a response burst, it may be difficult to determine accurately a clear beginning and end point for each behavior. For example, if one were counting the number of times a student tapped his pencil on his desk, would you count each tap as a contact between the pencil and the desk? Most times, a students tapping his or her pencil would tap multiple times in a very short period, making the counting of each individual tap very difficult to capture accurately.

Time sampling procedures were developed to ease the collection of data for behaviors that may be of longer duration, are continuous, occur at high frequencies, or when the recording of more than one behavior at the same time is desired. Time sampling consists of dividing an observation session into equal portions of time, or intervals, and recording target behaviors within each interval. For example, a 15-minute observation session might be broken into 60 15-second intervals. Each interval would be scored based upon the occurrence of the target behavior(s) within the interval according to the behavior's operational definition.

Time sampling requires the use of a cueing device. Repeatedly glancing at a wall clock or wristwatch in order to keep track of the intervals would detract too much attention away from the target student being observed. Thus, it is important when conducting time sampling to use a cueing device that offers audio cues when to record. One type of device is to use a prepared audio tape with recorded signals (i.e., beeps) that signify the start of each interval. Shapiro (2004b) provides instructions for making a time sampling audio tape. Another is to use a countdown timer that can be reset after each interval. A third option is to use a personal digital assistant that automatically maintains intervals for the observer (Shapiro, 2003).

Time sampling methods are a vital part of the direct observation repertoire because of their potential to simplify and make more efficient the data collection process. Because of the increased efficiency, it is more feasible for observers to collect data on a wider range of topographies and behaviors with a wider range of intensity (high frequencies, long durations), as well as collecting data on several different behaviors simultaneously. For example, the Behavior Observation of Students in Schools (BOSS; Shapiro, 2003, 2004a, 2004b) provides the observer with a feasible and reliable means to code active and passive academic engaged time through momentary time sampling, in addition to recording motor, verbal, and passive off-task behaviors through partial-interval time sampling during 15-second intervals. Hence, time sampling procedures provide a powerful method of collecting systematic and quantitative data on a number of behaviors at once.

It is important to remember that, unlike event, duration, or latency methods, time sampling provides only an *estimate* of the actual occurrence of behavior. Each form of time sampling results in an over- or underestimate of behavior. The results of a time sampling observation are usually reported in terms of the percentage of intervals scored. For example, suppose a student was on-task during 46 intervals of a 15-minute whole-interval observation with 10-second intervals. The results of this observation would report that the student was on-task approximately 51% of the *intervals observed*. Notice that it was *not* reported that the student was on-task 51% of the time—rather, only the percentage of intervals in which the behavior occurred throughout the interval. There are three methods of time sampling data collection: whole-interval, partial-interval, and momentary time sampling.

Whole-Interval Time Sampling

When using whole-interval time sampling, an interval is scored if the behavior occurs throughout the entire interval. Thus, if out-of-seat behavior is the behavior of interest, an interval would be scored if the student was out of his or her seat for the entire interval.

Whole-interval recording is appropriate for behaviors in which continuous performance of the behavior is desired (Watson & Steege, 2003), such as studying or playing with peers. Whole-interval time sampling also provides an approximate duration of the behavior by summing the number of intervals and multiplying by the length of each interval. One important point regarding whole-interval time sampling is that this method tends to underestimate the actual occurrence of the behavior (Saudargas & Lentz, 1986), especially if the intervals are long in duration. For example, if one were observing a student playing appropriately with toys, and the student stopped occasionally to glance around the room, one would record those intervals in which such glances occurred as the behavior not occurring. Thus, if one were using 10-second intervals, a simple glance away from the playing activity would render the interval as "behavior not occurring," when in reality the behavior had occurred for 8 of the 10 seconds of the interval. The result is an underestimate of the actual occurrence of the behavior.

Partial-Interval Time Sampling

When partial-interval time sampling is being employed, an interval is scored when the behavior occurs at any time during the interval. For example, if calling out was the behavior of interest, the observer would score a particular interval if the behavior occurred at any point during that interval. Note that only the interval would be scored, not how many times the behavior occurred during the interval. As in whole-interval time sampling, the shorter the intervals used, the more precise the estimate of the behavior is obtained. Note also that partial-interval time sampling tends to overestimate the actual occurrence of the behavior because some nonoccurrences of the behavior are ignored if they are juxtaposed to intervals when the behavior was observed (Lentz, 1988; Saudargas & Lentz, 1986).

Partial-interval time sampling is best suited for behaviors that occur at moderate to high rates (so that the interval procedure has the best chance of capturing the number of occurrences of the behavior) or those that may be of an inconsistent duration (Watson & Steege, 2003). Thus, many different behaviors would be amenable to this method. The power of partial-interval recording lies in its potential to provide the observer with a way to monitor several behaviors and score them during the same interval. For example, the label "off-task behavior" can encompass a wide variety of behaviors that the student might demonstrate characterizing himself or herself as "off-task." The practitioner may want to collect data regarding whether the student is displaying off-task behaviors of a more verbal (i.e., calling out, whispering to peer), motor (i.e., out of seat, tapping pencil), or passive (i.e., daydreaming, looking out window) nature. During each interval, the observer can observe the student for the presence of any of the three behaviors and, if present according to the operational definitions, score the behavior in an appropriate box. At the end of the observation, these data would provide an estimate of the frequency with which the student displayed each of the behaviors. The advantage of partial-interval recording is that behaviors such as on-task behavior that are often continuous and do not have easily discernible starting- and stopping-points can be accurately captured by this method. In addition, partial-interval recording can be an excellent procedure when the behavior is very high frequency and trying to count each instance of the behavior would not result in accurate data.

Although partial-interval recording can easily capture high-rate behaviors, the method often overestimates the actual occurrence of behavior, especially if a behavior is somewhat continuous. For example, if one is recording on-task behavior using partial-interval recording in 10-second intervals, a student who is on-task for only 2 seconds would be recorded as "on-task" for that interval when in reality he or she was off-task for 8 seconds and on-task for only 2 seconds. The final calculation of percentage of intervals in which the behavior occurs would then be an underestimate compared to counting the actual duration or frequency of the behavior.

Momentary Time Sampling

Momentary time sampling involves the scoring of an interval if the behavior occurs (or is occurring) precisely when the interval begins. For example, if on-task behavior was the behavior of interest, the observer would observe the student when the signal is given for the start of the interval. If the student was on-task at that moment, the observer would score the interval as on-task and ignore the behavior for the duration of the interval.

Momentary time sampling is appropriate for behaviors that occur at high frequencies or are continuous but when it is less feasible to continuously monitor them (Watson & Steege, 2003). Because the observer need only observe the behavior at the start of the interval, resources are freed to monitor other behaviors through the use of another method, such as partial-interval recording.

Momentary time sampling has been found to both over- and under-estimate the frequency of actual occurrence of behavior (Lentz, 1988; Saudargas & Lentz, 1986). Because the method is based on a recording of behavior only at an instant in time, it is a strategy likely to reduce the potential systematic over- and underestimation errors of whole- and partial-interval sampling. Although one cannot predict whether momentary time sampling will result in close estimates of actual occurrence of behavior, studies have shown that the error of estimation for momentary time sampling is less then other forms of time sampling (Lentz, 1988; Saudargas & Lentz, 1986).

Performance-Based Recording

Watson and Steege (2003) describe performance-based recording, which involves the rating of observed behaviors according to a predetermined scale. This type of recording is appropriate for instances when the behavior is observed firsthand but it is not feasible to record data at that moment. Instead, a rating of the behavior's frequency, duration, or latency is made when the observer is able to record. For this reason, performance-based recording is ideal for teachers to collect data themselves on their students' behavior.

Prior to an observation session, a criterion is developed on which behaviors will be rated. For example, a tantrum lasting less than 1 minute might be considered a "1," one lasting 1–4 minutes a "2," 5–10 minutes a "3," and more than 10 minutes a "4." Following a particular class period, the teacher would rate the observed tantrums according to the scale. As another example, fewer than three call-outs during a class period might be rated a "1," 3–5 rated a "2," 5–10 a "3," and so on. What performance-based recordings sacrifice in precision they recoup in conservation of resources. Providing teachers with a method of quantitative data collection allows evaluators to allocate their time elsewhere while still being able to obtain quantitative data from the cases in which they are consulting.

Permanent Product Recording

Permanent product recording involves the inspection of tangible or "permanent" materials completed by the student. Permanent products might include math worksheets, handwriting samples, essays or compositions, graffiti, or damaged or destroyed property.

Although permanent product inspection is not necessarily "direct" observation in that the behavior was not directly observed at the time it occurred, this method does, however, provide the practitioner with a means to observe directly the "results" of the behavior. This can provide important information regarding the frequency, intensity, and severity of a behavior. For students with spelling difficulties, permanent products of the student's recent spelling tests may provide information regarding typical or common spelling mistakes. Likewise, math worksheets may indicate what types of problems or what errors the student is commonly making.

Some behaviors, due to their nature, are practically impossible to observe at the moment they occur. Indeed, for many behaviors such as stealing, vandalism, or substance abuse students may make every effort *not* to be observed. However, inspection of the results of these behaviors soon after they occur can yield important information. Graffiti or vandalized property may indicate locations or times of day in which the behavior is more likely to occur. Records of the number of items reported stolen from lockers or other school areas can indicate the frequency of theft. Furthermore, inspection of damaged or destroyed property can help define the severity and seriousness of a particular problem behavior by recording the cost and extent of the damage inflicted.

Peer Comparison Data Collection

Collection of peer comparison data is accomplished with exactly the same methods in which data are collected with the target student. However, the observer may decide how much time or how many intervals to devote to peer comparison. Often, this decision is based upon the topography of the target behavior(s), number of behaviors being observed, and the number of peers from which data will be obtained. Skinner, Rhymer, and McDaniel (2000) describe two methods for collecting peer comparison data: simultaneous recording, which involves observing all students in a group at the same time, and discontinuous recording, which involves dividing time between observation of the target student and observation of peers. Both procedures work best within the use of a time sampling procedure. Simultaneous recording is best used with small groups of students grouped together in close physical proximity, such as part of a small group. Additionally, use of a time sampling method that does not require continuous monitoring is warranted, such as partial-interval or momentary time sampling. Discontinuous recording, on the other hand, allows the observer more latitude in the types of time sampling that can be used, as each interval is devoted to observing the target student or one of his or her peers. This method will yield more reliable data when a group of five or so students is identified and the observer rotates among these students at each peer comparison interval.

It is important when collecting peer comparison data to avoid using either the best-behaved or the most poorly behaved students in the class. A good idea is to talk to the teacher beforehand, asking him or her to identify a number of students whose behavior is considered "average." As mentioned earlier in this chapter, the collection of peer comparison data is a critical component of defining student problems, because it provides valuable insight regarding the overall ecology as well as general behavioral expectations of the classroom. Peer comparison data provide a context for the problem behavior; they supply a "normative base" upon which the severity of the student's behavior can be compared, a benchmark upon which goals can be developed, and a measuring stick on which progress toward the goals can be monitored.

BRIEF CASE EXAMPLES

Data from two cases are presented here. In one case, a fourth-grade student was referred because of an academic skill problem, specifically a problem in writing. The case illustrates how the systematic direct observation data collected for that case illustrated how behavioral problems evident during instruction were a function of the student's struggle with academic skills. The second case was a fifth-grade student who was referred primarily for behavior problems, verbal outbursts during class including inappropriate language, as well not completing homework, fidgety behavior, and banging his head in frustration on his desk. In this case, systematic direct observation data were used to better identify the functions of the behavior.

Ashley

Ashley was a fourth-grade student referred by her teacher because of poor academic performance in writing. In addition, her teacher, Mrs. Wachs, indicated that Ashley demonstrated a "significant lack of independence" in completing her work.

Systematic direct observations were made during two different types of writing instruction, selected in consultation with Mrs. Wachs. The first 15-minute observation was during whole-class instruction on the mechanics of writing poetry. Students were asked questions and provided feedback throughout the lesson and were expected to attend to both Mrs. Wachs and their own written products. In the second 15-minute observation, Ashley was given an independent writing assignment in which students were asked to provide additional details to their poetry. Mrs. Wachs then held a conference with her students about their individual writing.

Ashley was observed using the Behavioral Observation of Students in Schools (BOSS) (Shapiro, 2003, 2004b). The observational system recorded levels of academic engagement (active or passive) as a momentary time sample every 15 seconds, along with the nature of any off-task behaviors (passive, verbal, and motor) in a partial-interval format if they occurred during the 15-second interval. Additionally, randomly selected peers throughout the classroom were observed on the same behaviors every

fifth interval to provide peer comparison data. Finally, to determine if the
teacher was engaged in active, directed instruction toward the students, the
teacher's behavior was also recorded every fifth interval.

Results of the observations are shown in Table 9.1. During the whole-
class instruction, Ashley showed on-task behavior (addition of active and
passive engaged time) equivalent to her peers (Ashley and peers = 91.67%
of intervals). When Ashley was on-task, she tended to have more passive
engaged time, suggesting that she spent more time listening and paying
attention than actively participating in the activities. Likewise, she showed
almost no off-task behavior throughout the lesson. In contrast, during the
independent work activity Ashley had a substantially lower level of academic engagement (Ashley on-task = 22.91% of intervals; peers = 75% of
intervals) and had a very high level of off-task behavior. In particular,
Ashley often spent time pretending her pencils were talking to each other
and playing with them, instead of writing.

The systematic direct observation data for Ashley showed that the
teacher's perception that Ashley did not work independently was confirmed in the observation of her independent work period. At the same
time, the fact that Ashley fully attended to the group lesson and showed
levels of engagement equivalent to her peers suggested that under conditions where the teacher is in control Ashley may do much better in terms of
attention to task. Such a finding was a bit surprising to the teacher and suggested that the development of interventions for Ashley may be more successful if larger group activities were used. When independent work was to
be assigned, it was suggested to the teacher that Ashley might benefit from
working in smaller cooperative groups rather than alone.

These data were part of a larger assessment process that included a
more in-depth examination of Ashley's academic skill development to

TABLE 9.1. Percentage of Intervals Observed for Ashley and Peer Comparison
Students during Whole-Class and Independent Writing Assignments

	Whole-class instruction		Independent work	
Behavior	Ashley (48 intervals)	Peers (12 intervals)	Ashley (48 intervals)	Peers (12 intervals)
Active engaged time	4.2	16.7	14.6	41.7
Passive engaged time	87.5	75.0	8.3	33.3
Off-task motor	0.0	4.2	60.4	25.0
Off-task verbal	2.1	0.0	26.9	4.2
Off-task passive	2.1	0.0	2.1	4.2
Teacher-directed instruction		83.3		58.3

determine if her difficulties in writing were part of a performance (won't do) or skill (can't do) problem. While the full details of that assessment are beyond the scope of this chapter, it was determined that Ashley's written language skills were only slightly behind her expected level and much of the problem was a function of a performance deficit during independent work periods. Thus, the target for subsequent intervention was improving her work during independent skill activities and not on the specifics of writing mechanics.

David

David was referred by his teacher primarily because of his verbal outbursts in class. He would often make negative self-statements such as "I hate school," or "I'm stupid," in addition to occasionally using profanity. His teacher, Ms. Fritz, believed much of his behavior to be attention-seeking.

Systematic direct observation of David's behavior was conducted on two 20-minute occasions on two different days when, according to his teacher, the behaviors were most likely to occur. During these periods the number of negative self-statements ("I hate school," "I hate myself") and/or other verbal outbursts such as cursing were counted. In addition, the events immediately preceding and following the outburst were recorded. In addition, other incidents of disruptive behavior (tipping his chair, fidgeting in his seat) were counted.

The observations revealed that David had negative self-talk twice across each of the 20-minute observations. On three of the four occasions, another student commented to David about his self-talk, and in one case his teacher reprimanded him. The data suggested that these behaviors were likely attention-seeking responses. David tipped his chair three times and fidgeted four times during the observations. No responses to these behaviors from others were evident, suggesting that these behaviors were serving more of a self-stimulating function.

These data were part of a comprehensive psychological evaluation that examined other aspects of David's behavior. As a result, it was clear that David thrived on attention, especially one-on-one attention from peers. A recommendation for a peer tutoring program was made and found to be highly successful in reducing David's inappropriate self-talk. In addition, a daily goal of verbal outbursts was set for specific academic activities, with individual teacher attention as the contingent reinforcement. This intervention was also very successful in reducing David's inappropriate verbal outbursts. The case is an excellent example of how systematic direct observation was used in the process of conducting a functional behavioral assessment.

SUMMARY: USING SYSTEMATIC DIRECT OBSERVATION
IN THE PROBLEM-SOLVING PROCESS

Systematic direct observation provides an essential component of the problem-solving model. As one can see, there are a large number of options from which the practitioner can draw in conducting the observations. Each method of observation has its advantages and disadvantages, and while some methods can result in equally valid data for the same behavior, other methods may give erroneous results if the method is not carefully matched to the nature of the problem.

Figures 9.1 and 9.2 offer helpful guides for practitioners when choosing the method of systematic direct observation that will result in the data that will best reflect the nature of the problem. Figure 9.1 offers examples of the types of problems often encountered in school referrals. These problems are matched with the type of systematic direct observation that is best suited to capturing the data related to the problem. Certainly, it is recognized that some behaviors can be observed through multiple methods, and deciding which method is best must be done at the level of the individual practitioner who is conducting the assessment. However, the figure offers guidance to practitioners who may be less familiar with the many ways that these data can be collected.

Figure 9.2 offers a decision tree for guiding practitioners toward the right method in general. As one works through the decision process, the methodology that will most likely result in the most accurate type of systematic direct observation emerges.

Deciding which type of systematic direct observation to use is not always a simple decision. Many times, practitioners must also consider the costs versus benefits of the form of systematic direct observation that they have decided to use. For example, it may be that the best form of data collection is time sampling. However, time sampling requires that the observer be able to stay vigilant to the student being observed throughout an instructional period. The job requirements of those who typically conduct these assessments, such as school psychologists, may not allow the luxury of spending long periods of time observing in one setting. As such, the evaluator may have to trade the advantage of collecting time sampling data for the efficiency of a performance type of observation done by the teacher. Such decisions should be made carefully, considering the consequences of obtaining data that may not truly reflect the referral problem.

Despite the potential challenges of conducting systematic direct observation, these data represent the heart of the problem-solving process. The data are designed to complement all other forms of data collection, including those obtained through a process of interviewing teachers as well as through more formal informant reports such as rating scales. Together, the data from systematic direct observation and all other methods of data collection form the basis upon which the problem-solving process is built.

REFERENCES

Bergan, J. R., & Kratochwill, T. R. (1990). *Behavioral consultation and therapy*. New York: Plenum.

Boyajian, A. E., DuPaul, G. J., Handler, M. W., Eckert, T. L., & McGoey, K. E. (2001). The use of classroom-based brief functional analyses with preschoolers at-risk for attention deficit hyperactivity disorders. *School Psychology Review, 30*, 278–293.

Cone, J. D. (1978). The Behavioral Assessment Grid (BAG): A conceptual framework and a taxonomy. *Behavior Therapy, 9*, 882–888.

Daly, E. J., III, & Murdoch, A. (2000). Direct observation in the assessment of academic skills problems. In E. S. Shapiro & T. R. Kratochwill (Eds), *Behavioral assessment in schools: Theory, research, and clinical foundations* (2nd ed., pp. 46–77). New York: Guilford Press.

Daly, E. J., III, Witt, J. C., Martens, B. K. , & Dool, E. J. (1997). A model for conducting a functional analysis of academic performance problems. *School Psychology Review, 26*, 554–574.

Demaray, M. K., & Elliott, S. N. (1998). Teachers' judgments of students' academic functioning: A comparison of actual and predicted performances. *School Psychology Quarterly, 13*, 8–24.

DuPaul, G. J. (2003). Assessment of ADHD symptoms: Comment on Gomez et al. (2003). *Psychological Assessment, 15*, 115–117.

DuPaul, G. J., Power, T. J., McGoey, K. E., Ikeda, M. J., & Anastopoulos, A. D. (1998). Reliability and validity of parent and teacher ratings of attention-deficit/hyperactivity disorder symptoms. *Journal of Psychoeducational Assessment, 16*, 55–68.

DuPaul, G. J., & Stoner, G. (2003). *ADHD in the schools: Assessment and intervention strategies* (2nd ed.). New York: Guilford Press.

Feinberg, A. B., & Shapiro, E. S. (2003). Accuracy of teacher judgments in predicting oral reading fluency. *School Psychology Quarterly, 18*, 52– 65.

Fuchs, L. S., Fuchs, D., & Deno, S. L. (1985). Importance of goal ambitiousness and goal mastery to student achievement. *Exceptional Children, 52*, 63–71.

Goh, D. S., Teslow, C. J., & Fuller, G. B. (1981). The practices of psychological assessment among school psychologists. *Professional Psychology, 12*, 699–706.

Gresham, F., Watson, S. T., & Skinner, C. H. (2001). Functional behavioral assessment: Principles, procedures, and future directions. *School Psychology Review, 30*, 156–172.

Hutton, J. B., Dubes, R., & Muir, S. (1992). Assessment practices of school psychologists: Ten years later. *School Psychology Review, 21*, 271–284.

Kratochwill, T. R. (1985). Case study research in school psychology. *School Psychology Review, 14*, 204–215.

Lentz, F. E., Jr. (1988). Direct observation and measurement of academic skills: A conceptual review. In E. S. Shapiro & T. R. Kratochwill (Eds.), *Behavioral assessment in schools: Conceptual foundations and practical applications* (pp. 76–120). New York: Guilford Press.

March, R. E., & Horner, R. H. (2002). Feasibility and contributions of functional behavioral assessment in schools. *Journal of Emotional and Behavioral Disorders, 10*, 158–170.

Mash, E. J., & Terdal, L. G. (Eds.) (1997). *Assessment of childhood disorders* (3rd ed.). New York: Guilford Press.

Merrell, K. W. (2003). *Behavioral, social, and emotional assessment of children and adolescents* (2nd ed.). Mahwah, NJ: Erlbaum.

Ruth, W. J. (1996). Goal setting and behavior contracting for students with emotional and behavioral difficulties: Analysis of daily, weekly, and total goal attainment. *Psychology in the Schools, 33,* 153–158.

Saudargas, R. A., & Lentz, F. E., Jr. (1986). Estimating percent of time and rate via direct observation: A suggested observational procedure and format. *School Psychology Review, 15,* 36–48.

Scott, T. M., Nelson, C. M., & Zabela, J. (2003). Functional behavior assessment training in public schools: Facilitating systemic change. *Journal of Positive Behavior Interventions, 5,* 216–224.

Shapiro, E. S. (2003). *Behavioral Observation of Students in Schools* (computer software). Austin, TX: Psychological Corporation.

Shapiro, E. S. (2004a). *Academic skills problems: Direct assessment and intervention* (3rd ed.). New York: Guilford Press.

Shapiro E. S. (2004b). *Academic skills problems workbook* (rev. ed.). New York: Guilford Press.

Shapiro, E. S., & Heick, P. F. (2004). School psychologist assessment practices in the evaluation of students referred for social/behavioral/emotional problems. *Psychology in the Schools, 41,* 551–561.

Shapiro, E. S., & Kratochwill, T. R. (Eds.). (2000a). *Behavioral assessment in schools: Theory, research, and clinical foundations* (2nd ed.). New York: Guilford Press.

Shapiro, E. S., & Kratochwill, T. R. (Eds.). (2000b). *Conducting school-based assessments of child and adolescent behavior.* New York: Guilford Press.

Skinner, C. H., Rhymer, K. N., & McDaniel, E. C. (2000). Naturalistic direct observation in educational settings. In E. S. Shapiro & T. R. Kratochwill (Eds.), *Conducting school-based assessments of child and adolescent behavior* (pp. 21–54). New York: Guilford Press.

Skinner, C. H., Dittmer, K. I., & Howell, L. A. (2000). Direct observation in school settings: Theoretical issues. In E. S. Shapiro & T. R. Kratochwill (Eds.), *Behavioral assessment in schools: Theory, research, and clinical foundations* (2nd ed., pp. 19–45). New York: Guilford Press.

Wade, T. C., & Baker, T. B. (1977). Opinions and use of psychological tests: A survey of clinical psychologists. *American Psychologist, 32,* 874–882.

Watson, T. S., & Steege, M. W. (2003). *Conducting school-based functional behavioral assessments: A practitioner's guide.* New York: Guilford Press.

Wilson, M. S., & Reschly, D. J. (1996). Assessment in school psychology training and practice. *School Psychology Review, 25,* 9–23.

SUGGESTED READINGS

Shapiro, E. S. (2003). *Behavioral Observation of Students in Schools* (computer software). Austin, TX: Psychological Corporation.

This is a software program that runs on any PDA that uses the Palm operating system. The program is designed to facilitate the collection of school-based in-classroom behavioral data that are known to link to academic achievement outcomes. Some personal customization of the data collection system is possible, although the observational code used in the software is based on the code described by Shapiro (2004b).

Shapiro, E. S., & Kratochwill, T. R. (Eds.). (2000). *Conducting school-based assessment of child and adolescent behavior.* New York: Guilford Press.

This edited text provides a practitioner-oriented approach to conducting assessment of school-based problems. The text covers all aspects of the assessment process from interviewing through direct observation, through the use of rating scales and checklists. An excellent resource for practitioners, the text offers clear and useful case study information throughout to guide the practitioner in the assessment process.

Watson, T. S., & Steege, M. W. (2003). *Conducting school-based functional behavioral assessments: A practitioner's guide.* New York: Guilford Press.

This text is a practitioner-friendly description of the process of conducting functional assessments in schools. The book is packed full of forms and step-by-step methods for completing direct observations. Practitioners would find this text especially helpful to those who are not well skilled in conducting functional assessments of school-related problems.

CHAPTER 10

♦ ♦ ♦

Rating Scale Applications within the Problem-Solving Model

♦

R. T. BUSSE

It is a basic tenet of best practices that assessment should be a multiaxial enterprise to garner data from multiple sources, settings, and measures. Behavior rating scales have been validated as one useful method for meeting these best-practice goals in school and research-based assessment. In a traditional school-based assessment paradigm, rating scales most often are used for diagnostic and classification purposes such as special education placement, at which point their use ends. Ratings scales are not typically used to link assessment to intervention, nor, except for research applications, are rating scales used to evaluate intervention outcomes. The underuse of rating scales also is evident within the problem-solving and consultation literature, wherein assessment often relies on interview and observation methods. Thus, although rating scale methods may assist toward accounting for several aspects of behavior variance and can be used in an assessment-for-intervention model, rating scales often may be relegated to a classification role.

The primary purpose of this chapter is to provide a rationale and framework for the applications of rating scales within the problem-solving model. As part of a problem-solving approach, rating scale methods can be extended and applied to facilitate problem identification and definition, can be used in intervention implementation, and can be applied to evaluate intervention outcomes. Before exploring these applications, we will examine some basic assumptions and aspects of behavior rating scale technologies. But first, a brief caveat is warranted; given the scope and purposes of this book, there is insufficient space to delve into all aspects of rating scale technology and use. Where specific rating scales are included, they were selected for illustrative purposes. Suggested readings are offered at the end of the chapter for readers who wish to expand their knowledge base.

GUIDING ASSUMPTIONS
FOR RATING SCALE APPLICATIONS

Elliott and colleagues (Elliott & Busse, 2004; Elliott, Busse, & Gresham, 1993) provided several assumptions that set the stage for understanding the strengths and limitations of rating scales, and their subsequent applications. First, whether used for classification or in problem solving, well-designed rating scales possess sound psychometric properties, that is, they are reliable and valid assessment tools. Ethical users of rating scale methods must be familiar with the concepts of reliability and validity, particularly when extending scale applications, and users must be trained in interpreting rating scale scores and outcomes (American Educational Research Association, 1999).

Beyond this necessary knowledge base are unique aspects of rating scales that should be understood. Users should be aware that rating scales are more than a simple checklist or survey; rather, good rating scales are carefully constructed measures that typically assess behaviors across relative frequency rating dimensions (e.g., never, sometimes, always). For example, a parent may rate a behavior such as aggression as occurring "sometimes" as an indicator of relative frequency; little is known about the actual or absolute frequency. Moreover, rating scales essentially are summary observation measures of specific behaviors, or response classes of several related behaviors. Therefore, a key assumption in the use of rating scales is that raters' responses often are based on accumulated perceptions and observations of an individual across time and settings.

Two related assumptions are that ratings of behavior involve evaluative judgments based on the rater's standards for behavior, and that ratings are affected by environmental factors. Subsequently, ratings from multiple sources such as teachers, children, and parents may evidence only moderate agreement (Achenbach, McConaughy, & Howell, 1987; Ruffalo & Elliott; 1997). This aspect of rating scales is referred to as situation specificity because an individual's behavior often varies in relation to settings or situations, and a rater's standards for behavior influence his or her perceptions. As an obvious example, aggressive behavior may be tolerated while playing sports, but not in the classroom.

The final set of assumptions about rating scales relates to the decisions made pursuant to them. Rating scales can be used to make both norm-referenced and/or criterion-referenced decisions. Most published behavior rating scales adopt a norm-referenced approach in which a child's ratings are compared to a normative sample. Criterion-referenced applications may be more useful for decisions in problem-solving intervention because the comparison is some behavioral criterion rather a normative group. Both norm-referenced and criterion-referenced methods are useful, depending on the user's needs; the former is more useful for classification, the latter potentially for problem solving. Regardless of the use, each method should be subject to the social validity aspect of assessment, that is, the degree of importance and benefits to the individual and society (Messick, 1995). Specifically, if key participants in a problem-solving team disagree with the rating scale values, their use may be compromised.

OVERVIEW OF RATING SCALE CONCEPTS

Before moving to the larger topic of problem solving, it is useful to provide a brief overview of some key terms and concepts of rating scale technology. Rating scales can be roughly dichotomized as omnibus or behavior-specific scales. Omnibus scales are designed to measure a variety of behaviors and may be referred to as general purpose measures (Merrell, 2000). Omnibus scales typically provide an overall, or total, problem score that can be parsed into subscales that often are generically referred to as broad-band and narrow-band categories. The broad-band categories often are depicted as measuring either externalizing or internalizing behaviors, whereas the narrow-band categories are descriptive of specific behavior classes or clusters of behavior. For example, narrow-band scales of aggression or hyperactivity would be part of an externalizing broad-band scale, and narrow-band categories of depression or anxiety would be part of an internalizing broad-band scale. Behavior-specific scales, as the title implies, typically measure a discrete domain of behavior, such as social skills or self-concept.

Another concept relates to the informant from whom a scale is used to gather data. Some rating scales are designed to be completed solely by parents/caregivers, teachers, or by children in a self-report format, whereas other rating scales are designed to be completed by all three informants. Those scales that incorporate multiple raters provide for gathering what is known as cross-informant data. The decision of whom to include as a rater depends of course on the purpose of the assessment. It generally is considered best practice, however, to gather data from multiple informants to obtain a richer picture of a child's behavioral functioning across settings and situations. Using multiple informants also aids in consideration of the level of source and setting variances accounted for during an assessment.

There are several widely used, well-constructed cross-informant omnibus rating scales, such as the Child Behavior Checklist system (Achenbach, 2002), the Behavior Assessment System for Children (Reynolds & Kamphaus, 1992), and the Conners Rating Scale—Revised (Conners, 1997). There also are a large variety of well-constructed behavior-specific rating scales, some of which use a cross-informant format such as the Social Skills Rating System (Gresham & Elliott, 1990), and many well-constructed self-report measures such as the Reynolds Child Depression Scale (Reynolds, 1989). The choice of which rating scale to use depends on the referral issue and whether the scale is reliable and valid for its intended use.

RATING SCALES AS PROBLEM-SOLVING TOOLS

The sections on guiding assumptions and rating scale concepts provide a backdrop for exploring the applications of behavior rating scales in the problem-solving model. With these concepts in mind, we turn to an examination of some theoretical and practical issues regarding the applications of rating scales within the stages of problem solving for which they may be most useful.

Problem Identification and Definition

As defined in this volume, the problem identification and problem definition stages involve collecting data toward a decision as to whether a problem exists and justifies intervention, and to provide an operational or measurable definition of the problem. Given that a primary use of rating scales is diagnosis, it is reasonable to assume that rating scales will be useful in identifying problems. Indeed, rating scales can be useful in different aspects of problem identification. For example, it is often useful to administer a rating scale before meeting with a teacher or parent to facilitate subsequent interviews and to communicate prompt reaction to a referral. The information garnered from the rating scale may result in a more focused and efficient problem-solving interview. One might use an omnibus measure to gather data on a wider range of behaviors than those listed on an initial referral. Depending on the results, those data can be used to substantiate the problem definition, to identify potential problems that were not initially identified, and to validate that other behaviors are not of concern. The results of the ratings then can be compared and converged with data gathered during other assessment activities, such as interviews and observations. A behavior-specific rating scale can be similarly used if information from the referral or a file review indicates that a specific problem type is the only area of concern. Behavior-specific scales may be most useful after an initial problem identification interview to validate the significance of the problem during the problem definition phase.

The types of data included in the results of rating scales range from indicators of general behavior patterns to occurrences of specific behaviors and item analysis. For linking problem identification to problem definition, and ultimately to intervention, an item analysis is most useful. The broad-band categories are not as useful for problem specification—how does one translate "externalizing" into a specific behavior or intervention? Similarly, many narrow-band categories are too broad to facilitate specific problem definition. The category of "aggression" may help somewhat to refine the problem definition, but these larger response classes can consist of several behaviors. These categories are useful in an initial phase of data gathering and, as we will see later, in the problem solution stage. These issues are akin to what is known as the aptitude-by-treatment dilemma, a phenomenon often discussed in relation to intelligence tests, wherein assessment results that identify a larger class of behaviors typically have not been found to lead to specific interventions.

An item analysis involves examining individual items that are rated as a significant problem and comparing the ratings to behaviors of concern as identified in a referral or during other assessment procedures. As with the broader-scale applications, an item analysis has strengths and weaknesses. A particular strength is that individual items that support the referral concern(s) can be used to validate the problem definition. For example, consider a referral concern that is initially described as hyperactivity, which, during a problem-solving interview, is refined to a target behavior of being "out of seat." A related item rated as a significant problem on either an omnibus or behavior-specific hyperactivity scale can aid in justifying the concern and need for intervention. If the scale uses a cross-informant format, items can be compared across raters to ascertain the level of situational specificity, that is, whether the behavior evident is in only one or, rather, more settings. The major weakness of the item analysis approach is that single-item reliability and validity are not established. That is, the reliability and validity of rating scales primarily are based on clusters of items, such as broad- and narrow-band categories, and there is no strong research to validate the use of single items. One way to offset this weakness is to ensure that multiple assessment methods are employed, such as observations and interviews, and to examine the convergence of the results with the item analysis.

Another relative weakness of item analysis procedures relates to the level of treatment utility one can expect from their use. Some items are molar in nature, that is, they are broader in scope, whereas some items are molecular and as such are more specific. For example, an item such as "makes friends easily" is molar, whereas a more discrete item, "appropriately invites friends to play," is molecular. In general, molecular items are more specific and, as such, are more useful in problem definition. Individual items also exhibit the aptitude-by-treatment interaction dilemma or, more aptly, an item-by-treatment interaction dilemma. Thus, an item may aid in targeting a problem for intervention during the problem definition phase, but individual items do not directly lead to a specific intervention. This is a limitation to item analysis and a major reason why rating scales typically are not as useful in the exploring solutions phase of problem solving.

In the next two sections, we step away from the uses of published rating scales to describe extensions of rating scale methods that can be readily applied within the problem-solving model. We first explore the use of rating scale technology in monitoring treatment integrity during the implementing solutions phase, followed by expansions of rating scale methods in progress monitoring.

Implementation of Solutions

After a problem is defined in measurable terms, solutions are explored for the intervention implementation phase of problem solving. Interventions should be chosen that are linked to the assessment data and that have a research base to validate their use. This concept has become known as evidence-based intervention (Kratochwill & Stoiber, 2000). Once an intervention is selected, it is imperative that a specific plan or intervention protocol be devised that delineates each step or component of the intervention. A written intervention plan is important for several reasons. From a practical perspective, a written plan aids in validating an agreed-upon intervention, ensures that everyone involved is "on the same page," serves as a reminder or prompt to engage in the intervention and, just as importantly, removes potential problems with remembering the intervention steps. A written intervention plan also may enhance the level of treatment or intervention integrity. Intervention integrity refers to the degree to which an intervention is implemented as intended (see Chapter 15, this volume). If an intervention is not implemented as intended or as set forth in the evidence-based literature, it cannot be known whether intervention outcomes were the result of the intervention. Thus, if an intervention fails, it is not known which factors need to be explored further to solve the problem. Therefore, an important assessment component during the intervention implementation phase of problem solving is the monitoring of intervention integrity.

As explored in more detail in Chapter 15 of this volume, intervention integrity can be assessed through observations and by simply asking the intervention agent whether they are adhering to the intervention protocol. Observations of intervention implementation obviously are more direct, although it may not be possible to observe a useful length of the intervention if it takes place across a long time period or in other settings such as a child's home. Asking about adherence to an intervention may serve as a prompt, but it is a weak method of assessment because of reliance on a single summary memory or perception. A useful alternative procedure is to adapt rating scale methods for use as an intervention integrity monitoring tool.

Gresham (1989) presented an example of an intervention integrity assessment tool that combined an intervention plan protocol with a rating scale format. In the example, the steps of a response cost program were delineated along with a five-point rating of level of agreement for whether each intervention step was implemented as defined. This method of combining a written plan with a rating of integrity not only serves as an intervention protocol, but it also provides for an assessment of an intervention agent's adherence to the intervention plan. The data gathered from an intervention integrity assessment can be helpful toward ascertaining whether the overall treatment was implemented as intended, and the individual steps or items can be useful toward determining which steps were most problematic. For example, it may be that certain steps were more difficult to follow, were perhaps superfluous, simply forgotten, or the step(s) were deemed not useful or unacceptable. A follow-up interview can be conducted to assess potential reasons for failure to adhere to the intervention protocol. This intervention integrity rating scale format can be used by anyone involved in an intervention, for example, teachers, parents, consultants, or by the child in a self-monitoring intervention. The method also is useful for direct intervention such as individual or small group therapy. Finally, the method can be used as an observation tool to provide an index of interrater agreement for the level of adherence to an intervention plan.

A reproducible template for constructing an intervention integrity rating scale is found in Figure 10.1. One may choose to use the frequency rating employed on the scale, or choose to create another response format, such as level of agreement. This template provides for operationalizing the intervention components and provides a daily record of intervention integrity. It is recommended that the scale be offered with a rationale for its use. Most people understand the importance of following directions toward a desired outcome, whether it is taking medications, following a recipe, or engaging in a lesson plan. Because the use of an intervention integrity system probably will be a foreign notion, it is useful to use terminology that is readily understood by our clients. It also is important to consider that it can be difficult to remember to complete the rating form; therefore, it is useful to use daily "integrity reminders" such as phone calls, short notes, and face-to-face check-ins.

Student _____   Dates of Intervention _____

Teacher _____

It is important to clearly describe the steps of the plan and to rate how often you did each step every day. Place the number from 1 to 4 in the daily box squares that describes how often you did each step.

NEVER	SOMETIMES	MOST OF THE TIME	ALWAYS
1	2	3	4

	DAYS				
Intervention Steps	Mon	Tues	Wed	Thur	Fri
1.					
2.					
3.					
4.					
5.					
6.					
7.					
8.					
9.					
10.					

Comments about the plan and your ability to do the steps:

FIGURE 10.1. Intervention Worksheet. From Busse (2005). In R. Brown-Chidsey (Ed.), *Assessment for Intervention: A Problem-Solving Approach.* Copyright 2005 by The Guilford Press. Permission to photocopy this figure is granted to purchasers of this book for personal use only (see copyright page for details).

Problem Solution

The problem solution phase involves evaluating whether a given intervention(s) was effective and making a decision about whether the intervention should be continued. One of the major tasks in the implementing solutions and problem solution phases is progress monitoring. Indeed, as shown throughout this volume, ongoing assessment is part and parcel of the problem-solving model. This concept is in contrast to a traditional assessment-for-classification model, wherein assessment methods are used to define a problem, at which point the assessment ends. In problem-solving assessment, the methods used in problem definition are inextricably linked to the entire process, and, as such, the assessment tools we use are employed in ongoing assessment toward problem resolution. Thus, progress monitoring continues to involve best-practice assessment procedures, that is, gathering data from multiple sources, settings, and methods.

Rating scale outcomes can be used at different levels in a simple pre–post evaluation method or within an ongoing assessment procedure. If the problem behavior is part of a cluster or response class of behaviors, narrow-band or behavior-specific scales can be used to evaluate the effects of the intervention on a wider scale than assessment methods such as observations that typically focus on one or two behaviors. Broad-band scales probably are less informative and are overly time-consuming for progress monitoring; therefore, it is less likely they will be used in evaluating intervention outcomes.

When one uses rating scale scores to assess intervention outcomes, the primary task is to evaluate whether the changes are significant. One method is to compare pre- and posttest standards scores and then decide whether the magnitude of change is large enough to demonstrate significant progress. A simple method to evaluate effectiveness is whether the change is at or beyond one standard deviation. A more precise procedure is to use a method known as the Reliable Change Index (RCI). The RCI is a method that provides an effect size or indicator of change from pretest to posttest data that can be used to represent statistical as well as social or educational significance (Jacobson, Follette, & Revenstorf, 1984; Jacobson & Truax, 1991; Nunnally & Kotsche, 1983). The basic procedure involves subtracting one standard score from another and dividing by the standard error of measurement (SEM), which is the standard deviation of measurement error that is reported in a scale's technical manual. The method uses the logic of other statistics such as t-tests by examining the difference between scores in relation to a measure of variance.

There are several variations for calculating an RCI, some of which use more sophisticated variance terms, although in practice the basic procedure probably is most useful. The RCI can be used to provide an index of magnitude of change, such that an RCI of ≥ 1.6 indicates a strong, positive change, RCIs ≥ 0.6 to 1.5 may indicate moderate change, and RCIs ≥ -0.5 to 0.5 indicates no behavioral change. RCIs also may be negative, which would indicate that a behavior problem had worsened.

Another rating scale application for monitoring intervention progress is found in the method of Goal Attainment Scaling (GAS; Kiresuk, Smith, & Cardillo, 1994). GAS is a criterion-referenced approach to documenting intervention effectiveness. The basic methodology involves operationally defining successive levels of behavioral progress on a 5-point or 6-point scale, that is, -2 to $+2$, wherein -2 indicates that a behavior is much worse and $+2$ indicates significant improvement or behavioral goal was attained. For example, consider a student for whom work completion is defined as a target behavior. Baseline data indicate that the student's current rate of work completion is 40–60% (GAS rating 0). During the problem definition phase it is agreed that an increase to a rate of 61–85% would indicate progress toward the intervention goal (GAS = 1), and an increase to greater than 85% would indicate the intervention goal was attained (GAS = 2). A decrease to 30% indicates a moderately worse completion rate (GAS = -1), and a decrease to below 30% indicates the behavior has significantly worsened.

The GAS method is simple to use, readily understandable, and it can be used to gather baseline as well as intervention data as an ongoing progress monitor. Therefore, GAS also can be applied to problem identification and problem definition. GAS can be used with teachers, parents, and with children as a self-monitoring device. Depending on the need, the GAS method can be used for different evaluation intervals, ranging from hourly ratings to daily or weekly ratings. The method also can be used with item analysis results from a rating scale, wherein the item serves as the target behavior and goals are constructed around the item. The major steps in the effective use of GAS are to gather sufficient baseline data to construct the scale and to reach agreement on the definitions of goal attainment. It also is important to consider the evaluation integrity, whether the evaluation method is being consistently used, and whether it is used as intended. A reproducible GAS template is found in Figure 10.2.

RATING SCALE ASSESSMENT
FOR INTERVENTION SYSTEMS

Many commercially available rating scales include statements in the accompanying manuals that the scales are useful for designing interventions and for monitoring interventions. Few rating scale tools, however, actually provide a framework for accomplishing these goals, and still fewer provide research to support these claims. In this section, a handful of tools are

Student _____   Dates _____

Teacher _____

Behavioral Goal:

Goal Attainment Scale with Descriptions for Monitoring Change

+2 _____

    _____

+1 _____

    _____

0 _____

    _____

−1 _____

    _____

−2 _____

    _____

PROGRESS GRAPH

Rating										
+2										
+1										
0										
−1										
−2										
Dates										

Place an X in the box for your rating on each date

FIGURE 10.2. Goal Attainment Scale Worksheet. In R. Brown-Chidsey (Ed.), *Assessment for Intervention: A Problem-Solving Approach.* Copyright 2005 by The Guilford Press. Permission to photocopy this figure is granted to purchasers of this book for personal use only (see copyright page for details).

briefly described that employ a rating scale approach that may be useful in individual or group-based problem-solving applications.

Stoiber and Kratochwill (2001) developed a useful, commercially available tool that employs GAS ratings within a problem-solving-based model known as Outcomes PME: Planning, Monitoring, Evaluating. Outcomes: PME uses an evidence-based framework that facilitates the design, implementation, and monitoring of academic and behavioral interventions. The evaluation method combines GAS ratings with other assessment data and provides a method for evaluating multiple outcomes within a consensus-building framework that uses a rating scale application called convergent evidence scaling (Busse, Elliott, & Kratochwill, 1999; Elliott & Busse, 2004).

Another available set of tools is a series of separate rating scales and accompanying intervention manuals constructed by McCarney (e.g., McCarney, 1995) and published by Hawthorne Educational Services, Inc. These products include rating scales and intervention manuals for a variety of school-related concerns, including ADHD, adaptive behavior, emotional and behavioral disorders, and prereferral intervention. Overall, the rating scales may be adequate for screening purposes. Of interest here are the intervention manuals that attempt to link specific items to interventions. Although useful to some degree, the intervention manuals often contain an entire page of suggested interventions for each item and, as such, lack a certain level of specificity.

Goldstein and colleagues (e.g., Goldstein & McGinnis, 1997) created a series of social behavior small-group interventions called *Skillstreaming* that separately target preschool children, elementary school-age children, and adolescents. The *Skillstreaming* series uses a combination of self-report and teacher-report rating scales to identify specific social behaviors for intervention. Significant ratings are charted for each problem behavior and monitored during the intervention. For each item or skill, a specific intervention is provided. *Skillstreaming* comes in separate books for each age level. Each book contains reproducible assessment tools, the books are clearly written and easy to follow, and the intervention series has a research base to support its use.

Another useful rating scale tool that links assessment to intervention is the Social Skills Rating System (SSRS; Gresham & Elliott, 1990). The SSRS uses a parent, teacher, and child self-report cross-informant method to identify children's and adolescents' social skill strengths and deficits. The system includes an intervention record form that is linked to the results of individual ratings. A separate social skills intervention guide (Elliott & Gresham, 1991) provides for intervention procedures for each skill or item identified as a problem on the rating scales. The intervention guide also provides an excellent user-friendly overview of intervention planning and implementation issues.

The final rating scale system described here is somewhat unique because it targets academic behaviors rather than social or emotional concerns. The Academic Competence Evaluation Scales (ACES; DiPerna & Elliott, 2000) and the Academic Intervention Monitoring System (AIMS; Elliott, DiPerna, & Shapiro, 2001) provide an integrated assessment for intervention system that uses teacher and self-report ratings. The system combines a norm-referenced (ACES) with a criterion-referenced (AIMS) approach that can facilitate the problem-solving process. The progress monitoring system uses both Goal Attainment Scaling and a Reliable Change Index. The AIMS has additional positive features; the manual contains a useful section on evidence-based interventions to improve academic skills, and there is a Spanish version of the rating scale.

AN INTEGRATED SCENARIO

We turn now to an example of the applications of rating scales within the problem-solving model. This scenario is a case composite that was constructed for illustrative purposes; several specifics are abbreviated so that rating scales applications may be highlighted.

Scott Smith is a third grader who was referred to the school's problem-solving team (PST) by his teacher, Ms. Jones, because of her concerns about his escalating aggressive behaviors at school. Based on the referral concern, the PST assigned the school psychologist, Mr. Witmer, as the primary case manager. The problem identification phase proceeded with a file review that revealed that Scott had a history of aggressive behaviors, such as hitting and shoving other children. Because these were initially minor concerns, a brief building consultation team meeting was conducted when Scott was in second grade. The subsequent interventions included a parent conference, talking to Scott about his behaviors, sending him to the principal's office, and keeping him in the classroom during recess. Mr. Witmer recorded this information and subsequent data on an intervention summary form to keep track of data collection (see Figure 10.3).

After the file review, Mr. Witmer decided to administer the rating scales from the *Behavior Assessment System for Children* (BASC) in the interim while interviews and observations were being scheduled. Mr. Witmer chose the BASC because it employs an omnibus cross-informant system that would allow him to gather data on other potential behavioral and school-related behaviors and to gather data to validate the referral concerns. Ms. Jones completed the teacher rating scale. Mrs. Smith was provided with the parent scale, but she did not complete it.

The data from the teacher BASC showed an elevated standard score (mean = 50; standard deviation = 10) on the broad-band externalizing problems scale (62) and an average score on the internalizing problems

Student _____   Teacher _____

Referral Concern(s):

1. File Review Data
   Previous assessment results:

   Previous interventions and outcomes:

2. Current Assessment Data
   Interview data:

   Observation data:

   Test and other assessment data:

3. Problem Validation and Definition

4. Intervention Plan with Defined Goals

5. Intervention Assessment Data
   Intervention integrity:

   Progress monitoring data:

6. Problem Solution
   Problem solution data:

   Decision to modify or continue the intervention:

FIGURE 10.3. Intervention Summary Worksheet. In R. Brown-Chidsey (Ed.), *Assessment for Intervention: A Problem-Solving Approach.* Copyright 2005 by The Guilford Press. Permission to photocopy this figure is granted to purchasers of this book for personal use only (see copyright page for details).

scale (44). The school problems composite score was in the average range (42). On the adaptive skills composite, wherein lower scores indicate severity, the composite score was in the at-risk range (39). On the narrow-band scales, Ms. Jones's ratings resulted in one clinically significant score for aggression (72) and an at-risk score for social skills (38). The remaining narrow-band scores were within the average range.

Mr. Witmer conducted a conjoint problem-solving interview with Scott's mother and teacher. During the interview, Scott's behavior was described as a significant problem at school but not at home. They decided to define the problem behavior as physical aggression toward other children, including hitting, kicking, and shoving. Ms. Jones described the aggressive behavior as occurring in all school settings, with unstructured settings such as the playground being the most problematic. To gather further data for the problem definition phase, Ms. Jones and Mrs. Smith both agreed to complete a GAS rating for school and home. Mr. Witmer gathered observational data which, along with Ms. Jones's GAS ratings, validated the concerns seen at school. Mrs. Smith's GAS ratings revealed that Scott's aggressive behavior occurred in the home and community settings; however, she did not believe that Scott's aggression was a problem outside the school setting.

Mr. Witmer conducted an intervention planning interview with Ms. Jones; Mrs. Smith did not attend but agreed to continue collecting GAS data. Mr. Witmer and Ms. Jones agreed to implement an intervention that included a time-out procedure for aggressive behavior, coupled with a differential reinforcement procedure to increase Scott's appropriate social interactions. Mr. Witmer and Ms. Jones constructed a written plan for the intervention. To gather progress monitoring data, Ms. Jones agreed to continue with the GAS ratings and to complete an intervention integrity rating scale.

After two weeks of implementation, Mr. Witmer and Ms. Jones met to examine the data and to discuss whether the intervention was effective. Ms. Jones stated she had difficulty remembering and making the time to complete the intervention integrity ratings, but she stated she was adhering to the intervention. Her GAS ratings indicated some improvement, with an average daily rating of +1.2. Mrs. Smith's GAS ratings indicated little change at home, with an average rating of +0.44. An examination of the GAS ratings revealed that Scott's behavior had not changed during the first week of implementation but improved during the second week of implementation. It was agreed that the plan would stay in place for another week, at which time Mr. Witmer and Ms. Jones met to evaluate whether the improvement warranted discontinuation of the plan. Ms. Jones completed another BASC, which resulted in a lower aggression subscale score (60), and her GAS ratings for the week averaged +1.6. Mrs. Smith did not complete GAS ratings for the week, but stated that Scott's behavior had not changed. Mr. Witmer calculated a Reliable Change Index on the aggression subscale scores, which showed significant change at an RCI of +3 (72 − 60/ SEM = 4). Based on these data, Mr. Witmer and Ms. Jones decided that Scott's behavior had improved to a sufficient degree to discontinue the intervention.

Case Analysis

Before reading further, consider for a few moments the strengths and weaknesses of the assessment methods depicted in the case scenario. In particular, consider the rating scale applications: Which applications were appropriately used? What would you have done to improve the assessment?

Let us first consider which rating scale applications seem appropriate. Mr Witmer: (1) used an omnibus scale to facilitate a prompt reaction to the referral and to guide the interview; (2) combined interview and observation data with a narrow-band scale to assess aggressive behaviors; (3) used a GAS rating to gather multiple method data; (4) attempted to gather intervention integrity data; and (5) used the RCI to evaluate changes from pre- to postintervention.

Let us next consider what Mr. Witmer might have done to improve the assessment. Could he have used an item analysis to validate specific concerns? Could he have used GAS ratings to gather baseline data? Would it have been useful to use a specific-behavior scale to assess social skills and link the results to an intervention aimed at increasing prosocial behaviors? Would it have helped to follow through with assessment and intervention integrity reminders? Should a follow-up assessment have been conducted to evaluate whether the outcomes were maintained?

The response to each of these questions is "Yes"; however, this scenario depicts several realities that problem-solving personnel face in school settings. We often have difficulty gathering complete data, particularly when multiple sources are involved; therefore, we have holes in our assessment. This reality is one reason for gathering data in a multivariate framework in order to enhance the reliability and validity of our assessment and to offset the compromises one must make when attempting to gather data in situ. Another reality is the significant amount of time, effort, and resources required to engage in a complete problem-solving assessment. We must, however, approach problem solving with the same systematic methodology used in traditional school-based assessment. We often set up ourselves and our clients for failure in problem solving when specificity is lacking due to incomplete assessment practices. If the data are too general, the intervention vague, and follow-through lacking, the likelihood is high that the intervention will be ineffective.

SUMMARY

Rating scale applications possess several positive features that make them useful within a comprehensive problem-solving model of assessment and intervention. Rating scales are relatively cost-effective, they can be used for individual or group-based problem solving, they can be used to validate behavior specification, and rating scale methods can be applied to evaluate intervention outcomes. In short, rating scales are useful problem-solving tools.

Take-home points

- Be knowledgeable and ethical regarding rating scale uses.
- Rating scales are summary perceptions and observations of behavior.
- Ratings from multiple sources often only moderately agree.
- Choose rating scale tools to fit the assessment needs.
- Link assessment to intervention by using multiple sources and methods.
- Use GAS and RCI as multiple outcome indicators.
- Assess intervention and evaluation integrity.
- Remember to follow through and to follow up.

REFERENCES

Achenbach, T. M. (2002). *Achenbach System of Empirically Based Assessment*. Retrieved November 5, 2003 from the ASEBA website, *www. aseba.org/index.html*.

Achenbach, T. M., McConaughy, S. H., & Howell, C. T. (1987). Child/adolescent behavioral and emotional problems: Implications of cross-informant correlations for situational specificity. *Psychological Bulletin, 101*, 213–232.

American Educational Research Association (1999). *Standards for educational and psychological testing*. Washington, DC: Author.

Busse, R. T., Elliott, S. N., & Kratochwill, T. R. (1999). Influences of verbal interactions during behavioral consultations on treatment outcomes. *Journal of School Psychology, 37*, 117–143.

Conners, C. K. (1997). *Conners Rating Scales—Revised*. Toronto: Multi-Health Systems.

DiPerna, J. C., & Elliott, S. N. (2000). *The Academic Competence Evaluation Scales*. San Antonio: Psychological Corporation.

Elliott, S. N., & Busse, R. T. (2004). Assessment and evaluation of students' behavior and intervention outcomes: The utility of rating scale methods. In R. B. Rutherford, M. M. Quinn, & S. R. Mathur (Eds.), *Handbook of research in emotional and behavioral disorders* (pp. 123–142). New York: Guilford Press.

Elliott, S. N., Busse, R. T., & Gresham, F. M. (1993). Behavior rating scales: Issues of use and development. *School Psychology Review, 22*, 313–321.

Elliott, S. N., DiPerna, J. C., & Shapiro, E. S. (2001). *Academic Intervention Monitoring System*. San Antonio: Psychological Corporation.

Elliott, S. N., & Gresham, F. M. (1991). *Social skills intervention guide: Practical strategies for social skills training.* Circle Pines, MN: American Guidance Service.

Goldstein, A. P., & McGinnis, E. (1997). *Skillstreaming the adolescent.* Champaign, IL: Research Press.

Gresham, F. M. (1989). Assessment of intervention integrity in school consultation and prereferral interventions. *School Psychology Review, 18,* 37–50.

Gresham, F. M., & Elliott, S. N. (1990). *Social Skills Rating System.* Circle Pines, MN: American Guidance Service.

Jacobson, N. S., Follette, W. C., & Revenstorf, D. (1984). Psychotherapy outcome research: Methods for reporting variability and evaluating clinical significance. *Behavior Therapy, 15,* 336–352.

Jacobson, N. S., & Truax, P. (1991). Clinical significance: A statistical approach to defining meaningful change in psychotherapy research. *Journal of Consulting and Clinical Psychology, 59,* 12–19.

Kiresuk, T. J., Smith, A., & Cardillo, J. E. (Eds.). *Goal attainment scaling: Application, theory, and measurement.* Hillsdale, NJ: Erlbaum.

Kratochwill, T. R., & Stoiber, K. C. (2000). Empirically supported interventions and school psychology: Conceptual and practice issues: Part II. *School Psychology Quarterly, 15,* 233–253.

McCarney, S. B. (1995). *Attention Deficit Disorders Evaluation Scale—School Version.* Columbus, OH: Hawthorne.

Merrell, K. W. (2000). Informant report: Rating scale measures. In E. S. Shapiro & T. R. Kratochwill (Eds.), *Conducting school-based assessments of child and adolescent behavior* (pp. 203–234). New York: Guilford Press.

Messick, S. (1995). Validity of psychological assessment. *American Psychologist, 50,* 741–749.

Nunnally, J., & Kotsche, W. (1983). Studies of individual subjects: Logic and methods of analysis. *British Journal of Clinical Psychology, 22,* 83–93.

Reynolds, W. M. (1989). *Reynolds Child Depression Scale.* Odessa, FL: Psychological Assessment Resources.

Reynolds, C. R., & Kamphaus, R. W. (1992). *Behavior Assessment System for Children.* Circle Pines, MN: American Guidance Service.

Ruffalo, S. L., & Elliott, S. N. (1997). Teachers' and parents' ratings of children's social skills: A closer look at the cross-informant agreements through an item analysis protocol. *School Psychology Review, 26,* 489–501.

Stoiber, K. C., & Kratochwill, T. R. (2001). *Outcomes PME: Planning, monitoring, and evaluating.* San Antonio: Psychological Corporation.

SUGGESTED READINGS

American Educational Research Association. (1999). *Standards for educational and psychological testing.* Washington, DC: Author.

This book is essential reading for anyone who uses standardized assessments in school-based settings. The standards also are available online at *www.apa.org/science/standards.html.*

DeVellis, R. F. (1991). *Scale development: Theory and applications.* Newbury Park: CA: Sage.

This small volume is an excellent primer for those who are interested in rating scale construction.

Shapiro, E. S., & Kratochwill, T. R. (Eds.). (2000). *Behavioral assessment in schools: Theory, research, and clinical foundations* (2nd ed.). New York: Guilford Press.
Shapiro, E. S., & Kratochwill, T. R. (Eds.). (2000). *Conducting school-based assessments of child and adolescent behavior.* New York: Guilford Press.

These companion volumes combine theory and applications of school-based assessments that are useful within the problem-solving model. The chapters in each book by Merrell and by Eckert and colleagues provide excellent complementary coverage of rating scale applications.

CHAPTER 11

◆ ◆ ◆

Identifying and Validating Academic Problems in a Problem-Solving Model

◆

MARK R. SHINN

In a classic article on school-based consultation by Witt (1991) the analogy of pre-Copernican thought was used to describe typical school consultation practices. Witt contended that consultants are often thought of as the center of the consultative process, much akin to the pre-Copernican world view (i.e., that of Ptolemy) that the earth was the center of the universe. From this perspective, consultants possess an "expert" status that leads consultees to expect the solution to a problem to come *from* the consultants. Instead, Witt proposed a conception of consultation as less consultant-centered, with more emphasis on the various *interrelationships* among consultation variables.

Witt's use of the pre- and post-Copernican analogy in understanding consultation is helpful because it provides an illustration of how a particular phenomenon, whether it is the movement of planets or the consultation process, can be explained from very different perspectives. Often, not all perspectives are equally valid for a given phenomenon. When one view fails to explain the phenomenon adequately, a more satisfactory view may replace it. This change from one view to another is referred to as a paradigm shift (Kuhn & Horwich, 1993).

The identification and validation of academic problems within a problem-solving approach to special education service delivery also is a dramatic paradigm shift for some educators. I believe the use of pre- and post-Copernican analogies is helpful in understanding differences in how and why things are done differently in a problem-solving model. Current special identification policies and practices for students with academic problems typically are based almost exclusively on a disability model, where it is presumed that there is something *within the student* that is causing learning problems (Tilly, Reschly, & Grimes, 1999; Ysseldyke & Marston, 1999). For most students with severe achievement problems, this within-the-student problem is called a learning disability (LD). At the heart of the diagnostic assessment is the ability–achievement discrepancy. One or more ability test(s) and achievement test(s) are given, and, should a "severe" discrepancy be found, special education services eligibility is determined.

I liken this process to the pre-Copernican view of the universe, where the earth (i.e., the within-child disability) is the center of the planetary system, and all things, including how we provide remedial services, revolve around it. In contrast, the paradigm shift to a problem-solving model is similar to the shift the Copernican view required when the dominance of the earth (e.g., disability) in its explanatory power shifted to a different focus where the sun became central to the explanation of planetary motion. To play out this analogy, I will propose that the *general education achievement expectations within a particular context* (e.g., the school or school district) serve as the sun in explaining how students are identified and defined as having academic problems. Just as the Copernican view allowed for a more parsimonious explanation of the movement of the planets, I will suggest that problem-solving academic identification and validation practices are also more parsimonious than the disability-driven model and, as importantly, that the practices are more time-efficient, fair, and equitable for improving outcomes for *all students*.

PTOLEMY'S PRE-COPERNICAN SYSTEM

When reading this section on the background of Ptolemy's astronomical system, I encourage the reader to substitute the concept of "disability," especially in the context of a learning disability described in federal legislation and operationalized differentially in 47 of our 50 states (Reschly, Hosp, & Schmied, 2003). In approximately 150 A.D., after years of observing the movement of stars, the known planets, the moon, and the sun, the Greek astronomer Ptolemy formalized the astronomical proposition that the earth was the center of the universe. Ptolemy developed not a single "system" but a number of systems, one for each major celestial body (e.g., planet). Although the systems were not identical, they had a number of similarities. According to Ptolemy's systems, the major celestial bodies rotated around the earth. The planets were posited to move at a constant rate of speed around the earth, and mathematical predictions were made about where any given planet would be in relationship to the earth at a given time. An array of "powerful mathematical techniques" (Crowe, 1990, p. 32) were developed to account for these motions, with formulae and diagrams disseminated in more than 13 books that were estimated to take months to read. To reduce the complexity of the mathematics underlying planetary motions, Ptolemy produced his *Handy Tables*.

Although his model was frequently accurate, Ptolemy observed that sometimes the planets weren't where they were predicted to be in the sky. In fact, sometimes a planet not only was not where it was predicted to be but also appeared to be moving backwards. The model was compromised further when the size of the moon became difficult to explain based on his predictions. The moon often was smaller or larger than his formulae would predict. To deal with these difficulties, Ptolemy constructed an explanation of the movement of planets that was very complex. To account for differences in the size of the moon, he simply selected a formula that explained its size after the fact.

For nearly 1,300 years, this paradigm dominated the science of astronomy. To explain the ever expanding knowledge base and keep the paradigm consistent, however, more complicated and arbitrary details were added. As a result, the system became less and less satisfying. Contemporary perspectives on Ptolemy acknowledge his contribution to understanding and explaining astronomical phenomena in his day. However, some summations are relevant to consider. Among them are the following:

> The scheme became a victim of its own success. . . . For as long as it served its purpose, it implied a special status for the Earth—i.e., that it is permanently at the center of the Universe. What had begun as a descriptive convenience thus became a matter of singular significance. (*Encyclopedia Britannica*, 1982)

> The aim of Ptolemy's geometrical choices was the accurate description of the complicated motions in the sky. In this, he succeeded magnificently by *great cleverness*. What he did *not* seek was a unified picture of these motions. (Friedlander, 1985)

Ptolemy himself commented on the failure of a unified paradigm to explain the existing observed phenomena, stating that "I do not profess to be able thus to account for all the motions at the same time, but I shall show that each by itself is well explained by its proper hypothesis" (Friedlander, 1985).

Ultimately, 1,300 years later, Ptolemy's paradigm was rejected in favor of an alternative view. Critics (e.g., Hartmann, 1985) argued that part of the dissatisfaction with the pre-Copernican paradigm was *aesthetic*. The system(s) had become increasingly unwieldy and complicated. The dissatisfaction also was *intellectual*. Astronomers were displeased by the inaccuracies and inconsistencies in predictions. Finally, *obvious errors* had accumulated.

PRE-COPERNICAN IDENTIFICATION OF ACADEMIC PROBLEMS

Since its institutionalization as the mechanism for identifying and serving students with severe achievement needs as part of federal legislation in 1975, the within-child disability model has been criticized for its aesthetic and intellectual problems, as well as concerns about obvious errors. Most of these identification concerns have focused on the identification of students with severe academic problems within the category of learning disabilities, the largest single disability category in terms of numbers of students identified as eligible for special education services. This chapter cannot synthesize all of these concerns, but I will try to present some of the more obvious examples. For more detail on the insufficiency of the within-the-child disability-driven view with respect to learning disabilities, I recommend the reader review the reports, book chapters, and books in Table 11.1.

Aesthetic Concerns

That the current system of identifying students with academic problem is unwieldy and complicated is without question. Since inception, states have been entitled to specify a diagnostic criterion for each of the 13 federal disability categories because of a lack of national consensus. Although federal definitions provide states general guidance, the operationalization of these guidelines varies considerably. For example, in learning disabilities, the primary diagnostic components are the severe discrepancy between ability and achievement and attention to other potential causes of unexpectedly low achievement such as English language learning or attendance. However, "a consensus as to the best method to determine the discrepancy and criteria for what constituted 'severe' has never been achieved" (Reschly, Hosp, & Schmied, 2003, p. 5). Criteria vary from state to state and, significantly, across districts within states. Currently, 19 states specify the necessity of a severe ability–achievement discrepancy but make no attempt to define severity. As a result, local education agencies (LEAs) and schools develop their own criteria. In my own state of Illinois, I have observed at least five

TABLE 11.1. A Summary of Recommended Articles and Documents on Within-the-Child Disability-Driven Identification Practices with Students with Severe Achievement Needs

Publication	Comment
President's Commission on Special Education Excellence (2002)	Summary recommendations for improving service delivery, including assessment.
Learning Disabilities Roundtable (2002)	Summary report and recommendations from a number of major groups and constituencies regarding LD.
Lyon, Fletcher, Shaywitz, Shaywitz, Torgesen, Wood, et al. (2001)	A synthesis of the empirical database regarding LD identification, including the failures of the ability–achievement discrepancy model and recommendations for the future.
Stanovich (2000)	Stanovich's book that reviews his career's writing regarding reading, students with reading difficulties, and what is known about the role of ability in identifying LD.
Reschly, Hosp, and Schmied (2003)	A review of the history of LD identification practices from the perspective of federal and state definitions.
Shinn, Good, and Parker (1999)	A critique of identification of academic problems and solutions from a problem-solving perspective.

different methods and criteria for operationalizing this discrepancy, from simple discrepancies to regression formula discrepancies, ranging from 12 points to 22 points. Some states use very complicated mathematical formulae (e.g., estimated true scores, or 1.5 standard deviations of the *difference score*, which is not the same as a 1.5 standard deviation difference) that require the use of tables for each pair of instruments used. An illustration of the fundamental problems in the severe ability–achievement discrepancy approach is shown in Figure 11.1, adapted from Shinn, Good, and Parker (1999).

This figure represents the modeled distribution of scores between an ability and achievement test that correlates .67 and the consequences of identification using a 19-point discrepancy. Reading scores below 80 would be scores of very low readers. Students in Area A may be served in special education through the category of mental retardation. Students below the regression line have severe ability–achievement discrepancies, but it should be noted that *only some of them* (Area B) have severe reading problems. Additionally, a large number of students with severe reading problems (Area C) would *not* have a severe ability–achievement discrepancy and may not be eligible for special education. This situation creates a dilemma for educators.

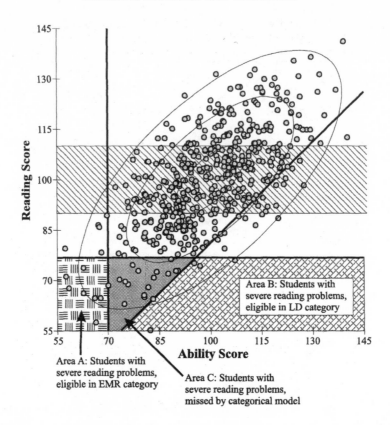

FIGURE 11.1. Joint frequency distribution of ability and achievement scores. From Shinn, Good, and Parker (1999). Copyright 1999 by Sopris West. Reprinted by permission.

Intellectual Dissatisfaction

Professional organizations such as the National Association of School Psychologists (NASP, 1994, 2003), National Association of State Directors of Special Education (NASDSE, 1994), National Association of Directors of Special Education (NASDE, 2002), and various national task forces (e.g., President's Commission on Special Education Excellence, 2002; U.S. Department of Education, 1994) have expressed intellectual dissatisfaction with the disability-centered identification model. This dissatisfaction is long-standing. For example, almost 20 years ago Reschly, Genshaft, and Binder (1987) surveyed NASP practitioners (*n* = 600), leadership staff (*n* = 139), and faculty members (*n* = 166) and reported that nearly two-thirds of practitioners agreed that students are classified as learning disabled so that services can be provided, *even though they are not really handicapped* (my emphasis). Nearly 90% of the NASP leadership expressed agreement with that statement. A similar proportion of practitioners (64%) agreed with the statement that too many students are classified as LD and placed in special education. Around 80% of the NASP leadership and school psychology faculty also agreed. More than 70% of practitioners and faculty and 90% of NASP leaders agreed that better regular classroom instruction would prevent many students from being classified as LD. Most recently, in response to proposed legislation, NASP (2003, p. 2) expressed intellectual dissatisfaction with current procedures, recommending that legal reforms:

1. Maintain current definition of LD in law (see Individuals with Disabilities Education Act of 1997), but change eligibility criteria in regulations.
2. Eliminate use of the scientifically unsupported ability–achievement discrepancy requirement.

Intellectual dissatisfaction also is shared by parents. In a recent survey of parents by the National Center for Learning Disabilities (2002), 82% of parents reported *total support* for replacing the wait-to-fail LD identification model. More than 85% of surveyed teachers also expressed "total support" for a change in identification practices.

Obvious Errors

Over the years, at least three interrelated errors concerning LD identification practices have revealed (1) that disability is not solely a within-student phenomenon but also is attributable to *where* the student lives; (2) students with severe achievement *needs must fail for considerable periods of time* (i.e., years) to become eligible (the "wait to fail" model); and (3) students *with severe achievement problems may be less likely to receive services* than students with less severe achievement needs. I will discuss the first of these obvious errors in more detail. The accumulated evidence about the obvious errors in (2) and (3) above, are discussed in more detail in the references cited in Table 11.1 and are illustrated, in part, in Area C of Figure 11.1.

The errors attributable to the within-the-child model, regardless of the school or community context, are long-standing in the professional literature and are acknowledged by practitioners as they try to understand why a student who has not been considered disabled for years in one school district is referred for special education within weeks of transfer to another school district. Practitioners also report the converse: students who have received special education in one district may be considered as not eligible for special education when they move.

Within the professional literature, Singer, Palfrey, Butler, and Walker (1989) examined the case records of individual students in five large school districts across the country. They looked at test results and records to determine whether a student labeled as disabled in District A would be identified similarly using the criteria of District B. They concluded that school districts

> differed in the percentage of students they identified as handicapped, the frequency with which they used various labels, the criteria used to define groups, and the functional levels of students given the labels. Consistency was greatest for those labeled hearing impaired and, to a lesser extent, physically/multiply handicapped and weakest for those labeled mentally retarded and emotionally disturbed; results for those labeled speech impaired and learning disabled fell between these two extremes. (p. 278)

Given the reported differences among states in LD criteria, one might expect that Singer et al. might observe significant disagreements in LD classification. Their observed rates of classification agreement between any two of the five districts ranged from 50 to 70.6%, with a total reported consistency of 64%. However, classification of students as mentally retarded (MR), a diagnostic category typically regarded as less controversial than LD, was *more inconsistent*. Agreement between pairs of districts' MR classifications ranged from 36.1 to 61.2%, with a reported total consistency of 54.1%.

More recently, Peterson and Shinn (2002) compared ability and achievement testing results of 48 grade 4 students labeled LD in high- and low-achieving communities in Minnesota, a state with an explicitly defined ability–achievement discrepancy criterion of 1.75 standard deviations using a regression approach. Only 56% and 67% of students with LD in the high- and low-achieving communities respectively met the state's ability–achievement criterion.

OTHER EXPLANATIONS
FOR IDENTIFICATION PRACTICES?

As long as there have been special education identification practices for students with severe academic needs based on use of a within-the-student ability–achievement discrepancy model, there has been a counterargument that the defining feature of these students is severe low achievement alone. Over 20 years ago, Ysseldyke and Algozzine (1983) argued that LD is best explained by a severe achievement discrepancy, suggesting that data indicated that students labeled LD were an identifiable subset of students performing poorly in school. The problem is *not* that the student is, for example, reading as well as an ability score would predict. Instead, in this view, students are determined eligible for special education services when their reading skills are significantly lower than other students' reading scores. I would label this alternative explanation as an *absolute achievement discrepancy* (AAD) model. An illustration of the AAD model is shown in Figure 11.2.

This explanation is *aesthetically more appealing.* Instead of making decisions based on a bivariate distribution of ability and achievement scores, which by its nature uses difference scores that may not be reliable or unusual (see Shinn et al., 1999, for more detail), the achievement alone approach is based on a univariate distribution of achievement. The severe discrepancy is operationalized as a discrepancy between average national achievement (e.g., 50th percentile) and actual student achievement on commercially available norm-referenced achievement tests. These "between-persons discrepancies" are more reliable and the degree of "unusual" (i.e., the percentage of students who would fall below a specific standard) can be debated, based on educational need and social values. Additionally, to many educators, this conception is more *intellectually satisfying.* One can interpret the results of the Reschly et al. (1987) survey of school psychologists as evidence of practitioners' *satisfaction* with an achievement-only

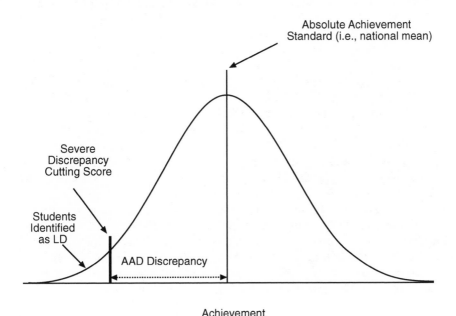

FIGURE 11.2. The absolute achievement discrepancy (AAD) model. From Peterson and Shinn (2002). Copyright 2002 by the National Association of School Psychologists. Reprinted by permission.

process, as nearly two-thirds of practitioners agreed that students are classified as learning disabled so that services can be provided, *even though the students are not really handicapped.*

The question arises, then, of whether the AAD model adequately explains school decision-making practices and whether "obvious errors" have accumulated. One can interpret a number of studies from different disciplines to provide empirical support for the AAD model. Shaywitz, Escobar, Shaywitz, Fletcher, and Makuch (1992) presented evidence that dyslexia represented the lowest end of the normal distribution of reading skills, and stated, "Dyslexia occurs along a continuum that blends imperceptibly with normal reading ability" (p. 148). A number of other studies conclude that identified students with LD are the *lowest*-achieving students (Gottlieb, Atter, Gottlieb, & Wishner, 1994; Gresham, MacMillan, & Bocian, 1996; Reynolds & Heistad, 1997; Shinn, Ysseldyke, Deno, & Tindal, 1986) compared to typically achieving students and low achievers. For example, Shinn, Tindal, Spira, and Marston (1987) compared the reading performance of three groups of students in a large urban school district: (1) students identified as LD in the area of reading, (2) low-achieving students receiving Title I, and (3) students receiving general education reading instruction only. On average, students with LD across grades 1–6 performed at the 3rd percentile relative to the reading achievement of general education students and significantly lower than Title I students who performed at about the 20th percentile. More than three out of every four students identified as LD performed below the 5th percentile of general education students.

A recent meta-analysis of 79 studies comparing LD and low-achieving students (Fuchs, Fuchs, Mathes, Lipsey, & Eaton, 2000; Fuchs, Fuchs, Mathes, Lipsey, & Roberts, 2001) lends strong empirical support to the AAD model. The largest and most consistent difference between school-identified LD students and low-achievinsg students was extreme low achievement with an effect size of .61. Students placed in special education programs for learning disabilities performed more than one-half standard deviation *lower* in achievement than their low-achieving counterparts.

The absolute achievement discrepancy model is aesthetically appealing, intellectually satisfying, and a number of studies provide consistent evidence in being able to explain school decision-making practices and reducing or eliminating two of the three obvious errors in the ability–achievement discrepancy model: (1) students *with severe achievement needs must fail for considerable periods of time* (i.e., years) to become eligible, the "wait-to-fail" model; and (2) students *with severe achievement problems may be less likely to receive services.* With respect to the former, the AAD model avoids the technical problems of the ability–achievement models and allows for reliable early identification of students with severe achievement needs (Fletcher, Coulter, Reschly, & Vaughn, in press; Simmons et al.,

2002). With respect to the latter, because the emphasis is on serving students with severe achievement problems and students are identified based on this same dimension, there would presumably be more equity in service delivery.

Despite the positive features of this model, it still fails to explain the effects of context and the consequences of students' disability status as a function of changing schools or school districts. Presumably, if the achievement-only discrepancy model were a satisfactory explanation for school decision-making practices, one would predict that there would be a relationship between the severity of achievement problems in communities and states and the number of students identified as eligible for special education. This relationship has not been established. In examining the achievement discrepancy data from the Peterson and Shinn (2002) article, one would expect that the students identified as eligible for special education from high- and low-achieving districts would achieve similarly, very low compared to the national achievement standard. This hypothesis was disconfirmed in the Peterson and Shinn (2002) study. When a severe achievement discrepancy was operationalized as 1.76 standard deviations below the national mean in reading, 81% of students from the low-achieving context met this criterion. However, only 22% of students from the high-achieving school districts met this same standard. Students placed in special education learning disabilities programs in the high-achieving school district read more like typically achieving students in the low-achieving district than they did students with LD in the low-achieving district. High-achieving students with LD performed more than 1 standard deviation higher on the Woodcock–Johnson Broad Reading Cluster than their LD counterparts in the low-achieving district.

A MORE PARSIMONIOUS EXPLANATION FOR IDENTIFICATION PRACTICES?

It should be noted that *both* the ability–achievement discrepancy and AAD explanations for special education identification of academic problems put the source of the problem solely within the student. The former, much like the pre-Copernican view of astronomy, provides a partial but grossly inadequate explanation for school-based identification practices. The latter appears to be a better explanation but still cannot adequately account for a number of common phenomena, especially the role of the community achievement context. In contrast to these two explanations, which Peterson and Shinn (2002) define as *absolute discrepancies*, they offer the concept of a *relative achievement discrepancy*. In this theory, schools identify students whose achievement is discrepant from the achievement expectations in a particular context (e.g., school, school district).

This explanation has the same positive attributes of the absolute achievement discrepancy theory (i.e., aesthetic appeal, intellectual satisfaction, and error reduction) and seems to provide a solution to the achievement context dilemma. Additionally, it *explains* the similarities in school-based LD classification outcomes for students with different levels of achievement when they are in high- and low-achieving contexts. In the Peterson and Shinn (2002) study, where both the ability–achievement and AAD models failed to provide high rates of classification of students as LD, when the criterion for a severe achievement discrepancy was 1.75 standard deviations from students from the same school, 85–95% of students from both communities met this standard.

PUTTING THE RELATIVE ACHIEVEMENT DISCREPANCY INTO PLACE: A PROBLEM-SOLVING PERSPECTIVE

In a problem-solving approach to identification of students with severe achievement problems, the relative achievement discrepancy (RAD) is a cornerstone of practice—or, using the astronomy metaphor, the center of the system. The *situation*, or context, is a prominent part of the definition of a problem. A problem is defined as a *discrepancy between what is expected and what is occurring in a given situation* (Deno, 1989). What *occurs* is the achievement level of the student for whom there are concerns. What is *expected* is the level of typical achievement of other students. The *situation* is the classroom, school, or school district context.

This *ecological perspective* requires that assessment for identification be multifaceted and not just focused solely on the student. Accurate assessment of students' academic performance is required, but also the expectations (i.e., the levels of performance of typical students) must be assessed. To measure the discrepancy, some level of local achievement norm is required (see Figure 11.3). To assess the situation, the level of concern (i.e., classroom, school, school district) must be identified, and information about the quality and implementation of curriculum and instruction must be obtained. The scope of assessing curriculum and instruction is beyond the scope of this chapter, and I will limit myself to discussing practices and issues regarding the assessment of students with concerns and expectations. For more information regarding assessment of instruction and curriculum, see Shapiro (2004).

Within the problem-solving perspective, although RAD provides a parsimonious explanation for school-based identification practices, some educators express concern about relying on the local situation or local norms to define an academic problem (Shinn & Bamonto, 1998). The concerns are stated like this: What happens to a low-performing student in a low-

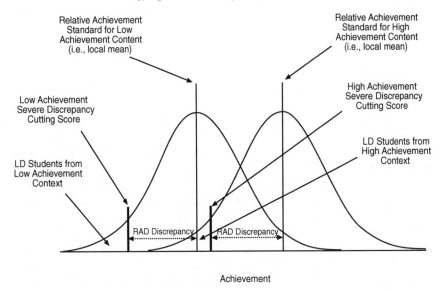

FIGURE 11.3. The relative achievement discrepancy (RAD) model. From Peterson and Shinn (2002). Copyright 2002 by the National Association of School Psychologists. Reprinted by permission.

performing school? My answer historically has been to point to our continued inability to separate individual student problems in terms of what Shapiro (2000) calls "small problems" from systems problems or "big problems." If *all the students* in a school have severe academic performance discrepancies, be they school district, state, or national achievement standards, the problems are not within the individual student but within the system and thus can only be addressed at that level.

Identifying Effective Interventions Is Central

Defining the problem situationally and obtaining data about the RAD is not the sole component in problem-solving identification practices, however. Four additional interrelated principles guide problem-solving assessment practices. First, the goal of problem-solving assessment is to *identify and validate effective instructional programs* that increase student achievement in the least restrictive environment. The goal is *not* just the identification of students. In other words, the identification of students is a means to identify effective interventions. The failure to do the latter renders the former meaningless. Thus, *successful intervention* is at the forefront of assessment and decision making.

Problem Solving Starts with Prevention

Second, prevention of academic problems is fundamental to a problem-solving model. Without this attention, problem solving, too, becomes a wait-to-fail model. In recent years, schools have become cognizant of the need for a multitiered intervention and prevention model such as the one shown in Figure 11.4. This figure, from Walker and Shinn (2002), shows the three-tier prevention model with an illustration as it applies to students with challenging social behavior. The first level of problem-solving, primary prevention, is designed to bring science-based validated interventions to *all* students as part of universal interventions. If these interventions are effective (e.g., a science-based reading program), then the needs of 80–90% of students can be met. However, even with effective universal interventions, some students will need more intensive or individualized programs to be successful (Deno, 1989). Secondary prevention, then, provides *selected interventions* (e.g., Title I reading programs) to meet the needs of at-risk students. However, even with effective secondary prevention programs, a small proportion of students will need more intensive, and likely more expensive, tertiary prevention programs. These *targeted interventions*, typically delivered through special education, have traditionally been the focus

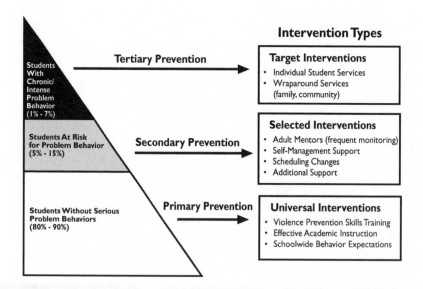

FIGURE 11.4. An illustration of the three-tiered intervention model. From Walker and Shinn (2002). Copyright 2002 by the National Association of School Psychologists. Reprinted by permission.

of our assessment process once concerns about student achievement are raised. A problem-solving model for students with achievement concerns, however, is based on building effective three-tiered intervention and assessment systems in proactive and linked ways. It is not just about finding new ways to identify students eligible for services at the tertiary prevention level.

The Importance of Educational Need and Benefit

The third fundamental principle of identification within a Problem-Solving model is that the entitlement decision (i.e., that the student needs special education) is based on the interaction of *severe educational need* and *educational benefit*. It is not the disability status, a within-person characteristic, that "confers" special education eligibility, but instead it is that there is a severe educational need that requires intensive or specialized intervention services beyond what can be provided in general education (i.e., supplemental aids and services) in order for the student to benefit from the instruction. The concepts of educational need and benefit have been implicit and explicit in both federal statutory law (e.g., IDEA '97) and case law (e.g., *Board of Education v. Rowley*, 1982) for a number of years. However, the concepts remain overshadowed by the pre-Copernican emphasis on finding the disability and determining eligibility.

In a post-Copernican view, educational need and benefit is at the forefront of decision making for *all students*. Accordingly, both these variables should be assessed explicitly, early, and continuously throughout a student's education. *Any* student with educational needs, regardless of severity, should be identified for instructional program adaptations as soon as possible. Only *some* of these students may require such extensive adaptations that they need special education in order to benefit (Deno, 1989). *Any* student who is not benefiting also should have their instructional program adapted when they are not progressing. Only *some* of these students may have such severe educational needs that they need special education in order to benefit (Deno, 1989).

The combination of severe educational need and insufficient benefit (e.g., rate of improvement) results in what currently is called a *dual discrepancy* (Fuchs, Fuchs, & Speece, 2002; Pericola-Case, Speece, & Eddy Molloy, 2003). For more than a decade, Iowa has implemented this dual-discrepancy approach in its statewide needs-based problem-solving model. As shown in Figure 11.5, adapted from the Heartland Area Education Agency (Tilly et al., 1999; Ikeda, Tilly, Stumme, Volmer, & Allison, 1996; Ikeda, Grimes, Tilly, Alison, Kurns, Stumme, et al., 2002), this problem-solving model is two-dimensional, with "intensity of problem" (educational need) and "amount of resources needed to solve problem" (benefit)

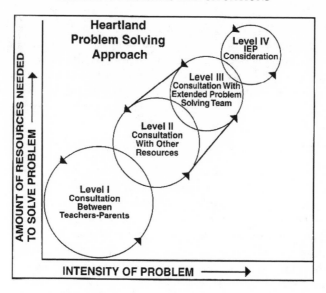

FIGURE 11.5. The Iowa problem-solving model based on educational need and benefit. From Tilly, Reschly, and Grimes (1999). Copyright 1999 by Sopris West. Reprinted by permission.

as the major axes. Problem-solving efforts are undertaken with *all* students, only some of whom require special education, in which the severity of the problem and the amount of resources needed to solve it are both high.

Assessment Systems That Fit Problem Solving

The fourth fundamental principle of identification within a problem-solving model is that *assessment data must fit the other design principles of problem solving.* That is, the assessment data must be able to (1) reflect the situation via relative achievement discrepancy (i.e., provide a "local norm"); (2) have an intervention focus (i.e., help identify effective interventions); (3) support a three-tiered prevention model; and (4) allow educators to make statements about severe educational need and benefit. The assessment system(s) also must be consistent across the three tiers of the prevention model so that a continuous database can be collected across levels of interventions and over time.

Implementation of a problem-solving model has been successful, in part, because curriculum-based measurement (CBM), a set of standardized and validated short-duration tests (Deno, 1985, 1986; Fuchs & Deno, 1991) in the basic skills of reading, mathematics computation, spelling, and written expression (Deno, 1985, 1986, 1989, 2003; Shinn, 1989, 1998), meets these assessment system needs. CBM consists of the following core testing strategies:

1. In reading, students read aloud from reading passages for 1 minute. The number of words read correctly constitutes the basic decision-making metric. Maze, a multiple choice cloze reading technique, also has been validated as a CBM testing strategy. The number of correct word choices per 3 minutes is the primary metric.
2. In spelling, students write words that are dictated at specified intervals (either 5, 7, or 10 seconds) for 2 minutes. The number of correct letter sequences and words spelled correctly are counted.
3. In written expression, students write a story for 3 minutes after being given a story starter (e.g., "Pretend you are playing on the playground and a spaceship lands. A little green person comes out and calls your name and . . ."). The number of words written, spelled correctly, and/or correct word sequences is counted.
4. In mathematics computation, students write answers to computational problems via 2- to 5-minute probes. The number of correctly written digits is counted.

CBM was developed more than 25 years ago in a program of research to provide special education teachers with a way to write objective individualized educational program (IEP) goals and continuously monitor progress in a formative evaluation model. See Deno (Chapter 2, this volume, and Deno, 2003) for more detail. To be useful in formative evaluation, CBM had to meet technical adequacy standards (i.e., be reliable, valid, and sensitive to improvement during short-term interventions) and be time-efficient so that special education teachers could monitor progress frequently (i.e., 1–2 times per week) without loss of large amounts of valuable instructional time. When students' rates of progress meet or exceed their expected rate of progress, with confidence educators can conclude that the students are benefiting and continue with the intervention. When students are not making their expected rates of progress, with confidence educators can conclude that students are not benefiting and change the intervention. A sample individual student CBM progress graph is shown in Figure 11.6.

Before the intervention began, the student showed approximately 50 words read correctly (WRC) per minute. A goal was written that the student would be reading 120 WRC by the end of the year if the intervention were effective. Results of the first intervention showed no significant improvement, and the intervention was changed so that the student might benefit. Program Change 1 produced a greater improvement rate, but the student's IEP team determined that this outcome was still less than the desired outcome, and Program Change 2 was implemented. The benefit of this change would be evaluated by using the same CBM method that was used in evaluating the previous interventions.

It became apparent early on in the program of CBM research that because such methods were time-efficient, easy to learn, and reasonably

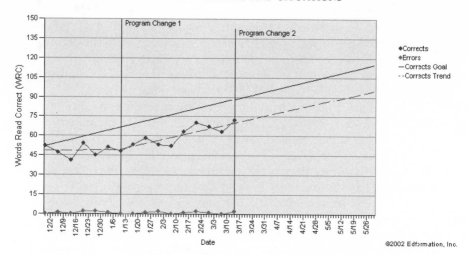

FIGURE 11.6. Frequent progress monitoring in reading CBM, showing actual rates of progress compared to expected rates of progress. From Edformation (2002). Copyright 2002 by Edformation, Inc. Reprinted by permission.

inexpensive, their use need not be limited to students with already identified severe academic problems and with the need for progress monitoring of IEP goals. CBM could be used in general education to develop local norms (Shinn, 1988), contribute to identification of students at risk or with severe achievement needs (Shinn & Marston, 1985), and aid in monitoring their progress (Marston & Magnusson, 1985).

In a problem-solving model, CBM is used as part of a tier 1 primary prevention program in benchmark assessment (see M. R. Shinn, M. M. Shinn, Hamilton, & Clarke, 2002, for more detail). All students are tested three times per year, and results are provided to general education teachers and teams for (1) universal screening to identify students' educational needs, (2) instructional planning, and (3) progress monitoring to determine benefit. A sample benchmark student graph is shown in Figure 11.7.

This box-and-whisker chart shows how the fourth-grade student compared to other fourth graders in reading at the fall benchmark assessment. Scores in the box correspond to the average range (25th–75th percentile). Scores in the bottom whisker (10th–25th percentile) are scores of below-average readers and suggest an "at-risk" status. Scores in the upper whisker are those of above-average readers (75th–90th percentile). This student's score of 60 WRC is significantly below the end of the lower whisker (10th-percentile) and suggests a student with a potentially severe educational need. If problem solving has not already taken place with this student, the benchmark results suggest a need to do so.

Benchmark assessment data in a problem-solving approach allow teachers to make decisions about *each* student's educational needs on an ongoing basis, beginning in kindergarten. Some students, like the one shown in Figure 11.7, may require intensive problem-solving interventions with a significant commitment of resources for the student to benefit. In contrast, the student in Figure 11.8 may not have severe educational needs. However, the future need for intensive supports would not be ruled out and would be evaluated objectively at the winter benchmark.

A theme in the post-Copernican model is the presence of both educational need *and* benefit as a cornerstone of decision making. A well-implemented problem-solving model is routinely providing information on both dimensions for *all* students. A second benchmark score allows educators to determine whether any student, regardless of need, is benefiting. For example, the student in Figure 11.9, is a student without severe educational need whose winter benchmark scores show benefit from the general education reading program. The fall benchmark reading score of 70 WRC improved to 95 WRC, a rate of improvement faster than that for typically achieving students.

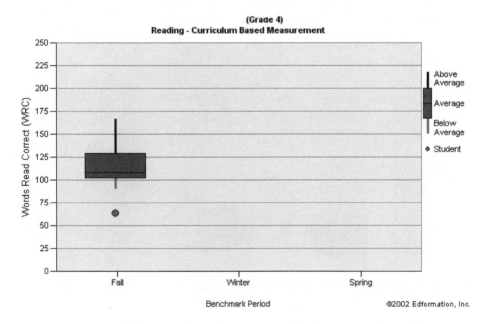

FIGURE 11.7. Fall benchmark reading CBM results showing student with severe educational need. From Edformation (2002). Copyright 2002 by Edformation, Inc. Reprinted by permission.

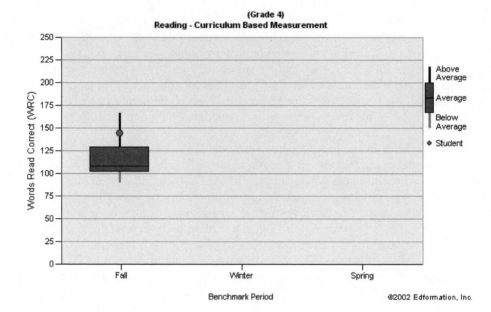

FIGURE 11.8. Grade 4 student without severe educational need compared to local peers. From Edformation (2002). Copyright 2002 by Edformation, Inc. Reprinted by permission.

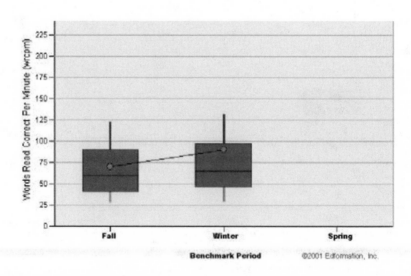

FIGURE 11.9. Grade 3 student without severe educational need who is benefiting from their educational program. From Edformation (2002). Copyright 2002 by Edformation, Inc. Reprinted by permission.

Identification of students' academic needs within a problem-solving model allows for evaluating the effectiveness of interventions that can be used *before* problems become severe. For example, the student in Figure 11.10 is an at-risk student whose teacher began problem solving with parents and team members based on the fall benchmark reading score. The intervention that was developed and implemented was effective. Winter benchmark scores show significant benefit from the reading intervention. The fall benchmark reading score of 40 WRC improved to 70 WRC, a rate of improvement faster than that for typically achieving students. Furthermore, the student's educational needs changed from being considered at risk to a student in the average range, albeit at the lower end of the distribution. This intervention would be continued and evaluated at the end-of-the year benchmark assessment, and might not require more intensive problem solving.

Finally, the benchmark assessment reading scores from a student with severe educational need who is not benefiting is shown in Figure 11.11. This student's reading CBM scores were significantly lower than general education counterparts at both the fall and winter benchmarks, *and* the rate of improvement was at a lower rate than that of other students. One would presume that the severe educational need in the fall would result in the initiation of problem solving. If the winter benchmark score were the outcome obtained as the result of level 2 problem solving, such as the Heartland Area model as shown in Figure 11.5, where intervention support

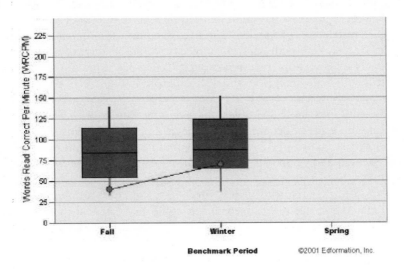

FIGURE 11.10. Grade 3 student with educational need who is benefiting from the reading intervention. From Edformation (2002). Copyright 2002 by Edformation, Inc. Reprinted by permission.

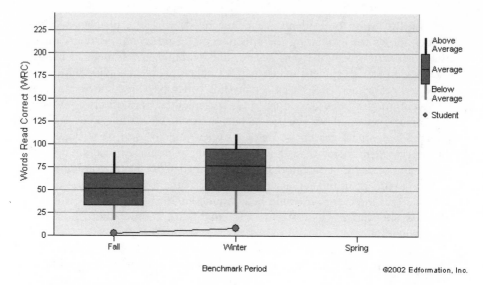

FIGURE 11.11. Grade 2 student with severe educational need who is not benefiting from the reading intervention. From Edformation (2002). Copyright 2002 by Edformation, Inc. Reprinted by permission.

is provided to the teacher by a building team, the intervention would be modified. Given the severity of the problem and the lack of benefit, it would be expected that the student may move to level 3 of problem solving, where a more intensive program that requires more resources and that may be more restrictive is provided. The need for more resource-intensive programs for a student with educational needs would be a *data-based decision* that is (1) a planned intervention using evidence-based practices; (2) implemented with high integrity; and (3) monitored frequently, preferably at least once per week.

Results of a level 3 problem-solving intervention with a third-grade student who was not benefiting from a level 2 problem-solving intervention are shown in Figure 11.12. In this case, a more intensive intervention was implemented and evaluated for about 10 weeks where progress was monitored weekly and compared to the team's expected rate of progress. These data showed that the student benefited from the intervention, and after a team meeting it was determined that it could be sustained by the general education teacher without further team support. Because level 3 intervention was effective, there was no demonstrated need for the intensive and more expensive interventions that would be required for special education eligibility determination, level 4 of problem solving. Had the results of progress monitoring of a level 3 intervention *not* shown benefits, again, the intervention might be modified and evaluated frequently by the team.

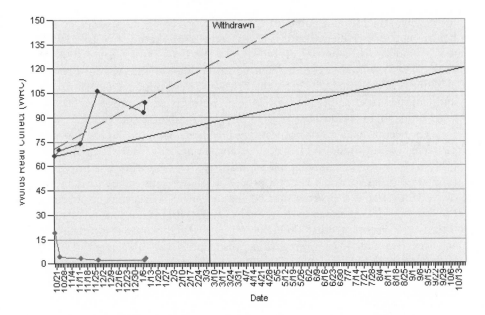

FIGURE 11.12. Frequent progress monitoring results from level 3 problem-solving intervention showing student benefit. From Edformation (2002). Copyright 2002 by Edformation, Inc. Reprinted by permission.

Alternatively, should the team believe that an intervention requiring significantly more resources and intensity was needed for the student to benefit, level 4 problem solving would be undertaken, in which special education eligibility is determined and an IEP is written.

Problem Solving and Response-to-Intervention Practices

It should be noted, then, that problem solving incorporates a *demonstrated response-to-intervention* (RTI) perspective in its decision making regarding special education identification. RTI is now offered as a legitimate method of identifying students as eligible for special education in national task recommendations (e.g., President's Commission, 2002) and legislation language in the reauthorization of IDEA. RTI is not the focus of this chapter for two reasons. First, although the incorporation of RTI language lends legal credibility and social validity to a problem-solving model, in many respects it has assumed a "life of its own" outside of the context of a problem-solving model. To me, without a change in worldview (i.e., shifting from a disability-driven perspective to a needs-based perspective), RTI has the potential to be a disconnected, procedurally driven process that diverts attention from the purpose of identifying effective interventions to identifying students as eligible for special education. We have observed this before in the "prereferral intervention" efforts of the mid- to late 1980s (e.g., Graden, Christenson, & Bonstrom, 1985; Graden, Christenson, & Casey, 1985), which too often devolved to "trying two interventions before eligibility is determined." Often, the "two interventions" were perfunctory and designed to expedite the process (e.g., notify parents, move a student's seat) rather than serious attempts to improve student achievement.

The second reason for not framing problem solving as RTI is that in a problem-solving model RTI is not a stand-alone, nor clearly demarcated, process. In a problem-solving model, *all students' education* is a response-to intervention process. It is not a procedure that begins only with a subset of students, but is a process that begins in general education by use of a three-tier model. As noted by L. S. Fuchs (2003), RTI is not new and can be traced as a recommended procedure to the 1982 National Academy of Sciences recommendations regarding disproportional placement (Heller, Holtzman, & Messick, 1982). Framing a problem-solving model as synonymous with RTI then, has the potential to shortchange the benefits to all students.

SUMMARY

In this chapter I set out to use the metaphor of pre- and post-Copernican thought to help the reader understand that implementation of a problem-solving approach to identification of academic problems was not just a different way of doing things but also a different way of thinking about academic problems. Problem solving is intended as a robust perspective whose "center" is different from prevailing special education identification practices. Rather than putting disability identification at the center of the process, the ambitious goal of problem solving is to identify effective interventions for *all students*. *Some* of these students may have severe educational needs that cannot be met without significant investment of resources beyond what can be provided by general education alone. Further, I have suggested that, regardless of the disability-centered perspective, schools currently make the judgments regarding severe educational need on the basis of the prevailing achievement context or the local achievement expectations. A problem-solving model just makes this implicit practice explicit, aligning what we say we do with what we actually do.

To conclude the metaphor, it should be noted that the shift from an earth-centered to sun-centered astronomical system took almost 1,500 years, in spite of considerable accumulated scientific evidence. The shift in focus was not without considerable controversy, where new astronomers were associated with paganism. Certainly, a shift to a problem-solving model also is controversial, and some critics have suggested that it jeopardizes special education (Fuchs, Mock, Morgan, & Young, 2003). As Crowe (1990) noted about post-Copernican thinking, the change in perspective "had profound implications that extended far beyond astronomy. . . . It raised deep and disturbing philosophical and theological issues" (p. 86). For some educators, a shift to a problem-solving perspective has required a reexamination of conceptions of disability, as well as the responsibilities of special *and* general education in meeting the needs of children. For others, however, this shift has enabled attention to be focused on the real challenges of trying to develop and implement effective interventions not for *some* students, but for *all*.

REFERENCES

Board of Education of Hendrick Hudson Central School District v. Rowley. (1982). 458, IS 176, 102 S.Ct. 3034, 73, L.Ed.2d 690, 5 Ed. Law Rep. 34, 1982.

Crowe, M. J. (1990). *Theories of the world from antiquity to the Copernican revolution.* New York: Dover.

Deno, S. L. (1985). Curriculum-based measurement: The emerging alternative. *Exceptional Children, 52,* 219–232.

Deno, S. L. (1986). Formative evaluation of individual student programs: A new rule for school psychologists. *School Psychology Review, 15,* 358–374.

Deno, S. L. (1989). Curriculum-based measurement and alternative special education services: A fundamental and direct relationship. In M. R. Shinn (Ed.), *Curriculum-based measurement: Assessing special children* (pp. 1–17). New York: Guilford Press.

Deno, S. L. (2003). Developments in curriculum-based measurement. *Journal of Special Education, 37,* 184–192.

Edformation. (2002). *Progress monitoring graph.* Retrieved August 1, 2004, from *www.edformation.com*

Encyclopedia Britannica (Vol. 18). (1982). London: Encyclopedia Britannica, Inc.

Fletcher, J. M., Coulter, W. A., Reschly, D. J., & Vaughn, S. (in press). Alternative approaches to the definition of learning disabilities: Some questions and answers. *Annals of Dyslexia.*

Friedlander, M. W. (1985). *Astronomy from Stonehenge to quasars.* Englewood Cliffs, NJ: Prentice-Hall.

Fuchs, L. S. (2003). Assessing Intervention Responsiveness: Conceptual and technical issues. *Learning Disabilities Research and Practice, 18,* 172–186.

Fuchs, L. S., & Deno, S. L. (1991). Paradigmatic distinctions between instructionally relevant measurement models. *Exceptional Children, 57*(6), 488–500.

Fuchs, D., Fuchs, L. S., Mathes, P. G., Lipsey, M. E., & Eaton, S. (2000). A meta-analysis of reading differences between underachievers with and without the learning disabilities label: A brief report. *Learning Disabilities: A Multidisciplinary Journal, 10,* 1–3.

Fuchs, D., Fuchs, L. S., Mathes, P. G., Lipsey, M. W., & Roberts, P. H. (2001, August 27–28). Is *"learning disabilities" just a fancy term for low achievement? A meta-analysis of reading differences between low achievers with and without the label. Executive Summary.* Paper presented at the Learning Disabilities Summit: Building a Foundation for the Future, Washington, DC.

Fuchs, L. S., Fuchs, D., & Speece, D. L. (2002). Treatment validity as a unifying construct for identifying learning disabilities. *Learning Disability Quarterly, 25*(1), 33–45.

Fuchs, D., Mock, D., Morgan, P. L., & Young, C. L. (2003). Responsiveness-to-intervention: Definitions, evidence, and implications for the learning disabilities construct. *Learning Disabilities Research and Practice, 18*, 157–171.

Gottlieb, J., Alter, M., Gottlieb, B. W., & Wishner, J. (1994). Special education in urban America. It's not justifiable for many. *The Journal of Special Education, 27*, 453–465.

Graden, J., Christenson, S., & Bonstrom, O. (1985). Implementing a prereferral Intervention system: Part II: The data. *Exceptional Children, 51*, 487–496.

Graden, J., Christenson, S., & Casey, A. (1985). Implementing a prereferral Intervention system: Part I: The model. *Exceptional Children, 51*, 377–387.

Gresham, F. M., MacMillan, D. L., & Bocian, K. M. (1996). Learning disabilities, low achievement, and mild mental retardation: More alike than different? *Journal of Learning Disabilities, 29*, 570–581.

Hartmann, W. K. (1985). *Astronomy, the cosmic journey.* Belmont, CA: Wadsworth.

Heller, K. A., Holtzman, W., & Messick, S. (1982). *Placing children in special education: A strategy for equity.* Washington, DC: National Academy Press.

Ikeda, M. J., Grimes, J., Tilly, W. D., III, Allison, R., Kurns, S., Stumme, J., et al. (2002). Implementing an intervention-based approach to service delivery: A case example. In M. R. Shinn, H. M. Walker, & G. Stoner (Eds.), *Interventions for academic and behavior problems: Preventive and remedial approaches* (pp. 71–88). Bethesda, MD: National Association of School Psychologists.

Ikeda, M. J., Tilly, W. D., Stumme, D., Volmer, L., & Allison, R. (1996). Agency-wide implementation of problem solving consultation: Foundations, current implementation, and future directions. *School Psychology Quarterly, 11*, 228–243.

Kuhn, T. S., & Horwich, P. (1993). *World changes: Thomas Kuhn and the nature of science.* Cambridge, MA: MIT Press.

Learning Disabilities Roundtable. (2002). *Specific learning disabilities: Finding common ground.* Washington, DC: U.S. Department of Education, Office of Special Education Programs, Office of Innovation and Development.

Lyon, G. R., Fletcher, J. M., Shaywitz, S. E., Shaywitz, B. A., Torgesen, J., Wood, F. B., et al. (2001). Rethinking learning disabilities. In C. E. Finn, A. J. Rotherham, & C. R. Hokanson (Eds.), *Rethinking special education for a new century* (pp. 259–287). Washington DC: Thomas B. Fordham Foundation.

Marston, D., & Magnusson, D. (1985). Implementing curriculum-based measurement in special and regular education settings. *Exceptional Children, 52*, 266–276.

National Association of Directors of Special Education. (2002). *NASDE Response to President's Commission on Excellence in Special Education.* Washington, DC: Author.

National Association of School Psychologists/National Association of Directors of Special Education. (1994). *Assessment and eligibility in special education: An examination of policy and practice with proposals for change.* Bethesda, MD: Author.

National Association of School Psychologists. (2003). *NASP Recommendations for IDEA reauthorization: Identification and eligibility determination for students with specific learning disabilities.* Bethesda, MD: Author.

National Center for Learning Disabilities. (2002). *Early help for struggling learners: A national survey of parents and educators.* New York: Author.

Pericola Case, L., Speece, D. L., & Eddy Molloy, D. (2003). The validity of response-to-instruction paradigm to identify reading disabilities: A longitudinal analysis of individual differences and context factors. *School Psychology Review, 32*, 557–582.

Peterson, K. M., & Shinn, M. R. (2002). Severe discrepancy models: Which best explains school identification practices for learning disabilities? *School Psychology Review, 31*, 459–476.

President's Commission on Special Education Excellence. (2002). *A new ERA: Revital-*

izing special education for all children and their families. Washington, DC: U.S. Department of Education.

Reschly, D. J., Genshaft, J., & Binder, M. S. (1987). *The 1986 NASP survey: Comparison of practitioners, NASP leadership, and university faculty on key issues*. Washington, DC: National Association of School Psychologists.

Reschly, D. J., Hosp, J. L., & Schmied, C. M. (2003). *Miles to go: State SLD requirements and authoritative recommendations*. Nashville, TN: National Research Center on Learning Disabilities.

Reynolds, M. C., & Heistad, D. (1997). 20/20 Analysis: Estimating school effectiveness in serving students at the margins. *Exceptional Children, 63,* 439–449.

Shapiro, E. S. (2000). School psychology from an instructional perspective: Solving big, not little problems. *School Psychology Review, 29,* 560–572.

Shapiro, E. S. (2004). *Academic skills problems: Direct assessment and intervention* (3rd ed.). New York: Guilford Press.

Shaywitz, S. E., Escobar, M. D., Shaywitz, B. A., Fletcher, J. M., & Makuch, R. (1992). Evidence that dyslexia may represent the lower tail of a normal distribution of reading ability. *The New England Journal of Medicine, 326,* 145–150.

Shinn, M. R. (1988). Development of curriculum-based local norms for use in special education decision making. *School Psychology Review, 17,* 61–80.

Shinn, M. R. (Ed.). (1989). *Curriculum-based measurement: Assessing special children*. New York: Guilford Press.

Shinn, M. R. (Ed.). (1998). *Advanced applications of curriculum-based measurement*. New York: Guilford Press.

Shinn, M. R., & Bamonto, S. (1998). Advanced applications of curriculum measurement: "Big ideas" and avoiding confusion. In M. R. Shinn (Ed.), *Advanced applications of curriculum-based measurement* (pp. 1–31). New York: Guilford Press.

Shinn, M. R., Good, R. H. I., & Parker, C. (1999). Non-categorical special education services with students with severe achievement deficits. In D. J. Reschly, W. D. I. Tilly, & J. P. Grimes (Eds.), *Special education in transition: Functional assessment and noncategorical programming* (pp. 81–106). Longmont, CO: Sopris West.

Shinn, M. R., & Marston, D. (1985). Differentiating mildly handicapped, low-achieving and regular education students: A curriculum-based approach. *Remedial and Special Education, 6,* 31–45.

Shinn, M. R., Shinn, M. M., Hamilton, C., & Clarke, B. (2002). Using curriculum-based measurement to promote achievement in general education classrooms. In M. R. Shinn, G. Stoner, & H. M. Walker (Eds.), *Interventions for academic and behavior problems: Preventive and remedial approaches* (pp. 113–142). Bethesda, MD: National Association of School Psychologists.

Shinn, M. R., Tindal, G., Spira, D., & Marston, D. (1987). Practice of learning disabilities as social policy. *Learning Disability Quarterly, 10*(1), 17–28.

Shinn, M. R., Ysseldyke, J., Deno, S. L., & Tindal, G. (1986). A comparison of differences between students labeled learning disabled and low achieving on measures of classroom performance. *Journal of Learning Disabilities, 19,* 545–552.

Simmons, D. C., Kame'enui, E. J., Good, R. H., III, Harn, B., Cole, C., & Braun, D. (2002). Building, implementing, and sustaining a beginning reading improvement model: Lessons learned school by school. In M. R. Shinn, H. M. Walker, & G. Stoner (Eds.), *Interventions for academic and behavior problems: Preventive and remedial approaches*. Bethesda, MD: National Association of School Psychologists.

Singer, J. D., Palfrey, J. S., Butler, J. A., & Walker, D. K. (1989). Variation in special education classification across school districts: How does where you live affect what you are labeled? *American Educational Research Journal, 26,* 261–281.

Stanovich, K. E. (2000). *Progress in understanding reading: Scientific foundations and new frontiers*. New York: Guilford Press.

Tilly, W. D., Reschly, D. J., & Grimes, J. (1999). Disability determination in Problem-Solving systems: Conceptual foundations and critical components. In D. J. Reschly, W. D. Tilly, & J. P. Grimes (Eds.), *Special education in transition: Functional assessment and noncategorical programming* (pp. 221–254). Longmont, CO: Sopris West.

U.S. Department of Education. (1994). *The national agenda for achieving better results for children and youth with disabilities*: U.S. Department of Education.

Walker, H. M., & Shinn, M. R. (2002). Structuring school-based interventions to achieve integrated primary, secondary, and tertiary prevention goals for safe and effective schools. In M. R. Shinn, H. M. Walker, & G. Stoner (Eds.), *Interventions for academic and behavior problems: Preventive and remedial approaches* (pp. 1–27). Bethesda, MD: National Association of School Psychologists.

Witt, J. C. (1991). Complaining, pre-Copernican thought, and the univariate linear mind: Questions for school-based consultation research. *School Psychology Review, 19*(3), 367–377.

Ysseldyke, J., & Algozzine, B. (1983). LD or not LD: That's not the question. *Journal of Learning Disabilities, 10*, 9–31.

Ysseldyke, J. E., & Marston, D. (1999). Origins of categorical special education systems and a rationale for changing them. In D. J. Reschly, W. D. Tilly, & J. P. Grimes (Eds.), *Special education in transition: Functional assessment and noncategorical programming* (pp. 1–14). Longmont, CO: Sopris West.

SUGGESTED READINGS

Shinn, M. R. (Ed.). (1989). *Curriculum-based measurement: Assessing special children.* New York: Guilford Press.

This volume offers a more in-depth treatment of CBM methods from the perspective of a number of authors.

Shinn, M. R. (Ed.). (1998). *Advanced applications of curriculum-based measurement.* New York: Guilford Press.

This book includes information on use of CBM with all grade levels and for students from diverse linguistic and cultural backgrounds.

CHAPTER 12

◆ ◆ ◆

The Role of Published
Norm-Referenced Tests in
Problem-Solving-Based Assessment

◆

RACHEL BROWN-CHIDSEY

Published norm-referenced tests (PNRTs) have long had a place in school-based assessment. Tests of IQ, academic achievement, visual–motor skills, and language have been used for many years in the United States as part of the process by which students are identified as needing specialized instructional supports. The history and legacy of such testing is mixed. IQ tests were originally developed in France to identify which students would benefit from instruction (Gould, 1981). Over the last century, a number of other types of tests have been developed as well (Salvia & Ysseldyke, 2003; Sattler, 2001). More recently, most U.S. states and the federal government have begun to require that students be tested on a regular basis in grades 3–8 (No Child Left Behind Act, 2003). Still, there is no guarantee that when students are tested with published instruments that their actual school performance will improve. Indeed, a number of problems with such tests have been identified (Jay, Heubert, & Hauser, 1999; Howell & Nolet, 2000; Viadero, 2003) including their inappropriateness for students with disabilities (National Center on Educational Outcomes, 2002; Shriner, 2000; Thurlow, Wiley, & Bielinski, 2003) and for those for whom English is a second language (Helms, 1997; Ortiz, 2002). This chapter will include information about published tests and suggestions for when to use them and when to rely on other assessment tools.

SOCIAL CULTURE OF TESTING PRACTICES

There appears to be a strong social validity to testing students. Since the publication of *A Nation at Risk* in 1983, the U.S. Department of Education as well as policymakers, state education agencies, and the public have placed increasing emphasis on using tests to monitor students' school progress (U.S. Department of Education, 1983). Certainly there have always been tests in schools, and some tests reveal important information about students' school progress. When used properly, certain tests can shed light on what skills and knowledge students have learned. In many instances, however, the tests chosen to learn more about a student's current abilities are not well matched to the type of decision being considered. For example, many decisions about whether a student needs special education services or should be retained are made on the basis of tests that do not reflect what the student has been taught (Berninger, 2002; Howell & Nolet, 2000). When a student is tested using an instrument that is not matched to what has actually been taught, there is a strong chance that the test results will be inaccurate (Salvia & Ysseldyke, 2003).

Despite the well-established limitations of PNRTs, these tests are used with great frequency to make important decisions about students' school futures. PNRTs are easily obtained, have clear directions, yield standardized scores, and are believed to be accurate for measuring students' skills. There is some evidence that there is greater social validity than other technical evidence to support the use of PNRTs (Elliott & Fuchs, 1997). All PNRTs have accompanying data related to their reliability and validity that the examiner is supposed to review before giving the test. In most cases, the statistical data are strong enough to justify the use of the test under certain circumstances. In other cases, however, individual students possess backgrounds different enough from the norming sample to preclude use of that test with those students (Ortiz, 2002). Although these are the standards published by the American Psychological Association (APA), National Association of School Psychologists (NASP), and National Council on Measurement in Education (NCME), anecdotal evidence reveals that practitioners are faced with difficulties when their schools own only one or two tests, have insufficient time for additional testing, or are unable to obtain culturally appropriate tests. These situations reflect the reality that many school professionals face. Nonetheless, just because a school owns a certain PNRT does not mean it should be given to all students in all circumstances. Instead, practitioners need to have a well-developed plan for determining when—and when not—to administer PNRTs.

DISCREPANCY AND "DISABILITY"

The most widely used application of PNRTs in schools is to determine whether a child has a so-called discrepancy between cognitive ability and academic achievement (Peterson & Shinn, 2002; Stage, Abbott, Jenkins, & Berninger, 2003). As discussed in detail in Chapter 11 of this volume, many school districts and state departments of education will provide special education services for a learning disability only if the student has an average or higher IQ score and below-average academic achievement. Although language was included in the 1997 and 2004 versions of the Individuals with Disabilities Education Act (IDEA, 1997; 2004) for districts to be allowed to use other methods to identify students with learning disabilities, most jurisdictions still use a discrepancy formula for this purpose. An exception is the state of Iowa, which has adopted problem-solving assessment methods on a statewide level (Reschly, Tilly, & Grimes, 1999).

As Shinn pointed out in Chapter 11, the major problem with discrepancy-based methods for determining the presence of a learning problem is that they are not very accurate. Specifically, there are three main ways that discrepancy calculation methods are likely to be flawed. First, the primary assumption that widely varying scores are atypical is inaccurate. Second, most of the time the two (or more) test batteries used for the discrepancy analysis were not conormed, so direct comparisons between the scores is inappropriate. Third, the tasks and skills included in the test batteries do not represent actual school assignments and activities, so the test scores may not represent what skills the student was actually taught and/or expected to learn. Each of these limitations will be discussed in turn.

Score Variation Is Normal

Although the basic premise behind the use of PNRTs, especially cognitive and achievement tests, is to learn whether a given student's scores vary significantly from what would be considered average for her age, it is rarely explained at individualized education plan (IEP) meetings that some score variation is normal. Indeed, it is well understood by statisticians that every time anything is measured some variation and error will be included in the score. For this reason, obtained scores are known as *estimates*. For most widely used PNRTs, there are data tables that summarize the expected variations in scores for people of different ages, sexes, and abilities. These tables are known as base-rate tables and provide examiners with information concerning whether an obtained score is meaningfully significant (Glutting, McDermott, Watkins, Kush, & Konold, 1997). Most psychoeducational reports omit any mention of the base rates, or expected frequencies, of specific score ranges. As a result, the scores reported and interpreted in many reports inaccurately estimate that a student has a clinically significant gap in aptitude and achievement scores when, often, the score spread is actually normal for students of that age. This is particularly true for younger students, for whom PNRTs are less reliable (Sattler, 2001).

A second issue related to score variation is the reporting and understanding of score ranges according to confidence intervals. The confidence interval is the range of scores above and below the obtained score estimate based on a certain level of statistical estimation. The confidence interval range indicates the lowest and highest estimated values of the student's score should he or she be tested again (Salvia & Ysseldyke, 2003). While many, if not most, practitioners report a confidence band for each test battery, they are not as frequently described in the narrative of the report, and they are rarely discussed at IEP meetings (Sattler, 2001). As a result of this practice, many decisions about a student's school future are made within a context in which the obtained score estimate is taken to be the absolute and true value of the student's current abilities. If, as pointed out above, the obtained score is actually off by a number of points, the students' real skills are not represented in the PNRT score results.

Different Norms Are Not Equivalent

A second major problem with PNRTs is that scores from different test batteries are not equivalent and should not be considered so. Despite this inequality, the scores from different batteries are often compared to determine whether a cognitive-achievement discrepancy exists. For example, a child might be given the Wechsler Intellectual Scale for Children (WISC) and the Woodcock–Johnson Tests of Achievement (WJ-ACH). The composite scores from these two batteries yield standardized scores with a mean of 100 and standard deviation of 15 points. Although these two tests are based on the same standardized metric, the norms developed for each test are not necessarily comparable (Salvia & Ysseldyke, 2003). Different students participated in each of the norming samples, and their unique characteristics contributed to the obtained scores (Lopez, 1997). Although there may be within-test covariance that can be controlled for when intrabattery comparisons are made, when cross-battery score comparisons are made, additional variation and error accumulate, and the extent to which the compared scores tell any meaningful information about a given student is very diluted.

There are two ways of getting around the problems with cross-battery test scores. One is to set higher, and more statistically conservative, score difference minimums for identification of a clinically meaningful score discrepancy. This is the method recommended by Flanagan and Ortiz (2001). Specific, and carefully designed, cross-battery assessment methods may be useful in certain evaluations; however, these should be designated a priori and used by all personnel in consistent ways in the school or district (Flanagan & Ortiz, 2001). A second way to deal with the inherent challenges in discrepancy analysis is to compare only scores obtained from conormed instruments so that additional measurement errors are reduced. Conormed instruments such as the Wechsler, Woodcock–Johnson, and Kaufman provide PNRTs that reduce some of the problems associated with score comparisons (Sattler, 2001).

Limited Instructional Utility

The third, and perhaps most compelling, limitation to PNRTs is that they offer very little information that can be used to develop improved instruction for students (Elliott & Fuchs, 1997; Howell & Nolet, 2000). As several researchers have shown, both the subtest and composite scores obtained on IQ and achievement tests provide very little information that can be used to design effective instruction (Kranzler, 1997; McDermott & Glutting, 1997). The limitations in what can be discerned from subtest analysis are present despite many years of effort to isolate specific trends and learning "styles" in students' subtest patterns (e.g., Kaufman, 1994). While general trends can be identified in an individual student's scores, these are broad patterns. Specific details about how and why a student thinks in a certain way cannot be learned from PNRT scores alone (McGrew, Flanagan, Keith, & Vanderwood, 1997). Instead, curriculum-based assessment methods are needed to show what the student has learned in comparison to what was taught (Berninger, 2002; Howell & Nolet, 2000; Shinn, 1989; Shinn, 1998).

Other Means of Disability Identification

The latest revisions to IDEA include a different method for identifying a learning disability. This method, known as Response to Intervention (RTI), involves implementing a variety of scientifically based instructional methods with students while monitoring their progress (National Joint Committee on Learning Disabilities, 2002). Those students who do not respond to good instruction over time are referred for a comprehensive evaluation to determine what is contributing to school problems. As noted by Shinn in Chapter 11, RTI methods have been around for a long time, although known by other names, such as regular education initiative, prereferral, and inclusion. All of these terms are ways of describing efforts to provide effective instruction for all students in the general education classroom before consideration of special education occurs. Neither problem-solving assessment nor RTI require or prohibit the use of any specific tests or methods. Instead, both of these models involve applying instructional methods and collecting data designed to resolve student school difficulties.

As noted by Shinn in Chapter 11, RTI and problem-solving assessment are not the same thing. Problem-solving assessment is a broad and general approach to students' school difficulties that situates the student in the context of the school community. Neither the student nor the school is to blame for the student's difficulties (Deno, 1985). Instead, it is the difference between what is expected at school and how the student actually performs that is the "problem." RTI is a policy initiative that attempts to apply problem-solving assessment and instruction in more systematic and concise ways (Brown-Chidsey, Loughlin, & O'Reilly, 2004; National Association of School Psychologists, 2003). Within the RTI model, students are identified as having a learning disability only after there are data to show that scientifically based instructional programs were not effective in remediating their learning needs (Fuchs, 2003; Fuchs, Mick, Morgan, & Young, 2003). Most field trials of RTI have used curriculum-based measurement (CBM) or other locally derived forms of assessment and data recording. These studies have shown that RTI methods are effective for resolving the learning difficulties of most children and providing important information about those who need additional instruction and/or assessment (Burns, 2002; Case, Speece, & Molloy, 2003; Speece, Case, & Molloy, 2003).

THE ROLE OF PUBLISHED TESTS IN PROBLEM-SOLVING ASSESSMENT

Although PNRTs have a number of limitations, that does not mean they should never be used. The appropriate use of published tests must be governed by students' needs. If a certain published test is identified to be the best and only way to determine a child's educational needs, then it could be used as part of an evaluation. Conversely, however, if there is no specific question or purpose guiding the use of a published test, it should not be used. Importantly, published tests should not be the first assessment conducted with a student. Instead, they should be the last in a series of assessment procedures, and used only if the other steps did not answer the question. In a problem-solving assessment model, there are a range of assessment procedures to consider (see Table 12.1). Each method must be considered according to whether it is likely to address the questions related to each stage of problem solving. Notably, published tests appear in Table 12.1 only at the problem definition stage. This is because PNRTs have limited capacity to contribute substantially at the other stages due to the problems discussed in this chapter. What follows next is a set of guidelines regarding when use of PNRTs would, and would not, be appropriate.

TABLE 12.1. Assessment Methods and Considerations Appropriate for Each Problem-Solving Stage

Problem-solving stage	Assessment methods	Considerations
Problem identification	Information report Interviews Direct observations	Who is the primary informant? What level of urgency is presented?
Problem definition	Interviews Direct observations Rating scales CBM FBA Published tests	What type of problem is being defined, and how much is it likely to undermine student performance? Is student eligibility for special instruction dependent on how the problem is defined? What risks are associated with imprecise problem definition?
Exploring Solutions	Survey-level assessment Functional behavior analysis	What empirically based methods have worked for similar problems in the past? How do consumers feel about the proposed solution (will they do it)?
Monitoring solutions	CBM Rating scales Interviews	What is the fastest and easiest means of recording student performance? How often should performance be measured? Who should do the recording?
Problem solution	Student performance at or above target level	How will we know when the problem is resolved? How can problem resolution best be documented?

WHEN TO USE PUBLISHED TESTS

The major guideline to follow regarding published tests is to use them if, *and only if,* other assessment procedures have been unable to identify, define, and solve the presenting problem. For most school-based problems, other assessment methods covered in this book will offer all the tools needed for all stages of problem-solving assessment for intervention. The considerations listed in Table 12.1 provide a few questions that the team should consider during each stage of problem solving. There are three situations related to problem definition that may call for the use of published tests: (1) widescale screening of all students, (2) when a student has a very mixed educational history, and (3) when a PNRT is mandated by law for identification and eligibility for services.

Screening

For certain screening assessments, PNRTs may offer the best tool to define which students are at risk for school difficulties and should be evaluated and monitored more closely. For example, most schools screen all students in the early grades on a wide variety of critical developmental milestones. These include vision, hearing, physical mobility, and preliteracy/numeracy skills. Due to the wide number of developmental domains included, as well as the need to conduct the assessments in a timely and organized manner, it may be helpful to use PNRTs for screening-level problem definition activities. The most likely moment when such activities occur is when students enter kindergarten. At this first point of contact with the school, it is helpful to identify and define which students may need additional and/or specialized services in order to be successful in school. Since all students are screened, problem identification activities are covered automatically; by screening all students, school personnel are engaging in primary prevention activities relative to commonly observed early childhood learning difficulties. Using a published early childhood developmental test enables school personnel to *define* the readiness of all students for the kindergarten curriculum by comparing all students against a common published standard.

There are some other assessment tools that may be useful for school entry problem-solving activities as well. For example, the Dynamic Indicators of Early Literacy Skills (DIBELS) provide a comprehensive and empirically based set of assessments for reading skill development (Good & Kaminski, 2002). While the DIBELS are a very powerful tool for literacy assessment, they cover only the language development domain, and schools need to screen all students in other domains as well (e.g., motor skills, behavior). Schools may choose to use a combination of screening tools that include the DIBELS as well as PNRTs so that all developmental areas important to school success are screened. One model for such assessment is the Problem Validation Screening developed by VanDerHeyden, Witt, and Naquin (2003).

Mixed Educational History

A second situation in which published tests may be the best tool for defining a problem is when a student has a very mixed educational history. For example, students who have attended a large number of different schools in a short period of time, who have been chronically absent, or whose school records are not available are likely to have gaps in their knowledge as compared to students who have more consistent educational experiences. Students who move around often or who are frequently absent from school are known to be at risk for school problems (U.S. Department of Education, 2002). As a result, the problem identification stage should be covered automatically when such students enroll at a new school. These students need swift definition of their school needs so that effective instruction can be provided as quickly as possible.

In such cases, PNRTs may provide the best tool to define the student's current educational standing as compared to a national sample of students. In this case, using a nationally norm-referenced test makes sense because the student does not have a common curriculum-linked educational history that can help define current skills and needs. Instead, a PNRT can offer a general overview of current skill levels and some idea of the student's current instructional level. Importantly, when PNRTs are used for this type of problem definition activity, they offer only hypotheses as to the student's skill levels. These hypotheses need to be checked and validated at the subsequent problem-solving stages when possible solutions and student progress are monitored.

Mandated by Law

The third situation in which the use of PNRTs may make sense is when existing regulations require that such a test be given for eligibility and service decision making. The most likely circumstance for such use is when a student may have mental retardation. The common standard and regulatory language regarding definition of mental retardation requires a multi-step assessment process (Brown-Chidsey & Steege, 2004). The minimum required components are an assessment of adaptive livings skills and behavior, assessment of cognitive abilities, and validation of onset prior to age 18. Of note, the American Association for Mental Retardation (AAMR) as well as a number of state and federal agencies include a numerical definition of MR that corresponds to the scores typically obtained on IQ tests. In certain jurisdictions, individuals will be eligible for specialized support services only if an IQ score of 70 or below is documented. For this reason, and until other pathways for obtaining such services are established, it is often necessary to administer an IQ test in order to define and substantiate that a student meets the criteria for mental retardation. Importantly, the IQ test cannot be the only assessment used, and the score must be interpreted in light of other information (Brown-Chidsey & Steege, 2004).

WHEN NOT TO USE PUBLISHED TESTS

Just as there are specific situations when PNRTs may be useful, there are a number of circumstances when they should not be used. Given that PNRTs should be used *only* if other assessment methods have not yielded a problem definition, the number of situations in which they should not be used is probably greater than the number when they could. For simplicity, two main assessment situations will be discussed here. PNRTs should not be used for either placement or instructional planning decisions.

Placement Decisions

Placement decisions are those moments when school personnel determine in which classroom or program a student will be enrolled. Due to the many limitations of PNRTs outlined in this chapter, they are very poor guides for placement decisions. The presence of measurement error as well as the lack of curriculum specificity in PNRTs means that they provide little guidance as to which classroom or specialized program is most likely to resolve a given student's school problem(s). Importantly, a number of legal cases have emphasized the inherent limitations in test scores for making placement decisions (Flanagan & Ortiz, 2002).

Instructional Planning

Similarly, test scores alone offer little guidance for instructional planning. As noted above, PNRTs yield general information about a student's relative skill development. They do not provide adequate precision to help teachers know which materials and teaching techniques a student needs to improve his or her skills (Shinn, 1998). For example, a student's obtained score range of 78–92 on either an achievement or cognitive test will not help a teacher know what reading materials are appropriate or if the student can add or subtract with regrouping. Instead, other assessment procedures are needed in order to discern the student's current instructional level. Even though PNRTs may be useful in a few problem definition situations, in the vast majority of cases, other methods such as CBM and FBA will provide more detailed and accurate information as to what instructional supports the student needs (Berninger, 2002; Brown-Chidsey, Davis, & Maya, 2003; Elliott & Fuchs, 1997).

Surgeon General's Warning

Reschly and Grimes (2002) have suggested that all PNRTs, and IQ tests in particular, should come with a "Surgeon General's warning" like those found on alcohol and cigarettes. The rationale for such a warning is that these tests have very serious potential negative side effects if used improperly; thus, warning consumers is vital to public welfare. Such a warning might be: "CAUTION: IMPROPER USE OF PNRT'S MAY LEAD TO INAPPROPRIATE INSTRUCTION AND NEGATIVE SCHOOL OUTCOMES FOR STUDENTS." The case made in this chapter is that published tests have inherent limitations that prevent them from being the universal best tool for school-based problem-solving activities. These limitations include the reality that, even when used minimally and in moderation, like tobacco and alcohol, there is *some risk* associated with the obtained scores. PNRT scores may under- or overestimate a student's current skills to such an extent that inappropriate and/or ineffective instruction is provided. Importantly, PNRTs are not able to be used for regular and frequent progress monitoring. In sum, PNRTs should be used sparingly, and with great care, only for certain specific purposes during problem definition activities. With that in mind, this chapter concludes with two case scenarios involving possible use of PNRTs.

CASE SCENARIOS

In order to demonstrate the features and limitations of published tests, two case scenarios are provided. In the first case, that of Bethany, a published test is used appropriately as part of the problem-solving activities related to her school needs. In the second case, Tim, PNRT use is sought but later ruled out, with other problem-solving methods successfully used instead.

Bethany

Bethany is 11 years old. She was adopted at 3 months by Bill and Theresa Washington. Little prenatal information about Bethany was available for her new parents. The adoption agency reported that she was delivered without complications but was reported to be small for gestational age. Theresa and Bill provided Bethany with a nurturing and rich early childhood environment. They read to her every day from an early age, but she met developmental milestones slightly later than expected. When Bethany was 3 years old, her parents enrolled her in a private preschool. Bethany made good progress, yet lagged behind the other students in the mastery of colors, letters, and numbers. Bethany excelled at music and art during her preschool years. At age 5, Bethany began half-day kindergarten. She made adequate progress during kindergarten and was promoted to first grade.

In November of her first-grade year, Bethany's teacher held a conference with her parents and told them she was very concerned about Bethany's lack of reading progress. The teacher recommended that Bethany participate in daily supplemental reading instruction through Title I. Her parents agreed, and Bethany received 30 minutes per day of additional reading instruction alongside the reading block in her classroom. The Title I instruction consisted of small-group intensive phonics and reading comprehension activities. By the end of first grade, Bethany was able to read at the 30th percentile when compared to other students in her school as evaluated with curriculum-based measurement (CBM). During the second grade, Bethany had similar trouble learning mathematics subtraction skills. She was provided with Title I math instruction for 30 minutes each day to supplement the classroom math lessons, and she developed adequate math skills by the end of second grade. Bethany's third-grade year was similar to first and second, and when she was provided with additional small-group instruction she was able to meet most grade-level expectations.

At the beginning of Bethany's fourth-grade year, her teacher, Ms. Marsh, used CBM to identify each student's baseline skills in reading and math. She used these data to plan instruction and help prepare the students for the statewide fourth-grade test in April. In November, Ms. Marsh asked to meet with Bethany's parents because of her concern that Bethany was not making much progress over her fall CBM levels. At the parent–teacher conference, Ms. Marsh reported that Bethany was making very slow progress despite receiving additional daily instruction in reading and math. Ms. Marsh also expressed concern about Bethany's difficulties transitioning between activities, following simple directions, keeping track of her belongings, and working independently. Mr. and Ms. Washington reported similar concerns about Bethany's home behaviors. They indicated that Bethany had to be given simple one-step directions for all tasks, supervised closely until a task was completed, and provided with assistance for most personal care activities such as dressing, bathing, preparing for bed, and eating. They reported that since the beginning of fourth grade Bethany had received fewer invitations to participate in social events with peers. Together, Ms. Marsh and Bethany's parents agreed that something more than just reading and math difficulties were affecting Bethany's overall development, and a comprehensive evaluation was needed.

After obtaining the Washingtons' written permission, a comprehensive psychological and educational evaluation of Bethany's skills was conducted. This evaluation included assessments of academic skills, observations of Bethany in several school settings, interviews with Bethany, her parents, and teacher, assessment of adaptive skills, and evaluation of cognitive abilities using a published norm-referenced test. Survey-level assessment using CBM revealed that Bethany was at the 10th percentile in oral reading, 4th percentile in silent reading, and 7th percentile in mathematics fluency when compared to benchmarks for other fourth-grade students in her school district. Verification of these scores with Bethany's scores on the Kaufman Test of Educational Achievement, 2nd Ed. (KTEA-2), revealed that she was at the 6th percentile in reading and 4th percentile in math when compared to a national sample of students her age. Observations of Bethany in her classroom, lunchroom, and on the playground revealed that she was on-task at a par with other students, but she completed much less work and relied on watching other students and asking the teacher to repeat directions in order to finish assignments and activities.

Bethany's adaptive living skills were assessed using the Scales of Independent Behavior—Revised (SIB-R). These teacher- and parent-completed rating scales revealed that Bethany had far fewer adaptive skills than other students her age. In particular, she was reported to need assistance with hygiene, dressing, and other self-care activities. Additionally, Bethany's social skills were reported to be considerably lower than other children her age. Based on these data, the brief version of the Woodcock–Johnson Tests of Cognitive Abilities, 3rd Ed. (WJ-III/COG), was completed. The brief WJ-III/COG includes three subtests and yields a Brief Intellectual Assessment (BIA) score. Bethany's BIA was 68, less than two standard deviations below average for a student her age. Bethany's scores on the three BIA subtests were evenly distributed, so it was interpreted as a valid brief estimate of her current cognitive abilities as measured by a published IQ test.

Taken together, the information gathered about Bethany suggested that she met the criteria for mental retardation. The evaluation report was given at an IEP meeting at Bethany's school, and it was decided by the team that she was eligible for special education services under the classification of mental retardation. Such a decision could not have been obtained without having administered all of the tests given during the comprehensive evaluation. In this situation, Bethany had been provided with high-quality instruction over a period of time when her academic achievement was monitored regularly using CBM. When it became clear that the interventions provided were not yielding the expected and desired performance for a fourth-grade student, it was decided to evaluate Bethany's needs in a more comprehensive fashion. Importantly, Bethany had made significant progress and achievement during her first years of school, having learned to read and do basic math operations. When the curriculum and expectations became more difficult in the fourth grade, Bethany was no longer able to meet those benchmarks at the same level as her peers. In this case, a comprehensive psychoeducational evaluation that included cognitive assessment was necessary and appropriate to identify Bethany's needs. Based on the findings of this report, a different educational program for Bethany was developed.

Tim

Tim Roberts is 12 years old and just started the sixth grade. This is Tim's first year in a new district; his family moved so that his dad, Bill, could take a new job in the aerospace industry. Tim's mom, Carol, is a bank teller. Tim is the oldest of three children. His family is of mixed Navajo, Hopi, and Anglo-European ancestry. In addition to moving for his dad's work,

Tim's family now lives closer to his maternal grandmother. Prior school records indicate that Tim made satisfactory progress in the small elementary school he previously attended. His new school is a middle school with more than 900 students in grades 6 through 8. In October of the current year, Tim's school advisor asked his parents to come in to the school for a meeting. The advisor, Mr. Johnson, reported that Tim was doing poorly in all his classes and wanted to discuss the situation. Tim's father could not attend the meeting, but his mother and grandmother agreed to meet with Mr. Johnson.

At the meeting, Mr. Johnson reported that Tim was receiving D's or F's in all his classes. The poor grades were due to incomplete and missing assignments, limited class participation, and poor test performance. When asked what extra efforts had been tried to assist Tim with his work, Mr. Johnson reported that he had tried to help Tim with his math homework during study hall but that Tim wanted to complete the problems differently than he was taught by the math teacher. Mr. Johnson reported that Tim rarely asks questions or asks for help and that he has few interactions with his classmates. Mr. Johnson asked Tim's mother to sign a permission form to allow Tim to be tested for a learning disability or depression. Tim's grandmother reported that she had helped Tim with a number of homework assignments and thought he had done a very good job; she asked what was wrong with the work he had done. Mr. Johnson reported that Tim had handed in some assignments but they were not done properly, and he had not yet handed in the correct work.

After conferring with her mother, Carol Roberts declined the testing permission. Then, she told Mr. Johnson that they would like to try other solutions before resorting to such testing. After some discussion, it was decided that Tim's teachers would make certain that he wrote all his assignments in a daily planner, his parents would check the planner each night, and assignments needing to be redone would also be written in the planner until completed. Tim's grandmother suggested that Tim's work be evaluated according to whether the answers were correct. Mr. Johnson agreed to this plan. In addition to the efforts to improve Tim's academic performance, a positive behavior support plan (PBSP) was written. This plan involved having Tim's teacher put a checkmark in his daily planner for each of Tim's positive social interactions. Tim's progress on the PBSP was to be monitored by having Mr. Johnson review and summarize the checkmarks at the end of each day during the study hall.

After the support plan for Tim had been in place for 2 months, Mr. and Ms. Roberts met again with Mr. Johnson. Tim's parents were delighted to hear that Tim was showing significant improvement in all school areas. His homework was being turned in on a regular basis, his test scores had improved, and he was interacting more often with his peers. Mr. Johnson asked if anything had changed in the home environment, and the Roberts indicated no. The Roberts did say that Tim reported being happier at school. They also said they were happy to know that Tim's progress had been facilitated without the use of additional testing.

Tim's case reveals how school improvement steps other than testing can, and should, be used before IQ or achievement tests are administered. Had he been tested using traditional discrepancy methods, Tim would have either qualified for special education services or not, but the steps put in place to improve his school performance would likely not have occurred. Instead, changes in the daily routines and expectations of the school personnel contributed to Tim's having a better idea of what was expected of him. Had Tim not made progress, additional instructional changes such as peer tutoring, more frequent progress monitoring, and evaluation of his homework completion methods could have been conducted. Only if Tim did not make progress consistent with the minimum expectations at his school would testing with PNRTs have been appropriate.

SUMMARY

This chapter provided a discussion and two case scenarios of the use of published tests in problem-solving-based assessment. PNRTs are a traditional and widely used part of many school-based assessments. Nonetheless, a large body of research has continually revealed that PNRTs have a considerable number of limitations, including error in measurement, curriculum insensitivity, bias against students of diverse linguistic and cultural backgrounds, and limited instructional applicability. Although there are a few situations in which PNRTs may be appropriate to use, they should be used only if other problem-solving assessment methods have not yet fully defined a problem and their use is likely to provide information beneficial to the child's current needs.

REFERENCES

Berninger, V. (2002). Best practices in reading, writing, and math assessment-intervention links: A systems approach for schools, classrooms, and individuals. In A. Thomas & J. Grimes (Eds.), *Best practices in school psychology IV* (pp. 851–866). Bethesda, MD: National Association of School Psychologists

Brown-Chidsey, R., Davis., L. & Maya, C. (2003). Sources of variance in curriculum-based measures of silent reading. *Psychology in the Schools, 40,* 363–377.

Brown-Chidsey, R., Loughlin, J. E., & O'Reilly, M. J. (2004, April). *Using response to intervention methods with struggling learners.* Mini-skills presentation at the 2004 Annual Conference of the National Association of School Psychologists, Dallas, TX.

Brown-Chidsey, R., & Steege, M. W. (2004). Adaptive behavior. In C. Skinner & T. S. Watson (Eds.), *Comprehensive encyclopedia of school psychology* (pp. 14–15). New York: McGraw-Hill.

Burns, M. K. (2002). Comprehensive system of assessment of intervention using curriculum-based assessments. *Intervention in School and Clinic, 38,* 8–13.

Case, L. P., Speece, D. L., & Molloy, D. E. (2003). The validity of a response-to-instruction paradigm to identify reading disabilities: A longitudinal analysis of individual differences and contextual factors. *School Psychology Review, 32,* 557–582.

Deno, S. L. (1985). Curriculum-based measurement: The emerging alternative. *Exceptional Children, 52,* 219–232.

Elliott, S. N., & Fuchs, L. S. (1997). The utility of curriculum-based measurement and performance assessment as alternatives to traditional intelligence and achievement tests. *School Psychology Review, 26,* 224–233.

Flanagan, D. P., & Ortiz, S. (2001). *Essentials of cross-battery assessment.* New York: Wiley.

Flanagan, D. P., & Ortiz, S. (2002). Best practices in intellectual assessment: Future directions. In A. Thomas & J. Grimes (Eds.), *Best practices in school psychology IV* (pp. 1351–1372). Bethesda, MD: National Association of School Psychologists.

Fuchs, D., Mick, D., Morgan, P. L., & Young, C. L. (2003). Responsiveness to intervention: Definitions, evidence, and implications for the learning disabilities construct. *Learning Disabilities: Research and Practice, 18,* 157–171.

Fuchs, L. (2003). Assessing intervention responsiveness: Conceptual and technical issues. *Learning Disabilities: Research and Practice, 18,* 172–186.

Glutting, J. J., McDermott, P. A., Watkins, M. M., Kush, J. C., & Konold T. R. (1997). The base rate problem and its consequences for interpreting children's ability profiles. *School Psychology Review, 26,* 176–188.

Good, R. H., & Kaminski, R. A. (Eds.). (2002). *Dynamic Indicators of Basic Early Literacy Skills* (6th ed.). Eugene, OR: Institute for the Development of Educational Achievement. Retrieved August 10, 2004, from *dibels.uoregon.edu/*

Gould, S. J. (1981). *The mismeasure of man.* New York: Norton.

Helms, J. E. (1997). The triple quandary of race, cultures, and social class in standardized cognitive ability testing. In D. P. Flanagan, J. L. Genshaft, & P. L. Harrison (Eds.), *Contemporary intellectual assessment: Theories, tests, and issues* (pp. 517–532). New York: Guilford Press.

Howell, K. W., & Nolet, V. (2000). *Curriculum-based evaluation: Teaching and decision-making.* Belmont, CA: Thomson Learning.

Jay, P., Heubert, J. P., & Hauser, R. M. (Eds.). (1999). *High stakes: Testing for tracking, promotion, and graduation.* Washington, DC: National Academy Press.

Individuals with Disabilities Education Act, 20 U.S.C. § 1400 *et seq.* (1997).

Individuals with Disabilities Education Act, 20 U.S.C. § 1400 *et seq.* (2004).

Kaufman, A. S. (1994). *Intelligent testing with the WISC-III.* New York: Wiley.

Kranzler, J. H. (1997). Educational and policy issues related to the use and interpretation of intelligence tests in the schools. *School Psychology Review, 26,* 150–162.

Lopez, R. (1997). The practical impact of current research and issues in intelligence test interpretation and use for multicultural populations. *School Psychology Review, 26,* 249–254.

McDermott, P. A., & Glutting, J. J. (1997). Informing stylistic learning behavior, disposition, and achievement through ability subtests—or, more illusions or meaning? *School Psychology Review, 26,* 163–175.

McGrew, K. S., Flanagan, D. P., Keith, T. Z., & Vanderwood, M. (1997). Beyond g: The impact of *Gf-Gc* specific cognitive abilities research on the future use and interpretation of intelligence test batteries in the schools. *School Psychology Review, 26,* 189–210.

National Association of School Psychologists. (2003). *NASP recommendations: LD eligibility and identification for IDEA reauthorization.* Bethesda, MS: Author.

National Center on Educational Outcomes. (2003). *Accountability for assessment results in the No Child Left Behind Act: What it means for children with disabilities.* Minneapolis: University of Minnesota, National Center on Educational Outcomes. Retrieved October 13, 2003, from *education.umn.edu/NCEO/OnlinePubs/NCLBaccountability.html*

National Joint Committee on Learning Disabilities. (2002). Achieving better outcomes—maintaining rights: An approach to identifying and serving students with specific learning disabilities. *NASP Communiqué, 31.*

No Child Left Behind Act of 2001, Public Law 107-115. (2001).

Ortiz, S. O. (2002). Best practices in nondiscriminatory assessment. In A. Thomas & J. Grimes (Eds.), *Best practices in school psychology IV* (pp. 1321–1336). Bethesda, MD: National Association of School Psychologists.

Peterson, K. M. H., & Shinn, M. R. (2002). Severe discrepancy models: Which best explains school identification practices for learning disabilities? *School Psychology Review, 31,* 459–476.

Reschly, D. J., & Grimes, J. P. (2002). Best practices in intellectual assessment. In A. Thomas & J. Grimes (Eds.), *Best practices in school psychology IV* (pp. 1337–1350). Bethesda, MD: National Association of School Psychologists.

Reschly, D. J., Tilly, W. D., III, & Grimes, J. P. (Eds.). (1999). *Special education in transition: Functional assessment and noncategorical programming.* Longmont, CO: Sopris West.

Salvia, J., & Ysseldyke, J. E. (2003). *Assessment: In special and inclusive education* (9th ed.). New York: Houghton Mifflin.

Sattler, J. M. (2001). *Assessment of children: Cognitive applications* (4th ed.). San Diego: Sattler.

Shriner, J. G. (2000). Legal perspectives on school outcomes assessment for students with disabilities. *Journal of Special Education, 33,* 232–239.

Shinn, M. R. (Ed.). (1989). *Curriculum-based measurement: Assessing special children.* New York: Guilford Press.

Shinn, M. R. (Ed.). (1998). *Advanced applications of curriculum-based measurement.* New York: Guilford Press.

Speece, D. L., Case, L. P., & Molloy, D. E. (2003). Responsiveness to general education instruction as the first gate to learning disabilities identification. *Learning Disabilities: Research and Practice, 18,* 147–156.

Stage, S. A., Abbott, R. D., Jenkins, J. R., & Berninger, V. W. (2003). Predicting response to early reading intervention from verbal IQ, reading-related language abilities, attention ratings, and verbal IQ-word reading discrepancy: Failure to validate discrepancy method. *Journal of Learning Disabilities, 36,* 24–33.

Thurlow, M., Wiley, H. I., & Bielinski, J. (2003). *Going public: What 2000–2001 reports tell us about the performance of students with disabilities* (Technical Report 35). Minneapolis: University of Minnesota, National Center on Educational Outcomes. Retrieved October 13, 2003, from *education.umn.edu/NCEO/OnlinePubs/Technical35.htm*

U.S. Department of Education, National Commission on Excellence in Education. (1983). *A nation at risk: The imperative for educational reform.* Washington, DC: Author.

U.S. Department of Education, National Center for Education Statistics (2002). *Digest of education statistics, 2001.* Retrieved July 8, 2003, from *nces.ed.gov/pubs2002/digest2001/tables/dt052.asp*

VanDerHeyden, A. M., Witt, J. C., & Naquin, G. (2003). Developmental and validation of a process for screening referrals to special education. *School Psychology Review, 32,* 204–228.

Viadero, D. (2003). Researchers debate impact of tests. *Education Week, 22*(21), 1–2.

SUGGESTED READINGS

Howell, K. W., & Nolet, V. (2000). *Curriculum-based evaluation: Teaching and decision-making*. Belmont, CA: Thomson Learning.

This book offers an overview of curriculum-sensitive assessment methods that can be used at all stages of the problem-solving process.

Salvia, J., & Ysseldyke, J. E. (2003). *Assessment: In special and inclusive education* (9th ed.). New York: Houghton Mifflin.

This volume includes a comprehensive review of contemporary assessment methods as well as the technical features of the most widely used published tests.

PART IV

◆ ◆ ◆

Identifying Solutions for School Problems

◆

CHAPTER 13

◆ ◆ ◆

Solution-Focused
Psychoeducational Reports

◆

RACHEL BROWN-CHIDSEY
MARK W. STEEGE

No assessment is likely to be useful until, or unless, the findings are communicated to those in a position to implement solutions. This chapter will provide information about how to write *solution-focused* psychoeducational reports. Information to be covered will include background on the scope and purpose of psychoeducational reports, the purposes of different types of reports, discussion of how solution-focused reports should be organized, and two sample reports incorporating the suggested format.

In traditional school assessment practices, the written report includes a summary of the evaluation conducted. Most of the time, the information contained in the report will be taken into consideration by the team considering whether and/or what type of special education services are needed. In such situations, the report comes near the end of the assessment process and may be looked at only at the team meeting and then put into the student's file. By contrast, solution-focused reports play a dynamic role in solution-focused assessment practices. Instead of one large summary report presented at the end of the assessment process, solution-focused assessment may involve several shorter reports that provide formative assessment results for the team to consider.

In order to demonstrate how solution-focused reports differ from more traditional report-writing practices, this chapter will start by reviewing certain report writing standards and practices. Next, the ways in which solution-focused reports differ from other styles of reports will be discussed. The sample solution-focused reports at the end of the chapter offer readers a chance to see how such a report format incorporates the elements of solution-focused assessment into formative assessment practices.

Although psychoeducational reports are an essential part of school psychology and special education practice, there are few resources available about how to write effective reports. Sattler (2001, p. 678) included a chapter on report writing and suggested that reports should contain the following nine sections:

1. Identifying information
2. Assessment information
3. Reason for referral
4. Background information
5. Observations during assessment
6. Assessment results and clinical impressions
7. Recommendations
8. Summary
9. Signature

These are fairly standard and typical sections likely to be found in most school-based psychoeducational reports. The major difference between Sattler's suggested elements and those found in solution-focused reports is that solution-based reports are formative assessment data while traditional reports are generally summative in nature.

Rather than suggest that all reports follow the same exact format, Tallent (1993) suggested that a flexible approach is best. Tallent also suggested that reports that are narrow in focus are best organized chronologically so that the order of events is easily understood by readers. While a chronological format may be useful to some, Ownby (1987) reported different results from studies of the usefulness of reports written for schools. Specifically, Ownby noted that reports that were organized by ability area(s), that included information about student strengths and weaknesses in behavioral terms, and that had explicit recommendations were the most useful to teachers (Ownby, 1987). Indeed, some researchers have found that educators generally find psychoeducational reports useless (Hoy & Retish, 1984). Hoy and Retish (1984) studied preferences between a traditional report format and one focused on identifying students' learning strengths. Study results revealed that the participants did not like either report very much, finding them both useless (Hoy & Retish, 1984).

A number of authors have pointed out the importance of consumer satisfaction in report writing (Lichtenberger, Mather, Kaufman, & Kaufman, 2004). Brenner (2003, p. 240) emphasized the importance of consumer interests and suggested that there are five steps that report writers can take to make their reports more useful to readers:

1. Reduce jargon.
2. Focus on referral questions.
3. Individualize content.
4. Focus on strengths.
5. Make concrete recommendations.

Brenner's five suggestions are often made to students first learning to write reports, but they are important reminders for all report authors. Indeed, the American Psychological Association Ethical Principles of Psychologists and Code of Conduct (2002) as well as the Principles for Professional Ethics of the National Association of School Psychologists (1997) include provisions related to readable and jargon-free reports. Nonetheless, report authors sometimes become so accustomed to certain terminology that they forget that general audiences such as parents and teachers may not be familiar with such terms. When report authors use words that are foreign to readers, the overall value of the report is diminished.

Another aspect of report writing heavily emphasized in training programs is the referral question. Yet, as noted by Brenner (2003), this is still sometimes overlooked by report authors. There are two reasons to make the referral question clear in the report. First, it helps to set the stage for the assessment activities. By stating the referral question early in the report, the nature and purpose of the assessment activities as they relate to the student's needs are clear (Lichtenberger et al., 2004). Second, if the referral question is stated at the outset of the report, all readers are alerted to how the assessment professional(s) interpreted the reason for referral. In some cases, there may be differences of opinion as to the nature of a student's school difficulties. When this occurs, multiple sets of assessment outcomes may be present. Then, even if report readers have different ideas about the student's needs, the specific nature of the obtained results is clear, and, if desired, alternative assessments may be conducted.

The importance of individualizing the content of assessment reports may seem obvious; yet, some reports are written so generically that they could apply to any number of students. Often, the elements of overly general reports are statements referring to unexpected or undesired assessment outcomes that the report author did not know how to interpret or summarize. When assessment findings are unclear or ambiguous, it is best to be clear about this ambiguity rather than cover it up with generic statements that could apply to many individuals. When overly broad language is used in a report, there is a danger that it will be interpreted by readers at face value even if it bears only minimal resemblance to the student. In such cases, the true nature and significance of the student's needs are masked or ignored. When a report author is not certain how to interpret or report certain results, this uncertainty should be stated. Then, if necessary, additional assessment activities can be conducted to examine the area(s) in question.

The importance of individualization of assessment reports is made apparent in cases when a student from a diverse linguistic, cultural, religious, socioeconomic, or ability background is evaluated (Dana, Aguilar-Kitibutr, Diaz-Vivar, & Vetter, 2002). In such circumstances, the unique nature of the student's needs is more likely to be obvious, but the implications from assessment activities may be harder to interpret. When group-specific norms, cultural standards, and linguistic variables are part of the assessment landscape, it is critical that report writers should not infer that the norms and standards applicable to the dominant culture are necessarily equally applicable to students from other backgrounds (Dana et al., 2002). Instead, the limitations of the assessment instruments and procedures need to be stated explicitly, and an interpretation of the results in light of the student's specific background provided.

Including information about a student's strengths is a report component often given lip service but not necessarily done in the systematic way that student deficits are reported. Brenner (2003) noted that the field of psychology does not have a strong history of citing student strengths in assessment reports partly because it has long been the tradition that identification of weaknesses is the primary goal of psychoeducational reports. By contrast, social workers have a long tradition of identifying and noting client strengths in their reports, and this is a report feature that consumers like (Brenner, 2003). Despite the emergence of individual strengths as an area of focus in psychology treatment methods, assessment reports continue to include few student strengths even when report writers are asked to include them (Brenner, 2003). Importantly, student strengths can play a role in intervention planning and implementation. For these reasons, more emphasis on student strengths in reports is needed.

The recommendation section of the report has long been identified as the most important to consumers; thus, the readability and usefulness of the recommendations is critical. Brenner (2003) suggested that reports need to include recommendations that are concrete and pragmatic. Research findings show that assessment report consumers want recommendations that are concrete, understandable, and feasible (Brenner, 2003). Additionally, it is important for recommendations to be linked to the referral question(s) so that potential solutions to the initial problem or concern are provided (Lichtenberger et al., 2004). To this end, it may be necessary to revise the referral(s) question so that the assessment activities address an answerable question for which there are known interventions to be recommended.

There are no national standards for evaluating psychoeducational reports such that readers might be able to refuse to read or accept those that are deficient. Nonetheless, examination of the existing studies on assessment reports provides some indicators of what constitutes a "good" report. The most common theme across the report studies is the importance of reader-friendly, consumer-based report writing practices (Brenner, 2003; Ownby, 1987). In the case of reports written for use in school settings, especially those related to special education, the language of the report must take into account the rules and regulations governing special education practices (Ownby, 1987). To assist those seeking to improve their report writing skills Salend and Salend (1985) offer a checklist that covers a wide range of elements likely to be found in school-based reports. This checklist may not include a report format that meets every evaluator's needs, but the idea of having a checklist is a good one. Whether designed by individual report writers or by a school-based team, such a checklist offers a systematic way for all report authors to verify that they have included all necessary items in each report they write.

A final aspect of traditional psychoeducational reports that is worth discussing is length. Some report authors are very concise, while others are quite wordy. Those researchers who have investigated the effects of report length on usefulness have found that longer reports are not necessarily better ones (Brenner, 2003; Donders, 1999; Salend & Salend, 1985; Tallent, 1993). Donders (1999) has noted that many assessment reports, especially neuropsychological reports, include very detailed accounts of every aspect of the obtained scores. Such detail is not necessarily helpful for most readers and, in many cases, prevents readers from getting the main ideas found in the report (Donders, 1999). When report writers focus too heavily on score details, they may confuse readers because they send a message that the score details are more important than the synthesis of the findings. For parents, teachers, and others who read such reports, complex descriptions of the scores may mask the "big ideas" meant to be conveyed by the report author. For this reason shorter reports may be better, especially in cases where continuous progress monitoring of student skill development over time can provide ongoing information about a student's school performance.

SOLUTION-FOCUSED PSYCHOEDUCATIONAL REPORT WRITING

Elements of Solution-Focused Psychoeducational Reports

The components that make up solution-focused psychoeducational reports match the stages of the problem-solving assessment model. Regardless of the solution stage, or the size and scope of the report, solution-focused

ıould be organized in such a way that they document
dividual student's needs are addressed by focusing on
here are two major types of solution-focused reports:
d *progress monitoring* reports. Outlines for evaluation
ing solution-focused reports are found in Tables 13.1
r. While these report outlines provide suggested for-
ılats and what information to include, these elements can be organized into
other report formats if that better suits the student's needs. Initial evaluation reports are more likely to contain the report elements listed in Table
13.1. Details about a student's outcomes after new programming has been
implemented could be included in progress monitoring reports with elements such as those in Table 13.2. In all cases it is important to identify
and clarify the referral question. For example, when the referral question is
stated in broad terms (e.g., "3-year reevaluation" or "to evaluate reading
problems") practitioners are advised to interview classroom teachers and/
or others to identify special areas of concern.

Identification of the Problem

The first section of a solution-focused evaluation report should include
three main components: (1) student identification information (e.g., name,
age, grade, classroom), (2) the date(s) when the problem was observed, and
(3) the name(s) and position(s) of those who identified the problem. These
three information elements provide the immediate context for the problem

---

TABLE 13.1. Solution-Focused Evaluation Report Outline

1. Identification of the problem
   a. Student's name, age, grade, classroom
   b. Date(s) when problem was observed
   c. Names and positions of those who identified the problem

2. Definition of problem
   a. Background information about student
   b. Current educational placement
   c. Present levels of performance
      • Student
      • Typically achieving peers
   d. Magnitude of differences between student's performance and
      what is expected
   e. Summary of problem definition

3. Possible solutions
   a. General education interventions
   b. Special education interventions

TABLE 13.2. **Solution-Focused Progress Monitoring Report Outline**

1. Intervention plan
   a. Student's name, age, grade, classroom
   b. Date(s) of meeting where problem was confirmed and intervention plan developed
   c. Names and positions of those who identified the problem

2. Progress monitoring activities
   a. Specific intervention activities to be implemented
   b. Days, times, and sequence of activities
   c. Outcome indicator(s) to be used to determine whether plan is working
   d. Personnel responsible for intervention implementation
   e. Date for next report and/or meeting

3. Intervention discontinuation
   a. Criteria to be met for program to end
   b. Persons to be involved
   c. Procedures to be used if student encounters more difficulties

identification stage of assessment. Problem identification is the stage when a student's school situation is perceived to be problematic by someone important in that student's life. The person who identifies that a problem exists could be a parent, teacher, bus driver, or the student him- or herself. It is important to include information about how, when, and by whom a school problem was identified because it validates that a concern has been raised about a student. In describing and validating the nature of the problem in the words and context of the person who reported the problem, no specific cause of the problem is identified or inferred. Instead, the basic chronological facts of how the problem came to be known are reported. This information then serves as the starting point for the second section of the report, the problem definition.

Definition of the Problem

This section of the report generally includes five major components: (1) background information about the student, (2) current educational placement, (3) present levels of performance (of both the student and peers), (4) magnitude of differences between the student's performance and what is expected, and (5) a summary of the problem definition. Each of these section components is important because collectively they serve as the framework around which the assessment and intervention activities are constructed.

Background Information

This subsection includes both academic and personal/medical information about the individual student. A good starting point for the background section is to provide a brief developmental history, including the student's prenatal, perinatal, and neonatal development. This information is generally gained from the student's parents, especially the mother. In cases where such information is not available from the parent(s), it may be obtained from prior testing reports or other related records. For some students, events or complications arising from pregnancy, delivery, or the first days of life may have a role in current problems. Accurate information from early childhood can provide a concise history of a child's lifespan development. If the student's early development was typical and no pregnancy or birth complications were reported, then the early development information moves quickly into discussion of attainment of the major developmental milestones such as walking and talking. There are expected typical developmental ranges for such milestones, and noting whether a child achieved such targets can be important. If a child met most or all but one milestone within the typical range, then there is less concern about diffuse developmental problems than if a number of milestones were attained later than expected or never.

In addition to early development information, it is important to include a history of any and all educational, medical, or related programs in which the student has participated. Such information can be summarized briefly but provides important information about the nature and scope of any past efforts to support or improve a student's long-term development. All together, the background information section sets the stage for understanding the nature and context of a student's school difficulties in light of past experiences.

Current Educational Placement

The background information section is followed by information about the student's current educational setting. This might be a general or special education program, but the name of the teacher(s), program purposes, and duration should be stated. Also included in this subsection is information about the types of activities usually employed in this setting. This section of the report provides information to the readers about what the student is currently being expected to do. It is impossible to determine whether a student's reported school difficulties are substantially different from his or her peers' if the typical daily expectations are unknown. If a student is already receiving specialized services, including special education, Title I, or other supports, descriptions of the exact instructional activities being provided to the student should be included. It is not sufficient to say that a student is receiving Title I instruction because it's impossible to know exactly what the student is doing during such lessons. Instead, the exact activities included in the Title I sessions should be reported.

Present Levels of Performance

Once the student's current placement is described, the extent to which his or her current skills and achievement vary from those of classmates can be evaluated. There are a number of methods by which the student's performance levels can be described. A summary of all the methods for defining student performance is outside the scope of this chapter; however, information about such methods can be found in other chapters in this volume. Regardless of the measurement tools used to define a student's performance, it is important that the scores be reported in such a way that the quality of the student's skills as compared to those of current classmates is identified. This can be done for all types of student behavior and skills, including academic achievement, behaviors, emotional responding, and social skills. Ideally, the student's scores are reported in the context of locally obtained benchmarks. Such benchmarks, or norms, are indicators of what level of skill or performance a typical student of the same age and grade would be expected to achieve.

For example, if a student has been referred for concerns about off-task behavior and attention, it would be necessary to report data related to the student's observed behaviors, as well as the behaviors of classmates under the same instructional conditions. Sometimes it is more appropriate to report a student's current performance in relation to normative benchmarks supplied by a published norm-referenced test. In such cases, it may be unnecessary to report the actual level(s) of typical performance because the obtained scores have been calibrated to document deviation from a normal score. For example, in the case of most cognitive assessment tests and many academic tests based on national norms, the obtained score is a standardized number with a mean of 10 or 100 and a set standard deviation. In such cases, the extent of a student's variation from the average score is documented in the score itself. In such cases it is best to include in the report a statement reminding the reader that the basis for comparing the individual student's score is a set of nationally published norms.

Magnitude of Differences between Student's Performance and What Is Expected

This section of the report provides important information regarding whether a student's current performance is close to that of peers or is dramatically different. An example of how this can be worded is "When compared to a national sample of students her age, Molly's math skills are in the average range." Alternatively, a statement regarding a student's classroom behavior might be "Bill was on-task 53% of observed intervals, while a randomly selected classmate was on-task 97% of observed intervals." Together with other assessment information such as interviews and record reviews, the information about a student's current performance compared with either local or national standards offers a way to document the extent of his or her deviation from what is expected. In cases where there is little or no difference between a student's scores or behaviors and average or expected levels, much less about the student's performance needs to be said. However, in cases where a student's performance levels are significantly different from what is expected according to local or national norms, more information about the student's actual performance should be included in the report. Such information may include subtest and cluster scores as well as documentation of specific behaviors during evaluation.

Summary of the Problem Definition

Together, the background information, current educational placement, present levels of performance, and magnitude of differences between student's performance and what is expected are used to document and define the presenting problem. Each of the above components of the problem definition is important because the determination of whether the identified "problem" is of sufficient magnitude to justify a different course of action can only be made when both the specific student difficulties and educational expectations are known. The problem definition summary should be stated in one or two sentences and provide situation-specific indicators of the problem. For example, for a student with reading difficulties, a problem summary could be "Information gathered from interviews, observations, testing, and work samples revealed that Nora's current reading skills are two grades lower than those of her classmates."

Possible Solutions

Once a specific problem definition summary is available, it is possible to develop ideas for solutions. Often, suggested remedies are provided in the evaluation report, although it is up to the individualized education program (IEP) team to decide exactly what, if any, special education services will be provided. Including suggested interventions in the report can help facilitate thinking and planning for implementation of solutions. Importantly, the set of recommended actions does not have to be limited to special education activities. It is very appropriate to include either, or both, general and special education interventions in the report.

General Education Interventions

A number of general education activities may be very helpful for students who have undergone an evaluation. These suggestions can be labeled as ideas that would be appropriate for implementation in the general education environment, so team members can consider ideas that include both less and more restrictive educational environments. For example, adjustments to seating arrangements, work completion procedures, consequences for behaviors, peer groupings, and use of assistive technology are all instructional adaptations that can be implemented in the general education classroom. Importantly, any improvements in school performance that a student experiences as a result of general education interventions may prevent the need for special education programming and a more restrictive classroom setting. Sometimes, a short-term small-group general education placement may be the best way to enhance a student's skills. For example, a number of studies have shown that targeted small-group reading instruction is very effective for improving student reading skills (Foorman, 2003). Not all general education supports have to be provided in large-group instructional settings. Title I programs supported by federal Elementary and Secondary Education Act (ESEA) funds are one example of small-group support that is part of general education.

Special Education Interventions

In some cases, general education adjustments are not adequate for the needs of a given student. If general education enhancements do not yield desired improvements in a student's school performance, then other supports should be used. In order for a student to receive special education instruction, he or she must be identified as a student with a disability, according to the federal and state special education regulations. Once an eligibility determination is made, special education services can be provided. It is never appropriate for one person to make an eligibility determination. This is the right and role of the student's educational team. Still, it may be helpful for the report to include recommendations related to specific types of instruction typically provided in special education programs. In particular, if a report has been completed as part of a student's reevaluation for special education services, then specific mention of recommended special education instruction is appropriate. Examples of special education interventions that might be included in report recommendations include individualized tutoring, very intensive behavioral support staffing ratios, highly specialized instructional settings such as therapeutic programs, and access to specialists uniquely related to the disability (e.g., sign language interpreters). An example of a solution-focused evaluation report is provided at the end of this chapter. Another example is the sample functional behavioral assessment (FBA) report found in Chapter 7.

Solution Monitoring Reports

If it is determined that a child's school problems are serious enough to justify some corrective action, an intervention program should be developed. For all interventions, both in general and special education, progress monitoring and intervention reporting should be done. An outline of the basic elements for solution monitoring reports is found in Table 13.2. Three main sections are recommended. First, the general findings of the evaluation report should be documented. Next, the intervention plan should be written out in sufficient detail that the teacher(s) who will be responsible for implementing it will know what to do. These details should include descriptions of specific activities, outcome indicators, personnel, and daily schedules (see Figure 13.1). A blank progress-monitoring graph for recording student performance data is found in Figure 13.2. As noted by Fuchs (1986, 1998), Fuchs, Fuchs, Hamlett, and Ferguson (1992), and Kratochwill, Elliott, and Callan-Stoiber (2002), interventions that are accompanied by detailed procedures as well as specific support for the staff who implement them are much more likely to be effective. In many school districts, the solution monitoring report may be the IEP; however, for interventions in general education, no IEP will be developed. For cases in which the intervention is extremely complex, the IEP may not afford adequate space for all details about the program. IEP team participants should determine whether the IEP will serve as the progress monitoring document or if a supplementary plan is needed. For all progress monitoring plans in both general and special education, there should be a specific date and time for the next team meeting as well as a description of the circumstances under which the program will be discontinued.

Due to the modular nature of solution-focused reports, it is possible that different personnel will contribute to and/or write certain sections of the report(s). When this is the case, it is important that each section author be identified and the source materials on which the section is based be clearly stated. Some personnel may prefer to write their own reports instead of contributing to a larger collaborative report. Others may choose to participate in a collaborative report that summarizes the findings from many activities.

SAMPLE SOLUTION-FOCUSED
PSYCHOEDUCATIONAL REPORTS

Two sample solution-focused reports are provided. The first is an evaluation report that covers the problem identification, definition, and generating solutions stages; this is more like traditional reports in that it includes

Student: _____ Case Manager: _____

1. Problem Definition
   Date of meeting when problem was defined: _____

   State the problem in the space here: _____

   _____

2. Intervention Activities
   Teacher/aide responsible: _____

   Specific teaching steps or methods: _____

   _____

   _____

   Frequency of instruction: _____

3. Progress Monitoring Activities
   Assessment method(s) used to track student's progress: _____

   _____

   Date for next report and/or meeting: _____

   Intervention discontinuation criteria: _____

   _____

FIGURE 13.1. Progress Monitoring Report Form. From Brown-Chidsey and Steege (2005). In R. Brown-Chidsey (Ed.), *Assessment for Intervention: A Problem-Solving Approach*. Copyright 2005 by The Guilford Press. Permission to photocopy this figure is granted to purchasers of this book for personal use only (see copyright page for details).

Student: _____   Case Manager _____

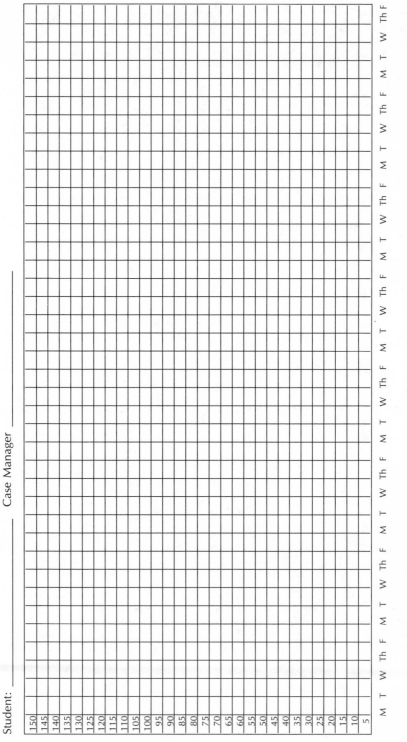

FIGURE 13.2. Blank progress monitoring graph. From Brown-Chidsey and Steege (2005). In R. Brown-Chidsey (Ed.), *Assessment for Intervention: A Problem-Solving Approach.* Copyright 2005 by The Guilford Press. Permission to photocopy this figure is granted to purchasers of this book for personal use only (see copyright page for details).

background information about the student as well as assessm(
results and proposed solutions. The second is a progress monito
that documents the same student's progress once daily reading
was provided.

Sample Evaluation Report

Student Information: Kyle Blake   *School*: Monroe Elementary
Date of birth: January 21, 1992   *Date of report*: March 23, 2003
Grade: 5   *School psychologist*: Steve
                                           Reynolds, NCSP

Referral Question/Statement of the Problem

On December 12, 2002, Kyle's mother, Barbara Blake, telephoned Kyle's
teacher, Monica Beaumont, and told her that Kyle had been unable to complete his homework for the third time that week. Ms. Blake reported that
Kyle has been complaining about school for many weeks, often becoming
hysterical and refusing to get on the bus in the morning.

Background Information

Kyle is the youngest of two children, and he lives with his mother and stepfather. His parents are divorced. His older sister (21) lives on her own.
Kyle's mother reported that her pregnancy with Kyle was healthy and
uncomplicated and that Kyle was born at full term via prescheduled Cesar-
ean. Kyle reportedly met all developmental milestones within normal limits. A review of Kyle's cumulative school record indicated that that he met
the criteria for kindergarten entry when he was screened at age 5 in his previous school district. There were no other records from Kyle's progress in
kindergarten, first, or second grade prior to enrolling at Monroe. Kyle's
quarterly and annual progress records from the second through fourth
grades indicated that he made satisfactory progress. All Kyle's teachers
reported both academic and social gains each year. Kyle has received assistance in reading through the Title I program since enrolling at Monroe.
Reports from the Title I teachers indicate that he has made some progress
in his reading skills, although they remain less developed than those of his
fifth-grade peers.

Current Educational Placement

Kyle is currently enrolled in the fifth grade at Monroe Elementary School.
He has attended Monroe since the second grade, when he moved from
Albuquerque. With the exception of Title I reading instruction, Kyle

receives all of his instruction in a general education classroom. The Title I program at Monroe uses the *Reading Recovery* curriculum, which involves having students work one-on-one with tutors who provide 30 minutes of instruction for the students each day.

Sources of Information Used to Evaluate Kyle's Present Levels of Performance

- Review of records
- Interviews with student and parent
- Classroom observation
- Woodcock–Johnson Tests of Cognitive Abilities, Third Edition
- Curriculum-based measures of reading
- Achenbach Child Behavior Checklist, Teacher Report Form, and Youth Self-Report

Reliability of Information

Kyle attended three sessions during the course of this evaluation. The sessions were held in a private office at Monroe School. Kyle came with the examiner willingly and indicated that he understood the purpose of the testing. Kyle worked on all testing activities diligently, appearing to do his best work. The test results reported below are believed to be accurate estimates of his true abilities on the skills tested.

Kyle's Current Level of School Performance

Kyle was interviewed to learn his perceptions of his current school and personal situations. In response to school-related questions Kyle reported that school was easier in third grade than it is now, but that he likes writing, once he gets an idea about what to write. He indicated that he does not have many friends at school, but there is one boy in his classroom who is his friend. When asked what would make school better for him, Kyle responded that he wishes his classroom were quieter and that there were more science lessons because he likes those the best. He also reported that he is experiencing difficulty in the area of reading. He specified that he has trouble sounding out words and understanding what he has just read.

Kyle's mother, Barbara Blake, was interviewed by telephone about her impressions of Kyle's current strengths and needs. In addition, Ms. Blake completed a student history form. In both the history form and telephone interview, Ms. Blake indicated that her greatest concern about her son right now relates to Kyle's fear of going to school. She reported that she felt that Kyle's classroom placement in the fifth grade was "not right for him." She indicated that she wonders whether the current classroom atmosphere is appropriate for Kyle and whether the current teacher really understands his needs. Ms. Blake also indicated that Kyle appears to learn best in one-on-one settings.

In order to learn more about Kyle's typical classroom behaviors, several classroom observations of Kyle were conducted. An initial observation was done during a math lesson from 10:45 to 11:50 A.M. The math lesson included three main components: teacher overview of plans and materials preparation, a game played in pairs or triads, and a whole-class discussion of the activities. Kyle was actively engaged in most components of the lesson, especially the first part when the students organized their notebooks. Kyle experienced a brief episode of difficulty finding a partner for the game, but this was resolved with teacher support. Kyle and his partner were active during the game but did not complete as much work as the other students in the room. Kyle was the least engaged during the summary discussion of the activity and did not participate as much in that activity. Kyle's general behavior during the observed math lesson was very similar to his classmates'.

Three additional observations were conducted with Kyle: a math worksheet activity, a science lab, and during independent reading time. These observations included use of a 6-second partial-interval recording procedure to measure academic engagement by Kyle and a representative sample of his classmates. Table 13.3 summarizes the observation data. The obtained data are reported as the percentage of intervals during which Kyle and his classmates were actively engaged in the target activity. The percentages revealed that Kyle was engaged more often (97%) than his peers (92%) in the science lab but less engaged during the math (67%) and independent reading (45%) activities.

Due to differences in the reported and observed difficulties Kyle was experiencing in school, additional assessment of Kyle's cognitive skills was conducted. For this reason, the Standard Battery and selected supplemental tests of the Woodcock–Johnson Tests of Cognitive Abilities, 3rd Ed. (WJ-III/COG), were given to Kyle to help learn more about his learning needs. Kyle's scores on the individual WJ-III/COG tests and cognitive skills clusters are given in Table 13.4. Even though the full WJ-III/COG Standard

TABLE 13.3. Percentage of Intervals during Which Kyle and Comparison Classmates Were Observed to be On-Task

Activity	Kyle	Classmates
Independent reading	45%	84%
Math worksheets	67%	88%
Science (lab)	97%	92%

TABLE 13.4. Kyle's Scores on the Woodcock–Johnson Tests
of Cognitive Abilities, 3rd Ed. (WJ-III/COG)

Test	Standard score	Confidence band	Percentile rank
Individual Tests			
Verbal Comprehension	88	79–97	21
Visual–Auditory Learning	77	69–84	6
Spatial Relations	79	69–88	8
Sound Blending	95	82–108	37
Concept Formation	78	70–85	7
Visual Matching	58	50–65	.2
Numbers Reversed	76	65–87	6
General Information	90	79–101	26
Retrieval Fluency	86	74–99	18
Picture Recognition	93	84–102	32
Memory for Words	87	75–99	20
Clusters			
Verbal Ability	89	81–96	22
Thinking Ability	75	69–82	5
Cognitive Efficiency	64	57–71	1
Comprehension–Knowledge	89	81–96	22
Long-term Retrieval	74	66–82	4
Visual–Spatial Thinking	82	74–91	12
Short-term Memory	79	70–88	8

Battery was administered, a General Intellectual Ability score is not reported for Kyle because there were too many significant differences among the individual WJ-III/COG test scores. The standard score is a norm-referenced measure of Kyle's performance compared to other students his age. It is based on an average of 100, with a standard deviation of 15. The confidence band shows the range of scores Kyle would be expected to earn if the same tests were given again. The percentile rank shows Kyle's relative standing when compared with others his age.

The scores for the WJ-III/COG indicate that Kyle's skills may fall in the broad average range; however, there was a great deal of variability among the individual test scores. For example, his scores on Verbal Comprehension, Sound Blending, General Information, Retrieval Fluency, Picture Recognition, and Memory for Words were all in the broad average range. This is in contrast to his scores on the Visual–Auditory Learning, Spatial Relations, Concept Formation, Visual Matching, and Numbers Reversed tests, where his scores were all in the below-average range. These score differences are somewhat explained by Kyle's pattern of performance on the tests comprising specific ability clusters. His scores on the combinations of tests measuring Verbal Ability, General Knowledge and Comprehension, and Visual–Spatial Thinking are all in the average range. Yet, his scores for Thinking Ability, Cognitive Efficiency, Long-term Retrieval, and Short-term Memory are all in the below-average range. This pattern of results may indicate that Kyle's cognitive skills are influenced by lower-than-average memory and thinking abilities.

In order to gain additional information about the nature of Kyle's reading skills, additional assessment was conducted using curriculum-based measurement (CBM) procedures. CBM items include oral reading passages for each grade level. Kyle completed a survey level assessment using CBM passages from the third through fifth grades. These passages are ones for which local benchmarks have been gathered so that there is a normative standard against which Kyle's reading performance can be compared. The passages were administered in reverse grade-level order so that he began with reading fifth-grade material and ended with reading third-grade material. The oral reading passages are grade-leveled stories that the student reads out loud for 1 minute while the examiner records which words are read correctly. Kyle's performance on the CBM passages is summarized in Table 13.5.

The oral reading scores show how many words Kyle read in 1 minute, how many were incorrect, and the total number of words read correctly. The CBM results suggest that Kyle is currently reading at the third-grade level. This is identified in the CBM scores in that his score on the fifth- and fourth-grade passages fell below the range expected of fifth- and fourth-grade students but in the range for third-grade students. Of note, Kyle's error rate while reading orally is fairly high. A reader, of any age, needs to be able to decode and comprehend about 95% of what is read. With errors as high as 5 to 10, it appears that Kyle's current reading fluency and accuracy are significantly weaker than that which is expected of a fifth-grade student. Qualitative analysis of Kyle's reading errors revealed consistent patterns. For words that Kyle did not know by sight, he used phonological decoding strategies to "sound out" the word. Thus, Kyle's reading strategies appear to be appropriate, and his errors reflect great difficulty with managing fluent, quick decoding of unknown words and understanding what he is reading.

In order to get an idea of how Kyle's general psychological profile compares to other boys his age, a set of norm-referenced questionnaires

TABLE 13.5. Kyle's Curriculum-Based Measurement Results

Level	Total words	Errors	Total correct	Benchmarks
Grade 5	48	10	38	99–157
Grade 4	63	6	57	89–140
Grade 3	75	5	70	54–115

were given to Kyle, his mom and stepdad, and his teacher to complete. The Achenbach Child Behavior Checklist (parent form), Teacher Report Form, and Youth Self-Report were all completed and returned to the examiner for scoring. Each of the questionnaires includes over 100 items about a child's general emotional and psychological functioning. The combined responses can be scored and compared to identify similarities in a child's current state of functioning as compared to other children of the same age. The scores obtained from the questionnaires about Kyle are summarized in Table 13.6. The T score is a standardized score with an average of 50 and a standard deviation of 10. Kyle's ratings of his own psychological well-being indicate that he is experiencing much worse internalizing symptoms than other boys his age. Such symptoms include feeling sad much of the time, having few friends, and experiencing frequent fears. His externalizing and total scale scores were not elevated. Kyle's mother and stepfather reported scores that were very similar to Kyle's, with an internalizing score 1 point higher than Kyle's rating, but nonelevated externalizing and total scores. Kyle's teacher—Mrs. Carlson's—ratings of Kyle revealed that his classroom behaviors and well-being are in line with those expected of a boy of Kyle's age for both internalizing symptoms (e.g., anxiety) and externalizing behaviors (e.g., aggression, misconduct).

Summary of Kyle's Current School Performance

The information collected as part of this psychological evaluation suggests that Kyle is a student of average to perhaps below-average abilities who is experiencing certain symptoms of anxiety and poor school performance. Observation of Kyle in his current classroom setting revealed that he was actively engaged in the assigned activities much less often than his peers during math and reading, but very engaged during a science lab. Kyle's performance in the area of reading appears to be lower than that of other fifth-grade students at Monroe. Kyle and his parents reported elevated levels of internalizing symptoms such as depression and anxiety; however, such indicators were not found in teacher responses to the same items.

TABLE 13.6. Kyle's Achenbach Child Behavior Checklist (Parent Report Form), Teacher Report Form, and Youth Self-Report Results

	Parent (CBCL)	Teacher (TRF)	Kyle (YSR)
Internalizing Behaviors	74[a]	57	73[a]
Externalizing Behaviors	53	58	58
Total Scale	59	53	56

[a]Statistically significant score.

Possible Solutions

GENERAL EDUCATION SOLUTIONS

Kyle's current placement in a general education classroom appears appropriate. He does not appear to be making progress in the Reading Recovery Title I program. Another Title I reading instruction program should be considered. Specifically, Kyle's reading rate is lower than his grade-level peers. A reading fluency program such as *Great Leaps* or *Read Naturally* may help Kyle increase his reading speed. In addition, Kyle would be likely to benefit from organizational supports to help him be able to get the most out of daily classroom learning activities. Specifically, a positive behavioral support plan that helps Kyle to map out and organize his daily activities and that rewards him when he participates actively in instructional activities is likely to help him stay on track with daily assignments and academic goals.

SPECIAL EDUCATION SOLUTIONS

No special education solutions for Kyle's school difficulties are recommended at this time. If the outlined general education and other solutions are not successful, then special education services may be considered at a later time.

OTHER SOLUTIONS

Kyle may benefit from a daily schedule used at home to organize his time. Such a schedule could be linked with specific goals and activities for improving his school performance such as designated homework completion times and rewards for meeting improved behavior goals.

Sample Progress Monitoring Report

Student: *Kyle Blake*   Case Manager: *Steve Reynolds, NCSP*

1. Problem Definition

   Date of meeting when problem was defined: *March 30, 2003*

   State the problem in the space here: *According to CBM scores, Kyle's current reading skills are at the third-grade level.*

2. Intervention Activities

   Teacher/aide responsible: *Monica Beaumont*

   Specific teaching steps or methods: *Kyle will read one passage from the fifth-grade* Great Leaps *reading fluency program five times each day.*

During the first reading, aloud, Kyle will be timed by Ms. Pressley. Kyle will read the passage three more times silently. On the fifth reading— again, aloud—Ms. Pressley will time Kyle again. Kyle's goal is to read every fifth-grade passage in 1 minute or less.

Frequency of instruction: *Kyle will participate in repeated reading practice every school day for 10 minutes.*

3. Progress Monitoring Activities

Assessment method(s) used to track student's progress: *Kyle's oral reading fluency rate on the* Great Leaps *passages will serve as daily indicators of progress* (see Figure 13.3).

Date for next report and/or meeting: May 24, 2003

Intervention discontinuation criteria: *When Kyle's ORF is at the fifth-grade level.*

SUMMARY

This chapter has included information concerning solution-focused report writing. Traditionally, psychoeducational reports have included information about a student's problems and deficits. Rarely has such information been useful in developing interventions designed to resolve student difficulties. Solution-based reports incorporate all five elements of the problem-solving model and help teachers, parents, and students have a clear problem definition that is based on the student's current performance as compared with the school's expectations. By organizing such reports around the stages of the problem-solving model, all report readers can be clear about who identified the problem, how it has been defined, what solutions have been tried, and what steps are recommended next. Importantly, solution-focused reports may include several parts developed and written by multiple informants over time. Problem evaluation reports help to clarify the problem before specialized instruction is provided. Progress monitoring reports provide information about a student's progress once an intervention has been implemented.

REFERENCES

American Psychological Association. (2002). Ethical principles of psychologists and code of conduct. Retrieved May 29, 2004, from *www.apa.org/ethics/code2002.html*

Brenner, E. (2003). Consumer-focused psychological assessment. *Professional Psychology: Research & Practice, 34,* 240–247.

Dana, R. H., Aguilar-Kitibutr, A., Diaz-Vivar, N., & Vetter, H. (2002). A teaching method for multicultural assessment: Psychological report contents and cultural competence. *Journal of Personality Assessment, 79,* 207–215.

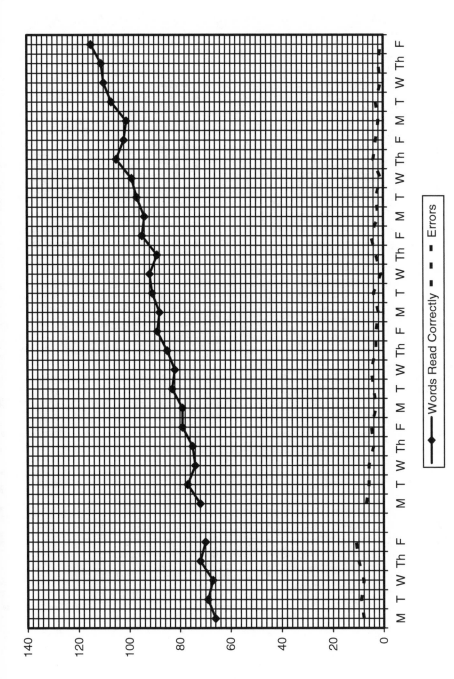

FIGURE 13.3. Kyle's progress monitoring graph.

Donders, J. (1999). Pediatric neuropsychological reports: Do they really have to be so long? *Child Neuropsychology, 5,* 70–78.

Foorman, B. (Ed.). (2003). *Preventing and remediating reading difficulties: Bringing science to scale.* Baltimore: York Press.

Fuchs, L. S. (1986). Monitoring progress among mildly handicapped students: Review of current practice and research. *Rural and Special Education, 7,* 5–12.

Fuchs, L. S. (1998). Enhancing instructional programming and student achievement with curriculum-based measurement. In J. Kramer (Ed.), *Curriculum-based measurement: Examining old problems, evaluating new solutions* (pp. 17–48). Hillsdale, NJ: Erlbaum.

Fuchs, L. S., Fuchs, D., Hamlett, C. L., & Ferguson, C. (1992). Effects of expert system consultation within curriculum-based measurement, using a reading maze task. *Exceptional Children, 58,* 436–450.

Hoy, M. P., & Retish, P. M. (1984). A comparison of two types of assessment reports. *Exceptional Children, 51,* 225–229.

Kratochwill, T. R., Elliott, S. N., & Callan-Stoiber, K. (2002). Best practices in school-based problem-solving consultation. In A. Thomas & J. Grimes (Eds.), *Best practices in school psychology IV* (pp. 583–608). Bethesda, MD: National Association of School Psychologists.

Lichtenberger, E. O., Mather, N., Kaufman, N. L., & Kaufman, A. S. (2004). *Essentials of assessment report writing.* Hoboken, NJ: Wiley.

National Association of School Psychologists. (1997). Principles for professional ethics. Retrieved May 29, 2004, from *www.nasponline.org/certification/ethics.html*

Ownby, R. L. (1987). *Psychological reports: A guide to report writing in professional psychology.* Brandon, VT: Clinical Psychology Publishing.

Salend, S. R., & Salend, S. (1985). Writing and evaluating educational assessment reports. *Academic Therapy, 20,* 277–288.

Sattler, J. M. (2001). *Assessment of children: Cognitive applications* (4th ed.). San Diego: Sattler.

Tallent, N. (1993). *Psychological report writing* (3rd ed.). Englewood Cliffs, NJ: Prentice-Hall.

SUGGESTED READINGS

Sattler, J. M. (2001). *Assessment of children: Cognitive applications* (4th ed.). San Diego: Sattler.

This book offers a very comprehensive treatment of all aspects of assessment including information on report writing. Although not organized in a problem-solving format, the report writing information does cover the basic elements and provides information about what must be covered in psychoeducational reports.

Lichtenberger, E. O., Mather, N., Kaufman, N. L., & Kaufman, A. S. (2004). *Essentials of assessment report writing.* Hoboken, NJ: Wiley.

This book includes information on many aspects of report writing, including technical and mechanical features of formal English, ways of displaying scores, and how to handle situations when the results are ambiguous. Even though this book is not organized around the problem-solving format, it does provide a good introduction to report writing for new professionals.

CHAPTER 14

♦ ♦ ♦

The Administrative Role in Transforming Schools to Support Problem-Solving-Based Assessment for Educational Intervention

♦

MARY LYNN BOSCARDIN

The role of administrators, including special education directors, principals, curriculum supervisors, and superintendents, in introducing, guiding, selecting, and supporting the use of problem-solving-based assessment for educational intervention is important to the success of students with disabilities. Administrators equipped with the knowledge and skills to support the implementation of scientifically based instructional practices of teachers are poised to be effective advocates of improved educational outcomes of all students. In this chapter, we examine two ways in which administrators facilitate the development, adoption, use, and evaluation of problem-solving-based assessment for educational interventions within the school culture. One considers refocusing the administrator role from one of manager to one of effective instructional leader. The other focuses on key leadership strategies for establishing best practices to improve the instructional practices of teachers and the educational outcomes of students with disabilities. These two venues should serve to transform the leadership mission.

LEGISLATIVE BACKGROUND

The role of the administrator of special education has evolved from child advocate to compliance monitor and legal counsel since the passage of Public Law 94-142, the Education for All Handicapped Children Act in 1975. Following the passage of this landmark legislation, diligent administrators sought to develop programs in the public schools where few had existed. Gerber (1996, p. 156) characterized special education's purpose as challenging the status quo: "Special education's focus and priorities challenge schools to produce a radical form of social justice: equality of educational opportunity for students who are sometimes characterized by extreme individual differences." Administrators of special education are the individuals who have been primarily responsible for advocating and ensuring both legal compliance and the implementation of instructional strategies that would be of benefit to individual students with both mild and extreme differences.

The No Child Left Behind Act (NCLB, 2001), while imbuing many of the values of special education, supports the identification and use of evidence-based practices. The Individuals with Disabilities Education Act (IDEA, 2004) requires that students' individualized education plans (IEPs) complement general curricular frameworks so that each student with a disability has the opportunity to access the general curriculum and participate in statewide assessments in order to meet state standards. With the passage of NCLB, the reauthorization of IDEA, and the publication of *A New Era: Revitalizing Special Education for Children and Their Families* (President's Commission on Excellence in Special Education, 2002), focus has shifted to outcome measures related to state-mandated curricula for all students, including students with disabilities. The President's Commission recently heralded the NCLB legislation as the "driving force behind IDEA reauthorization" (p. 7). However, a critical question remains: Will better alignment between the *systems* of special and general education provide *students* with a greater opportunity to learn or with a diminished opportunity to receive the individually appropriate instruction they need to grow into productive adulthood?

These latest directives ask special education administrators to play an even more important role by promoting collaboration among general and special education teachers and administrators to assure that high-quality programs are accessible to all students regardless of ability (Boscardin, 2004; Lashley & Boscardin, 2003). Special education directors are being asked to work more closely with school principals and related administrative staff, such as curriculum directors, school psychologists, and guidance counselors, to assist in the development of a working knowledge of the law and research-based interventions that make the curriculum accessible to students with disabilities. The emphasis on collaboration in the legislation could not arrive at a more opportune time.

REFOCUSING THE ADMINISTRATIVE ROLE

Historically, the special education director has been in charge of the educational programming for students who meet the eligibility criteria to receive special education instruction. Goor (1995) captures the professional management qualities of flexibility, advocacy, and collaboration in noting that the typical administrator of special education must "be a facile communicator, proficient manager, astute politician, and strategic planner . . . advocating for the best possible services, empowering staff, acknowledging the needs of parents, and collaborating with other administrators" (p. 3). According to Lashley and Boscardin (2003), the role of the special education administrator is shifting:

> Special education administrators are now at a crossroads in the field. Their challenge will be introducing flexibility to how the curriculum is conceptualized, advocating for access to the general education curriculum and assessments with appropriate accommodations and modifications, and promoting collaboration between general and special education teachers and administrators to assure that high quality education programs are accessible to all students. (p. 3)

Not only has the role of the special education administrator changed with time, but also the role of the general education administrator has changed. With the advent of site-based managed schools, building-level administrators are challenged to redefine their roles in ways that promote positive results for students with disabilities through evidenced-based instruction. In practice, principals are the instructional leaders for all students, including students with disabilities, rather than building- or district-level managers for general education (Coyne, Kame'enui, & Simmons, 2004).

Murphy (2001) recommended that the field of educational leadership be recultured by highlighting "the centrality of learning, teaching, and school improvement within the role of the school administrator" (p. 15). Murphy identified four content areas supported by the leadership literature as essential to restructuring the organization of preservice administration programs: (1) developing caring and supportive behaviors and dispositions;

(2) acquiring knowledge of variables influencing change; (3) encouraging collegiality and collaboration; and (4) understanding the ethical and moral foundations of leadership.

Recent empirical work (Gronn, 2000; Leithwood, Steinbach, & Ryan, 1997; Polite, 1993; Wallace, 2002) has focused on school restructuring, but little is known about the distribution of leadership tasks and activities related to special education. Distributed leadership models might alter the process for determining district and school goals and involve staff assuming various leadership roles. Such change also might be at odds with the legal requirements of IDEA. The challenge for administrators will be to redefine the leadership mission, transforming the dual system of general and special education administration to a distributed system of leadership that collaboratively supports the use of proven practices to achieve schoolwide and districtwide improvement for students with disabilities, as well as for all the students in their charge.

Skrtic (1995) noted that the individually oriented "adhocracy" (p. 763) that promotes collaborative and individualized special education programming is in direct contradiction to the bureaucracy that governs centralized and efficiency-oriented general education programs. Skrtic (1995) explained how the collision of these values results in a dual system of education, one for general education students and one for special education students. At this juncture, one might ask how the problem-solving model can be implemented in a way that would not fuel the dual system about which Skrtic (1995) speaks. How might a problem-solving-based approach to this situation make the most sense and yield the best results for students over time?

The employment of Deno's (1995) problem-solving model aids in the development of caring supportive behaviors that are of benefit to all students, including those with disabilities. The problem-solving model empowers others to bring about important changes through identification, acquisition, allocation, coordination, and use of social, material, and cultural resources necessary for teaching and learning (Spillane, Halverson, & Diamond, 2001). Team collaboration is one of those activities that promotes distributed leadership. This collaborative effort, be it building-based support teams or IEP teams, engages a variety of actors (e.g., teachers, specialists, parents, administrators) and artifacts (e.g., classroom work samples, portfolios, assessment results), culminating in the sharing of language, theories of action, and interpretive schema used to make instructional decisions about learning outcomes. Problem-solving-based educational leadership exemplifies a school culture in which all perspectives and voices are valued as part of a process of identifying and defining the learning issues. The distributed leadership approach exemplifies a professional level of caring where ownership and commitment for student learning and instruction is spread among numerous actors.

The use of Deno's (1995) problem-solving model for assessment is key to acquiring knowledge of variables influencing change that will result in positive learning outcomes and improved instructional practices. By gathering the important teaching and learning artifacts embedded in formal accounts of day-to-day practice that are not smoothed over, it is possible to understand what it is we think we do as being separate from actual practice (Spillane et al., 2001). It is the difference between the espoused and reality. The development of effective interventions relies on objective discussion of student performance over a variety of tasks as well as an understanding of the resources necessary to implement needed supports.

For the problem-solving model to be an effective means of assessment and intervention, flexibility, collegiality, and collaboration among the varied actors are essential for the development of knowledge from practices that is context-sensitive and task-specific (Spillane et al., 2001). Distributive leadership is an important gateway for developing collegiality and collaboration among the various intervention teams intended to support teaching and learning. Cohen and Ball (1998) could not have captured the importance of collegiality and collaboration any better when they stated, "The capacity to produce worthwhile and substantive learning is a function of interaction among elements of the instructional unit, not the sole province of any single element" (p. 5). Each actor's willingness to forgo ownership of any particular perspective is critical to successfully implementing a problem-solving approach that focuses on the whole student and not just discrete aspects of performance.

Moral Leadership

Educational leadership does not occur in a moral vacuum, although the current centralizing, rational–technical, compliance-oriented approach to educational governance and the inherent cautiousness of public educators discourage many prospective educators from engaging in moral discourse (Lashley & Boscardin, 2003). The singular focus on compliance with the law when determining services often excludes questions about social justice. Are the educational decisions being made about students with disabilities moral ones that everyone can be certain are ethical and just decisions? Because the education of students with disabilities is filled with examples of injustice, discrimination, inequality and inequity, and denial of dignity, those in leadership roles are in a pivotal position to provide rich opportunities for discussions about moral leadership through use of the problem-solving model. This model offers a contextually sensitive environment for this conversation. The moral and ethical discussions about students with disabilities accomplish two purposes: (1) they provide teachers with an understanding of how difference has been dealt with (that is, through discrimination) in American schools, and (2) they provide the opportunity to think differently about difference and discrimination and the influence each has on instruction. These learning experiences can act as an introduction to the problems of difference and discrimination that serves to better contextualize the diversity of individuals with disabilities. Merely possessing a particular categorical disability does not mean sameness for all within that category, extending the discussion of difference to race, ethnicity, sex, socioeconomic status, and sexual orientation of those with disabilities.

LEADERSHIP STRATEGIES
FOR ESTABLISHING BEST PRACTICES

Educational outcomes always have been important, but with the advent of evidenced-based methods that ask for proof of increased performance, they have taken on even greater significance. Newly introduced initiatives will have to endure close scrutiny to determine whether the instructional interventions selected produce increased educational outcomes. This intense scrutiny has ushered in a renewed interest in the dimensions of instructional leadership at the school and district levels that has an impact on outcomes for high- and low-achieving students, particularly students with disabilities. Tied to these student-focused instructional leadership dimensions are dimensions of leadership at the school and district levels that have an impact on the improved performance of teachers responsible for their instruction. How administrators affect the learning contexts at the school and district levels will be considered in this section.

If we accept Crockett's (2003) thesis that "a scientific orientation in schools fosters (a) clear intentions in setting priorities, (b) knowledge-based decisions, (c) instructional flexibility and appropriate instructional groupings, and, (d) strong professional bonds among teachers," then we must acknowledge the need for a major shift in the roles of administrators in supporting instructional programs for students with disabilities.

Attending to Basic Team Tasks and Setting Clear Priorities

When forming any type of team or collaborative relationship, attending to basic housekeeping tasks is a necessity if the priorities identified are to be successfully adopted. These basic team tasks, according to Smith and Stodden (1998), include identifying group members, determining team leadership roles and responsibilities, establishing ground rules and operational procedures, creating or reaffirming the collective vision, listing desired outcomes, and developing an action plan for each desired outcome.

Administrators who attend to the basic team tasks will facilitate the ease with which the problem-solving approach is implemented. The challenge of setting clear priorities is substantially diminished when desired outcomes and action plans for the team or collaborative group are determined prior to attempting to implement the problem-solving model. If the implementation of problem-solving-based assessment for educational intervention is to be embraced by teachers, administrators must be able to clearly define their expectations. A series of sequentially developed team activities, akin to the flow evident in Deno's (1995) model, must be implemented to ensure successful adoption.

Encouraging Knowledge-Based Decisions

Administrators who promote knowledge-based decisions and evidence-based instruction to solve educational problems will produce enhanced educational outcomes for students and improved instructional practices for teachers. The introduction of Deno's (1995) problem-solving-based model is an optimal method for ensuring consistency of application by staff. Providing professional development activities that introduce each stage with clear definitions, illustrated examples, and multiple opportunities for practice is one way to produce consistency in application. Having supervisors available for coaching those applying the problem-solving methods in their daily practices supports appropriate adoption of the model. Administrators can foster knoweldge-based practices by requiring that all instructional activities be grounded in some form or prior evidence of efficacy. Additionally, they can insist that data on all interventions be collected regularly and used as part of future team meetings and decisions.

The Importance of Instructional Flexibility

Although Deno's model is synonymous with a series of procedural steps that lead to evidence-based instructional interventions, the process is not intended to be plagued by structural rigidity. Rather, instructional flexibility is needed if the solutions are to be successful, making it less likely that educational placement will be confused with educational programs (Sharp & Patasky, 2002). Administrators are pivotal to assisting teachers in making the curriculum accessible to students through the use of problem solving by emphasizing the importance of instruction being the best tool for improving student performance. Administrators must help teachers re-engineer instructional material and the learning environment if the curriculum is to become accessible to students with disabilities. This may require varied instructional groupings or alternate settings reflective of their pedagogical practices. The problem-solving model is intended to encourage creativity and flexibility for teachers as they think about the best methods and settings for student learning.

Creating Strong Professional Bonds among Teachers

Administrators have a unique opportunity to provide the support and understanding necessary to cultivate an environment that contributes to the retention of a high-quality teaching force. By promoting collegial and collaborative environments where the decision making is based on the implementation of a problem-solving paradigm by general and special educators, it is possible for administrators to create a nurturing, caring, and positive environment that contributes to the improvement of educational outcomes for all students and the instructional practices of teachers.

To accomplish this task, it is important to consider the principles by which teams operate. By using Smith and Stodden's (1998) nine principles of teaming, administrators can help teams:

- Develop a shared/collective vision.
- Promote empowerment of all members.
- Engage in shared decision making.
- Demonstrate synergistic energy.
- Use diversity as a necessary part of creativity and collaboration.
- Fully include people affected by change(s).
- Facilitate the self-determination and personal growth of team members.
- Operate within an ecological context.
- Assume a dynamic and fluid quality.

Administrators who are able to demonstrate these principles will be able to guide others through the curriculum frameworks and support specialized instruction, which ultimately should lead to improved educational outcomes for students and greater success for teachers.

CASE EXAMPLES

Two cases are presented in this section to illustrate how the problem-solving model might be introduced by using a distributed leadership approach. Even when school leaders work separately but interdependently in pursuit of a common goal, leadership practice can be stretched across the practice of two or more leaders.

Example 1

Consider by way of example the participation of the principal and special education director in a reevaluation meeting. At this meeting the principal and director of special education along with the other team members, which include the parents, classroom teacher, special education teacher, speech and language therapist, school psychologist, and school counselor/ social worker, will collaborate to produce an instructional program that meets the educational needs of the student with disabilities. Like most team meetings, each team member possesses critical information about the effects of instruction on the educational outcomes of the student; however, not all these assessments may be evidence-based (e.g., classroom teacher anecdotes about student performance in lieu of work examples, or the professional, non-data-based, judgments of related services personnel). The special and general education personnel are aware of the problem-solving model through various professional development opportunities, but supervised coaching of its use has not occurred to facilitate implementation for developing curriculum interventions.

The two administrators at this point could revert to past practices and make unilateral decisions, or they could seize this opportunity to forge instructional change. At this point, the administrators choose to model appropriate use of the problem-solving model for the reevaluation team. The administrators would want to proceed sequentially, defining and clarifying each step and providing examples of each stage as needed. In terms of the instructional planning for the new IEP, the administrators would ask each team member to suggest specific evidence-based methods and ways of measuring progress toward goals. The success of the intervention resulting from the reevaluation meeting is dependent on the collegiality, collaboration, and flexibility of the group. The administrators, in this case, use distributive leadership to cultivate these qualities, using the full participation of each team member as the catalyst.

Example 2

In our second example, two different leadership styles send mixed messages to teachers. Meredith, the principal, maintains a friendly and supportive relationship with teachers, visits classrooms frequently, and uses the clinical supervision model to provide consistent feedback to teachers on instructional issues. She talks to teachers prior to her observation to determine areas of focus, observes their classroom instruction, and follows up with a postobservation conversation. Rarely, however, is there discussion of the problem-solving model during supervision meetings. The special education director, Jahmal, on the other hand, functions more as an authority figure with a much more formal relationship with his staff, who refer to him as "Doctor." He oversees special education programs and budgets for this district, reviews compliance issues, and makes final determinations about the quality of special education teachers' and related personnel's instructional practices. The two administrators have had the problem-solving model introduced to them during administrative professional development seminars and think they would like to implement it.

In this example, the administrators may choose to combine their expertise and integrate their roles and alter meeting expectations, which could be interpreted to mean it will not be "business as usual." The administrators decide to use both the clinical supervision model and the already in place building-based support teams, otherwise known as child study teams, to introduce and implement the problem-solving model (see Chapter 4, this volume). Using these teams has an advantage because they can simultaneously be used as an opportunity for team members to elevate their commitment to one another and the team. To begin the metamorphosis, the administrators ask teams to identify or adopt a shared vision. Simulated cases are used to introduce the steps of problem solving that lead to the implementation of evidence-based interventions. Once teams begin working toward the same goal, members are queried about their experience with the problem-solving process and the need for diversity of thought to creatively and collaboratively arrive at possible solutions.

By noting how different each of the simulated cases is from the others, the administrators are able to help team members understand that a dynamic and fluid ecological context is needed for the problem-solving model to operate successfully. In this example, the administrators created a situation in which teams learn that if they commit themselves to this model, each member, almost by default, begins to engage in self-determination and personal growth that naturally evolves into individual and group empowerment. In this second example, the principal can employ the clinical supervision model to reinforce the use of the problem-solving model by staff, and by becoming more collaborative the director of special education would reshape his or her role as one of instructional leader rather than authority figure.

CONCLUSION

The challenge for administrators will be to redefine the leadership, transforming the dual system of general and special education administration to a distributed system of leadership that collaboratively supports the use of proven practices to achieve schoolwide and districtwide improvement for students with disabilities, as well as for all the students in their charge. In an era of instructional accountability, it is imperative that administrators be able to transform schoolhouses into places that support positive outcomes for students with disabilities and foster the use of evidence-based instructional practices by teachers. Two ways of creating supportive administrative roles are to shift the administrative role from one of manager to one of instructional leader, and to use leadership strategies to establish effective evidence-based instructional practices that improve the educational outcomes for all students, including those with disabilities. Administrators have a critical role to play in supporting the use of a problem-solving model for educational intervention.

REFERENCES

Boscardin, M. L. (2004). Transforming administration to support science in the schoolhouse for students with disabilities. *Journal of Learning Disabilities, 37,* 262–269.

Cohen, D. K., & Ball, D. L. (1998). *Instruction, capacity, and improvement* (CPRE Research Report Series, RR-42). Philadelphia: University of Pennsylvania, Consortium for Policy Research in Education.

Coyne, M. D., Kame'enui, E. J., & Simmons, D. C. (2004). Improving beginning reading instruction and intervention for students with learning disabilities: Reconciling "all" with "each." *Journal of Learning Disabilities, 37,* 231–239.

Crockett, J. B. (2004). Taking stock of science in the schoolhouse: Four ideas to foster effective instruction. *Journal of Learning Disabilities, 37,* 189–199.

Deno, S. (1995). School psychologist as problem solver. In A. Thomas & J. Grimes (Eds.), *Best practices in school psychology III* (pp. 471–484). Washington, DC: National Association of School Psychologists.

Education for All Handicapped Children Act, 20 U.S.C. §1400 *et seq.* (1975).

Gerber, M. M. (1996). Reforming special education: "Beyond inclusion." In C. Christensen & F. Rizvi (Eds.), *Disability and the dilemmas of education and justice* (pp. 156–174). Philadelphia: Open University Press.

Goor, M. B.(1995). *Leadership for special administration: A case-based approach.* Fort Worth, TX: Harcourt Brace.

Gronn, P. (2000). Distributed properties: A new architecture for leadership. *Educational Management and Administration, 28,* 317–338.

Individuals with Disabilities Education Act, 20 U.S.C. §1400 *et seq.* (1997).

Individuals with Disabilities Education Act, 20 U.S.C. §1401 *et seq.* (1999).

Individuals with Disabilities Education Act, 20 U.S.C. §1400 *et seq.* (2004).

Lashley, C., & Boscardin, M. L. (2003). Special education administration at a crossroads. *Journal of Special Education Leadership, 16,* 63–75.

Leithwood, K., Steinbach, R., & Ryan, S. (1997). Leadership and team learning in secondary schools. *School Leadership & Management, 17,* 303–325.

Murphy, J. (2001, November). The changing face of leadership preparation. *The School Administrator,* 14–17.

No Child Left Behind Act, 20 U.S.C. §6301 *et seq.* (2001).

Polite, M. (1993). *A case of distributed leadership: Middle school transformation beyond initial transition.* Paper presented at the annual meeting of the American Educational Research Association, Atlanta (Eric Document No. ED360733).

President's Commission on Excellence in Special Education. (2002). *A new era: Revitalizing special education for children and their families.* Washington, DC: Office of Special Education and Rehabilitative Services. Retrieved February 23, 2003, from *www.ed.gov/inits/commissionsboards/whspecialeducation/*

Sharp, K. G., & Patasky, V. M. (2002). *The current legal status of inclusion.* Horsham, PA: LRP Publications.

Skrtic, T. M. (1995). The organizational context of special education and school reform.

In E. L. Meyen & T. M. Skrtic (Eds.), *Special education and student disability: Traditional, emerging, and alternative perspectives* (pp. 731–791). Denver: Love.

Smith, G. J., & Stodden, R. A. (1998). Handbook for improving special needs programs and practices through quality partnerships: The nine principles of teaming. In P. D. Kohler, S. Field, M. Izzo, & J. Johnson (Eds.), *Transition from school to life: A workshop series for educators and transition service providers.* Champaign, IL: Transition Research Institute.

Spillane, J. P., Halverson, R., & Diamond, J. B. (2001). Investigating school leadership practice: A distributed perspective. *Educational Researcher, 30*(3), 23–28.

Wallace, M. (2002). Modeling distributed leadership and management effectiveness: Primary school senior management teams in England and Wales. *School Effectiveness and School Improvement, 13,* 163–186.

SUGGESTED READINGS

Burrello, L. C., Lashley, C., & Beatty, E. E. (2000). *Educating all students together: How school leaders create unified systems.* Thousand Oaks, CA: Corwin Press.

The authors call for an end to the piecemeal strategy of including students in one classroom, one grade level, or one school at a time. Instead, this work presents ways in which administrators, school leaders, and the community can collaborate on decisions to implement personalized education plans, accountable curricular outcomes, and appropriate instructional adaptations.

Some of the key concepts include:

- Schools embracing special services personnel
- The roles of the community and other stakeholders
- Reconceptualizing schools based on learner-centered principles
- Program evaluation and incentives
- Brain and holographic design as a framework for complex adaptive systems
- Collaboration between school administrators and teachers
- Adapting curriculum and instruction

Effective leadership strategies are presented that enable administrators to better manage the cultural imperative of equity and excellence for all students. They further support the plan for unified schools through case studies and a program evaluation self-study guide.

Murphy, J. (2005). *Connecting teacher leadership and school improvement.* Thousand Oaks, CA: Corwin Press.

This book synthesizes theoretical, empirical, and practice-based literature in order to provide a comprehensive look at what is known about teacher leadership and what works to support it. The first part of the book explores the core concepts of teacher leadership, while the second part shows readers how to establish the context in their school or district to cultivate and support teacher leaders.

A vital piece of equipment in the school improvement toolbox, this book covers such important topics as:

- The principal's critical role in supporting teacher leadership
- Cultivating teacher leadership through professional development
- Overcoming organizational barriers that hinder teacher leadership
- How teacher leadership can help advance school improvement efforts

The ideological and empirical basis of teacher leadership is examined through a comprehensive model of change strategy in an effort to help teachers and principals create productive relationships that will strengthen our nation's schools.

Spark, D. (2004). *Leading for results: Transforming teaching, learning, and relationships in schools*. Thousand Oaks, CA: Corwin Press.

This textbook consists of 26 short, interactive essays to aid leaders in reflecting on change and committing to action. School leaders are shown how they can be accountable and achieve meaningful results for schools, districts, and their personal lives. Incorporating cutting-edge theories about improving the quality of leadership, teaching, and student learning, ideas are transformed into action to help administrators:

- examine assumptions and produce results-oriented thoughts, words, and actions;
- deepen understanding of important issues related to the interpersonal challenges of change; and
- engage in next-action thinking and applying what they have learned.

CHAPTER 15

♦ ♦ ♦

Treatment Integrity Assessment within a Problem-Solving Model

♦

LISA HAGERMOSER SANETTI
THOMAS R. KRATOCHWILL

The purpose of this chapter is to explain the role of treatment integrity assessment within the "implementing solutions" stage of a problem-solving model. Treatment integrity is the degree to which an intervention is implemented as planned (Yeaton & Sechrest, 1981). The purpose of assessing treatment integrity is to determine whether all of the components of an intervention are being implemented as planned on a consistent basis so that appropriate conclusions can be made about its effectiveness.

Let's take, for example, the case of Ms. Holden, an elementary school teacher who is frustrated with Tommy, who is often disruptive in class. Dr. Sawyer, the school psychologist, consults with Ms. Holden and develops the following intervention plan: Ms. Holden will (1) monitor Tommy's behavior during each instructional period, (2) chart the level of behavior on a goal chart created by Dr. Sawyer and Ms. Holden, and (3) provide Tommy with a reward for prosocial behavior above the specified criterion on a daily basis. After 2 weeks of implementing the intervention, a distraught Ms. Holden stops by Dr. Sawyer's office and gripes that she is not seeing consistent improvement in Tommy's behavior, doesn't know if Tommy's behavior will ever improve, and thinks he may require special education services. Based on Ms. Holden's report, Dr. Sawyer concludes that the intervention was ineffective and develops a new intervention plan that includes significant negative consequences for Tommy's disruptive behavior. Had Dr. Sawyer and Ms. Holden assessed treatment integrity throughout the intervention, as they did for Tommy's behavior, they would have realized that Ms. Holden was not consistently implementing all of the intervention components. Such treatment integrity data would have allowed them to revisit the feasibility of the intervention plan before Ms. Holden became frustrated and a punitive intervention was considered. As you can see from this example, the information gained from treatment integrity assessment can help school personnel evaluate the functional relationship between the implementation of an intervention and changes in a target behavior or skill.

The remainder of this chapter will provide more detailed information about treatment integrity and its assessment. The chapter begins by providing information on how treatment integrity evolved as a methodological concern as well as how researchers have addressed treatment integrity assessment in the intervention outcomes literature. Next, factors related to treatment integrity, methods of assessing treatment integrity, and strategies to increase treatment integrity are discussed. Finally, a case example illustrating a treatment integrity assessment within the problem-solving process is presented.

THE EVOLUTION OF TREATMENT INTEGRITY AS A METHODOLOGICAL CONCERN

Only recently has treatment integrity come to the forefront as an important methodological consideration in the social and behavioral sciences (Moncher & Prinz, 1991). Early psychotherapy researchers paid virtually no attention to the quality, uniformity, nature, or amount of psychotherapy provided (VandenBos & Pino, 1980). Generally, researchers pooled "treated" patients together for data analysis and provided only vague descriptions of the treatments under study (VandenBos & Pino, 1980). Descriptions of the treatments were often all-encompassing categorical labels (e.g., psychoanalytic or client-centered) or described according to the name of the individual (e.g., Rogers or Erikson) who pioneered the therapy approach (Moncher & Prinz, 1991).

Hans Eysenck's (1952) article "The Effects of Psychotherapy: An Evaluation" challenged the complacency of the mental health community by questioning the efficacy of psychotherapy (VandenBos & Pino, 1980). For the first time, there was a demand for accountability in psychotherapy research. Since that time, there has been a dramatic increase in the use of accountability procedures in intervention research. Intervention integrity is now championed from many corners, including the U.S. Congress, insurance companies, and consumer groups (Fireman, 2002; VandenBos & Pino, 1980). Thus, it is not surprising that a wide range of perspectives within the social and behavioral sciences (i.e., researchers in the areas of learning disabilities, social skills intervention, special education programs, and school-based behavioral consultation) have come to recognize the importance of treatment integrity assessment as "best practice."

WHY TREATMENT INTEGRITY ASSESSMENT IS A METHODOLOGICAL CONCERN

Treatment integrity assessment allows practitioners to make valid conclusions about the functional relationship between the implementation of an intervention and changes in student performance. Failure to ensure high levels of treatment integrity results in threats to the validity of interventions. There are four types of validity that allow researchers and practitioners to draw conclusions from intervention trials: (1) internal validity, (2) external validity, (3) construct validity, and (4) statistical conclusion validity.

Although it is generally assumed that an intervention agent implemented an intervention as planned, it is possible that he or she altered the intervention plan in a way unknown to anyone else and thus compromised internal validity (i.e., conclusions about the degree to which changes in the dependent variable can be ascribed to the manipulations of the independent variable). Such alterations have been coined "therapist drift" by Peterson, Homer, and Wonderlich (1982) and could have positive, negative, or neutral effects. For instance, an effective but poorly implemented intervention could be considered ineffective as a result of modifications in implementation. On the other hand, an ineffective intervention may be deemed effective as a result of adjustments in implementation unknown to anyone aside from the intervention agent.

In terms of external validity (i.e., conclusions about the extent to which the causal relationship between the independent and dependent variables generalizes to conditions beyond those of the experiment), it is difficult, if not impossible to replicate, evaluate, and generalize an intervention that is poorly defined, described, or implemented. To this effect, treatment integrity assessments are useful in that they require an operational definition of the intervention components and can therefore provide guidance for others who attempt to replicate the intervention. Construct validity (i.e., conclusions about the higher-order constructs represented by the persons, treatments, outcomes, and settings studied) is also influenced by treatment integrity. Without an operational definition of intervention components, it is difficult to rule out potential confounds that could affect the interpretation of the causal relationship between the intervention and student outcomes.

Intervention effectiveness data can also be influenced by the integrity with which an intervention was implemented. Inconsistent implementation or deviations in implementation can result in lower effect sizes, currently the most common metric for reporting intervention effectiveness, thus threatening the statistical conclusion validity of an intervention study (Gresham, MacMillan, Beebe-Frankenberger, & Bocian, 2000). Together, the four main types of treatment validity incorporate the core desired features of interventions. In order for an intervention to be demonstrably valid, it needs to be implemented with consistency and accuracy.

TREATMENT INTEGRITY ASSESSMENT IN THE INTERVENTION OUTCOMES LITERATURE

Recognizing that treatment integrity assessment is essential to drawing valid conclusions regarding intervention effectiveness, we now examine how researchers in the social and behavioral sciences have addressed treatment integrity in the treatment outcomes literature. Several reviews of treatment integrity in outcome literature (Gresham, Gansle, & Noell, 1993; Gresham et al., 2000; Peterson et al., 1982) have been conducted in recent years. Although each provides valuable information regarding the prevalence and quality of treatment integrity data in outcome literature, the results of these reviews are limited by their inability to be directly compared to one another due to differing methodologies and areas of focus.

Peterson and colleagues (1982) conducted one of the earliest and most influential reviews of treatment integrity assessment. They reviewed all of the experimental articles published in the *Journal of Applied Behavior Analysis (JABA)* from the journal's inception in 1968 (Volume 1, Number 1) to 1980 (Volume 13, Number 3). The type of treatment integrity assessment reported in each article was rated in terms of three categories: (1) some form of assessment reported; (2) no assessment was reported, but it was deemed unnecessary; or (3) no assessment was reported, and an assessment was deemed necessary. Likewise, the intervention definition reported in each article was rated in terms of three categories: (1) an operational definition was reported; (2) no operational definition was reported, but it was deemed unnecessary; or (3) no operational definition was reported, and a definition was deemed necessary. Data resulting from these ratings indicated that a majority of the experimental articles rated did include a definition of the intervention; however, they did not include treatment integrity assessment even when there was a high risk of inaccurate implementation.

Among the articles that included operational definitions, only an average of 16% (range 3–34%) also included a check on the accuracy of the implementation of the independent variable (Peterson et al., 1982). Thus, it appeared that researchers were more likely to operationally define interventions than assess their implementation. Nonetheless, it is important to note that over the 12-year span a slight increase in the percentage of experimental articles including treatment integrity assessment was evident.

In an effort to update the work of Peterson et al. (1982), Gresham, Gansle, and Noell (1993), reviewed experimental studies conducted with children and published in *JABA* between 1980 and 1990. Studies were considered to include an operational definition of the intervention if it could be replicated based on the description provided, while the treatment integrity assessment was rated in terms of three categories: (1) yes (quantitative data were provided); (2) monitored (mentioned assessment but no quantitative data were provided), and (3) not mentioned. Results of the review indicated that just under one-third (54 studies) of the 158 child studies provided an operational definition of the intervention. Furthermore, 25 studies (15.8%) assessed and reported levels of treatment integrity, 14 studies (8.9 %) reported monitoring treatment integrity but did not provide quantitative data, and the remaining 75.3% of the studies did not report treatment integrity data. The mean level of treatment integrity for the 25 studies that did report treatment integrity data was 93.8% (range 54–100%), with over half reporting 100% integrity.

Using the same coding criteria, Gresham, Gansle, Noell, Cohen, and Rosenblum (1993) reviewed experimental school-based studies published in multiple journals between 1980 and 1990. A large plurality (48.6%) of the school-based intervention studies reviewed utilized two or more interventions. Of the 181 studies reviewed, 35% (64 studies) provided an operational definition of the intervention(s). Only 14.9% (27) of the 181 studies were reported as having formally assessed and reported levels of treatment integrity for the independent variables, while 18 studies included treatment integrity monitoring but provided no quantitative data. The mean level of treatment integrity for the 27 studies that did include integrity assessment was 96.9% (range 75–100%).

In an effort to further extend this line of research and evaluate the extent to which treatment integrity is assessed in the learning disabilities intervention research, Gresham et al. (2000) reviewed articles published in three learning disabilities journals between January 1995 and August 1999. Of the 65 intervention articles reviewed, 18.5% (12 articles) assessed and reported treatment integrity data. Approximately one-half of the intervention studies reviewed alluded to or qualitatively described treatment integrity, but provided no numerical data regarding the number of treatment components implemented. Treatment integrity was not addressed in over 30% of the learning disabilities intervention articles reviewed.

Together, these reviews demonstrate a general lack of treatment integrity assessment in the intervention outcomes literature. Approximately 30% of the articles in the reviews (barring Peterson et al., 1982, which did not provide exact figures) provided an operational definition of the intervention, and fewer than 20% of the articles in these reviews reported treatment integrity data. Although not all of these reviews are directly comparable due to methodological differences, the absence of attention to treatment integrity assessment within intervention research is clear. One potential reason why treatment integrity has not been assessed may in part be due to the lack of knowledge about *how* it should be assessed. Understanding the construct of treatment integrity is an essential first step toward its assessment.

CONCEPTUALIZATIONS OF TREATMENT INTEGRITY

Yeaton and Sechrest (1981) provided one of the first conceptualizations of the interrelationship between treatment strength, integrity, and effectiveness and emphasized the importance of this interrelationship to treatment planning and execution. In their conceptualization, the authors emphasized four points. First, they stressed the importance of choosing theoretically strong interventions independent of knowledge of the outcome of the treatment in any given case. Choosing a theoretically strong intervention alone, however, may not be sufficient to increase the likelihood of treatment efficacy, as it is possible for a theoretically strong intervention to be ineffective if it is poorly implemented. Simply stated, "No amount of care in research design and statistical analysis can compensate for carelessness in planning and implementing treatments" (Yeaton & Sechrest, 1981, p. 161).

Second, the authors stated the importance of considering the *correlation* between a treatment's strength and the level of treatment integrity. In general, it is assumed that any decrease in treatment integrity will result in decreased treatment strength and effectiveness, and therefore treatments need to be implemented perfectly at all times. Although this is likely to be true for some treatments, it is possible that some treatments are more "immune to degradation" than others (Yeaton & Sechrest, 1981). Knowing what components of a treatment are essential to effectiveness is powerful and possible, if treatment integrity is monitored throughout implementation.

Third, the authors emphasized that treatment implementation is not a unitary concept. Whereas monitoring treatment implementation is essential to knowing a treatment's level of integrity, areas related to treatment implementation such as the complexity of the intervention and the professional competence of the treatment agent should also be taken into account. A complex, time-consuming, challenging treatment demanding multiple participants is likely to result in problems obtaining and maintaining high levels of treatment integrity (Yeaton & Sechrest, 1981). Furthermore, the authors proposed that highly skilled individuals may have more consistent levels of integrity across treatments whereas individuals with less training may have more variable integrity levels across treatments due to the varying complexity of the interventions. Finally, the authors noted that when a lapse in integrity is identified through monitoring of treatment implementation, contingencies might be used as a strategy to increase and maintain high levels of treatment integrity. Specifically, although physical or financial contingencies may not be necessary immediately or in every case, the authors noted that researchers and clinicians may need to utilize them toward the goals of treatment integrity, treatment effectiveness, and valid conclusions.

This early conceptualization of treatment integrity called upon researchers and clinicians to consider the importance of treatment integrity for the purpose of guaranteeing the appropriate level of integrity for every treatment. Such a guarantee requires (1) planning treatments with the appropriate strength, (2) being aware of factors related to the treatment that may influence treatment integrity, (3) implementing treatments with high levels of integrity, (4) monitoring integrity throughout implementation, and (5) using strategies such as contingencies to encourage high levels of implementation.

Gresham (1989) provided a second conceptualization of treatment integrity focusing predominately on factors that appear to be related to treatment integrity in school settings. According to this conceptualization, school professionals may be able to improve the level of integrity with which an intervention is implemented by considering these factors when developing an intervention plan:

1. Complexity of the treatment.
2. Time required to implement the intervention.
3. Materials or resources necessary to implement the intervention.
4. Number of intervention agents needed.
5. Motivation of the intervention agent(s).
6. Perceived and actual effectiveness of the intervention.

Complexity of the Treatment

The level of treatment integrity is directly related to the complexity of an intervention. For instance, an intervention that requires simultaneous use of multiple strategies may overwhelm the intervention agent and result in low treatment integrity. Therefore, if a range of equally strong intervention options exist, it is preferable to choose a less complex intervention. Likewise, if a complex, multifaceted intervention is necessary, it may be beneficial to introduce the central intervention components first, adding on layers of intervention strategies only once the intervention agent becomes fluent with the core components.

Time Required to Implement the Intervention

A lack of time is the most common reason provided by teachers for not implementing an intervention (Happe, 1982). The amount of time it takes a teacher to implement an intervention is influenced by other factors, such as the complexity of the intervention (i.e., the more complex the intervention, the more time it will require to implement). Therefore, it is important to consider the interaction among factors in addition to the factors themselves. In addition to the time required for the intervention itself, the competing demands of the intervention environment need to be considered.

Materials/Resources Necessary to Implement the Intervention

Understanding how to implement an intervention is a basic resource required to implement an intervention with a high level of integrity. Results from a recent line of research (Sterling-Turner, Watson, & Moore, 2002; Sterling-Turner, Watson, Wildmon, Watkins, & Little, 2001) indicated that direct training procedures, such as modeling and rehearsal feedback, were associated with higher levels of treatment integrity. Interventions that require materials or resources that are not readily available in a school setting (e.g., commercially packaged intervention materials) or to an intervention agent within the school setting (e.g., 4 hours weekly to conduct a one-to-one intervention) can decrease the intervention agent's ability to attain or maintain a high level of intervention integrity. When special or external resources are provided for an intervention (e.g., via a grant or a community agency partnership), it is especially important to consider how the intervention could be sustained should the resources be removed.

Number of Intervention Agents Needed

Interventions that require multiple agents are likely to be more complex, which require more time, and are therefore less likely to be implemented with a high level of integrity. For example, if two teachers job share, and the teacher present in the mornings has high integrity and the afternoon teacher has low integrity, the overall integrity will be lower than if only the first teacher could have served as the intervention agent. On the other hand, interventions that require multiple intervention agents are likely to have more strength and may generalize more across settings.

Motivation of the Intervention Agent(s)

How motivated an intervention agent is to bring about change is also important to consider. For instance, if a teacher requests assistance with a student in the hope that the student will be removed from the classroom, he or she may not be highly motivated to implement an intervention with a high level of integrity as compared to a teacher motivated to keep the student in his or her classroom. Even teachers who want to keep a student in their classroom may be unmotivated to implement an intervention with a high level of integrity if he or she (1) is not trained to implement the intervention, (2) does not believe in the theoretical underpinnings of the intervention, or (3) cannot easily incorporate the intervention into daily classroom activities.

Perceived and Actual Effectiveness of the Intervention

Previous research in the area of treatment acceptability (e.g., VonBrock & Elliott, 1987) suggests that the more effective an intervention is, or is perceived to be, the higher the level of treatment integrity (Gresham, 1989). Therefore, when developing an intervention plan, it is important to gauge the teacher's perception of or previous experience with that intervention. If the teacher, for whatever reason, does not believe that a particular intervention is going to work before implementation begins, it is less likely that the teacher will implement it with a high level of integrity. Conversely, if a teacher finds the intervention plan acceptable and quickly sees positive results, he or she is more likely to continue implementing it with a high level of integrity.

Once an intervention plan is developed with these factors in mind, the next step is to assess treatment integrity throughout implementation and intervene when the assessments indicate that it is being implemented with a low level of integrity.

METHODS TO ASSESS TREATMENT INTEGRITY

Treatment integrity can be assessed via indirect or direct methods. Indirect assessments can take many forms such as self-reports, behavioral rating scales, and behavioral interviews (Gresham, 1997). Teacher self-report measures can be completed at the end of the day and are often used to assess treatment integrity. Such measures require (1) an operational definition of each intervention component, (2) a framework for rating each intervention component (e.g., Likert scale, free response), and (3) the completion of the scale after implementation (see Figure 15.1). Teacher self-report measures, however, may result in reactive effects resulting in either an over-

Date: __ / __ / __ Class: <u>4th Grade Homeroom</u>

Teacher's Name: <u>Mrs. Becker</u> School: <u>Brighton Elementary</u>

Directions: The individual implementing this intervention is to complete this form at the end of every day regarding how they implemented the intervention during *that* day.

1. Intervention implemented by (check one): ☑ Teacher ☐ Other: _____

	Strongly Disagree				Strongly Agree
2. I described the response cost lottery system to the class.	1	2	3	4	⑤
3. I displayed and described the rewards that students could receive in the lottery.	1	2	3	4	⑤
4. I placed a 3 × 5 inch card on top of each student's desk.	1	2	3	4	⑤
5. I taped the card on three sides with one side open.	1	2	3	4	⑤
6. I inserted four slips of colored paper inside each card, using different colors for each student.	1	2	3	4	⑤
7. I removed slips for each card whenever a student violated a class rule.	1	2	③	4	5
8. I restated the class rule whenever a student violated the rule.	①	2	3	4	5
9. I placed the remaining tickets in the lottery box after lottery time concluded today.	1	2	3	④	5
10. I conducted the drawing for the winner today (Friday only).	1	2	3	4	⑤
11. The winner was allowed to select a reward (Friday only).	1	2	3	4	⑤
12. Intervention implemented in homeroom classroom.	1	2	3	4	⑤
13. Intervention implemented during instructional time.	1	2	3	4	⑤
14. Intervention implemented with entire class.	1	2	3	4	⑤

15. The lottery was in effect for: (< ½ hour)   ½ hour   > ½ hour

16. Intervention implemented once today.	1	2	3	4	⑤

☐ No deviations from the intervention plan

☑ I deviated from the intervention plan in the following ways:

<u>Was not consistent in recognizing violations of class rules. Restated the class rules</u>
<u>only at the end of the lottery session.</u>

FIGURE 15.1. Example of a self-report treatment integrity assessment.

or and underestimation of the level of treatment integrity. Other options include using behavioral rating scales or interviews; the length and complexity of such methods may make routine assessment of treatment integrity difficult.

Teacher self-monitoring (i.e., simultaneously implementing an intervention and assessing integrity) has not received a lot of attention from researchers as a viable direct measure of treatment integrity, as it may be incompatible with the implementation of an intervention. Direct observation is the most commonly used direct method to assess treatment integrity. Directly observing treatment integrity is identical to systematically observing any behavior in applied settings, and therefore factors such as the number of observation sessions and the reactivity of observations need to be taken into consideration (see Foster & Cone, 1986). Direct observation of treatment integrity requires (1) an operational definition of the intervention components, (2) a record of the occurrence or nonoccurrence of each component, and (3) a calculation of the percentage of treatment components implemented (see Figure 15.2).

The results of a study by Wickstrom, Jones, LaFleur, and Witt (1998) demonstrate the potential pros and cons of assessing treatment integrity via observation and self-report. This study examined the treatment integrity of 27 teachers participating in behavioral consultation. Treatment integrity was assessed with three measures of varying methodological rigor: (1) the Baseline and Intervention Record Form (BIRF), a teacher-completed rating scale; (2) a stimulus product; and (3) direct observation. Mean integrity for the least rigorous method, BIRF, was 54%. The presence of stimulus materials increased the mean integrity to 62%. Observations of treatment use, however, indicated that the mean percentage of target behaviors followed by the appropriate consequence was only 4%. The authors note that, while these disparate results could be influenced by issues such as measurement error or missed observations, it is also important to consider that they could be dependent on the method of assessment utilized. Thus, when interpreting outcome research, one should consider not only *whether* treatment integrity was assessed but also the type of measure used and how it may influence resulting treatment integrity data. Likewise, using multiple methods of assessment and examining assessment results for convergent findings in a practice setting will provide the richest information about how completely and consistently an intervention is being implemented.

Determining how completely and consistently an intervention is being implemented requires that the assessment consider all of the components of a specific intervention. Although some manualized interventions include treatment integrity assessment measures (e.g., see Webster-Stratton & Reid, 2003), there are currently no published all-purpose treatment integrity assessment measures. As a result, a different treatment integrity assessment must be created for each intervention implemented. Although this sounds

Date: __ / __ / __   Class: <u>4th Grade Homeroom</u>   School: <u>Brighton Elementary</u>

Teacher's Name: <u>Mrs. Becker</u>   Consultant: <u>Ms. Raterman</u>

Directions: The consultant will complete this form during a 30-minute observation of Mrs. Becker's 4th-grade class during instructional time. Any alterations to the intervention protocol will be in last column.

	Yes	No	Description of any alterations to the intervention plan:
1. Intervention agent was Mrs. Becker.	☑	☐	
2. Intervention implemented in homeroom classroom.	☑	☐	
3. Intervention implemented during instructional time.	☑	☐	
4. Intervention implemented with entire class.	☑	☐	
5. The lottery was in effect for 30 minutes.	☐	☑	*Only implemented for 20 minutes*
6. Intervention implemented once today.	☑	☐	

	Low Integrity				High Integrity	
7. Described the response cost lottery system to the class.	1	2	3	4	⑤	
8. Displayed and described the rewards that students could receive in the lottery.	1	2	3	4	⑤	
9. 3 × 5 inch card on top of each student's desk.	1	2	3	4	⑤	
10. Card taped on three sides with one side open.	1	2	3	4	⑤	
11. Four slips of colored paper inside each card (different colors for each student).	1	2	3	4	⑤	
12. Slips removed contingent on rule violations.	1	2	③	4	5	
13. Teacher restates rule contingent on violation.	①	2	3	4	5	*Restated rules only one time*
14. Remaining tickets placed in lottery box.	1	2	3	④	5	
15. Drawing occurs on Friday.	1	2	3	4	⑤	
16. Winner selects reinforcer on Friday.	1	2	3	4	⑤	

FIGURE 15.2. Example of a direct observation treatment integrity assessment.

like a daunting task, it need not be, because treatment integrity assessments can be created in a straightforward manner by completing the following three steps: (1) define the intervention; (2) define the basic who, what, when, and where aspects of the intervention plan; and (3) divide the intervention into specific components, each with its own assessment plan.

Define the Intervention

First, define the intervention in terms of its specific verbal, physical, temporal, and spatial parameters. For example, an investigation by Mace, Page, Ivancic, and O'Brien (1986) provides an excellent illustration of the definition of a time-out procedure:

> (a) Immediately following the occurrence of a target behavior (temporal dimension), (b) the therapist said "No, go to time-out" (verbal dimension), (c) led the child by the arm to a pre-positioned time-out chair (physical dimension), and (d) seated the child facing the corner (spatial dimension). (e) If the child's buttocks were raised from the time-out chair or if the child's head was turned more than 45 degrees (spatial dimension), the therapist used the least amount of force necessary to guide compliance with the time-out procedure (physical dimension). (f) At the end of two minutes (temporal dimension), the therapist turned the time-out chair 45 degrees from the corner (physical and spatial dimension), and walked away (physical dimension). (cited in Gresham, 1997, p. 104)

Defining variables in such a detailed manner will enable the individuals who designed (e.g., school psychologist) and implemented (e.g., teacher) the intervention to have a common understanding of how the intervention is to be implemented.

Define the Implementation Details of the Intervention Plan

Second, define the basic information about the intervention plan including (1) who will implement the intervention, (2) where, when, and how often the intervention components will take place, (3) how long the intervention session will last, and (4) who will receive the intervention. If any specialized materials are needed for the intervention, these should be described as well.

Divide the Intervention into Specific Components and Plan Their Assessment

Third, divide the intervention components into steps that retain the specific behavioral information included in the intervention definition. Next, describe each intervention component in terms of (1) how implementation will be assessed, (2) how frequency of implementation will be assessed, (3) how the duration of implementation will be assessed (e.g., free response, multiple-choice time ranges), and (4) how deviations from the original implementation plan will be assessed (e.g., have implementation agents check a box indicating a deviation and obtain a specific description).

In addition to constructing a treatment integrity assessment, it is essential to consider the psychometric properties of the assessment. Gresham (1989) proposed that the behavioral concept of measurement accuracy may be the most pertinent psychometric principle in evaluating treatment integrity. Accuracy refers to how sensitive a measure is to what is true about the behavior in question. This method lends itself to treatment integrity assessments, as the components necessary for accuracy-based assessment align with the guidelines set forth for treatment integrity assessment. For instance, for a measure to be accurate, an operational definition must be provided for each component prior to use of the measure. These definitions provide a "gold standard" against which data from the use of the measure can be compared to obtain a percentage of components implemented as intended.

Monitoring treatment integrity using multiple methods will provide reliable data to analyze the functional relationship between the implementation of an intervention and change in a student's progress. Ideally, all interventions would be implemented with 100% integrity, and as a result all students who received interventions would make great gains. However, in reality, not all interventions are implemented with a high level of integrity, and not all interventions, even when implemented with high integrity, result in student progress. In the latter case, the psychologist may need to return to the "exploring solutions" stage of the problem-solving process and select another intervention, taking into account its evidence base and the likelihood of its being implemented with a high level of integrity. Another possibility is that one may need to return to the "problem identification" stage of the problem-solving process to reevaluate the accuracy of the identified problem. When treatment integrity assessment data indicate that an intervention is not being implemented completely and consistently, the first step is to intervene with the treatment agent to increase his or her level of implementation, therefore affording the student an opportunity to benefit from the intervention.

PERFORMANCE FEEDBACK TO INCREASE TREATMENT INTEGRITY LEVELS

A recent line of research indicates that performance feedback can be utilized as an intervention to increase the levels of treatment integrity of school-based interventions. When using performance feedback as a strategy, school psychologists analyze treatment integrity and student performance assessments and provide the intervention agent with written and/or verbal constructive feedback. The feedback is intended to shape the intervention agent's implementation of the intervention and result in the intervention agent's being able to implement the intervention with increased proficiency and effectiveness.

Witt, Noell, LaFleur, and Mortenson (1997) evaluated the relationship between performance feedback and treatment integrity. In a multiple-baseline design study, four teachers were trained to implement an intervention for a student with an academic performance deficit. The intervention was designed so that each step of the intervention resulted in a permanent product, allowing the researchers to track the teacher's treatment integrity without the bias that may be present in self-report or direct observation methods. Teachers were provided with all of the necessary materials to carry out the intervention and were provided with both didactic and in-vivo training on how to implement the intervention. The results of the study demonstrated that teachers' treatment integrity was perfect immediately following training but decreased rapidly during posttraining baseline, with no teacher maintaining treatment integrity above 80% for longer than 2 days. Performance feedback included the consultant presenting the teacher with a graph of both the student's score on a daily worksheet and the teacher's treatment integrity as well as a brief discussion of missed intervention steps. When daily performance feedback was implemented, both treatment integrity and student outcomes improved. After performance feedback was removed, treatment integrity again declined but did so more slowly than during the posttraining baseline. All of the students' academic performance increased with the introduction of the intervention, and three of the four students' performance increased further with improved treatment integrity.

These results have been replicated several times. Noell, Witt, Gilbertson, Ranier, and Freeland (1997) used a similar design and found that teachers' treatment integrity was perfect for only a few days following training and then decreased. Furthermore, they found that treatment integrity increased immediately when performance feedback was introduced. Mortenson and Witt (1998) extended this line of research further with a follow-up study in which the schedule of performance feedback was decreased from once daily to once weekly. Using a similar design, results indicated that all but one teacher's implementation dropped several days after training, and for those whose integrity declined, treatment integrity increased immediately when performance feedback was provided. Sanetti and Kratochwill (2004) used a similar design and found that teachers' implementation decreased within a week of training but increased after completing a daily treatment integrity rating scale, which resulted from the Treatment Integrity Planning Protocol (TIPP). The TIPP is a process of both planning and creating a treatment integrity assessment for any school-based intervention based on both conceptual frameworks of treatment integrity. These results indicate that other methods of providing process data may be as effective as daily or weekly structured meetings.

Interestingly, Noell et al. (2000) found that brief daily meetings typically did not maintain high levels of treatment integrity similar to the more structured performance feedback meetings used in previous research. However, the brief meetings were moderately to highly effective for some teachers; therefore, the type and intensity of follow-up needed to increase and maintain treatment integrity may vary across intervention agents.

CASE SCENARIO

Ms. Smith, a second-grade teacher at Chestnut Hill Elementary School, approached the school psychologist, Dr. Delaney, regarding Ken, a student who is having difficulty reading. As part of the problem identification stage, Dr. Delaney met with Ms. Smith to collect specific information about Ken's difficulties with reading. At this meeting, Ms. Smith reported that she believed Ken recognized words in isolation about as well as his peers, but that it seemed to take him much longer to read connected text. As a result, Ken often had difficulty finishing assignments in the time allotted. As a result, Ken was never able to engage in any of the activities on the "I'm Finished!" list, which included playing math games on the computer, his favorite activity.

Dr. Delaney agreed to observe Ken during class and administer some brief reading measures to determine his current level of performance in basic reading skills. During the observation, Ken was very attentive to Ms. Smith's lesson and subsequent directions for an independent seatwork assignment. Although the assignment did not require a lot of reading, Ken appeared to spend a lot more time than his peers on the sections that required reading. He was the only student who did not complete the assignment before it was time for art class. Ken's scores on the Dynamic Indicators of Basic Early Literacy Skills (DIBELS; Good & Kaminski, 2002) indicated that his knowledge of the alphabetic principle was at grade level (DIBELS Nonsense Word Fluency = 53, in the "established" range), yet his oral reading fluency was below grade level (DIBELS Oral Reading Fluency = 22, in the "at-risk" range). Furthermore, Ken was able to read 33 of the 46 second-grade Dolch Sight Words, indicating that his knowledge of sight words was at grade level.

Dr. Delaney and Ms. Smith met a second time to review the assessment information and further define the problem. Together they determined that there was a discrepancy between Ken's oral reading fluency rate and that expected of second-grade students and that the discrepancy was large enough to warrant an intervention. After considering several intervention options, Dr. Delaney felt that repeated oral readings would be both effective for Ken and feasible in Ms. Smith's classroom. Dr. Delaney agreed to create the monitoring forms that would be necessary to implement the intervention and to continue administering the DIBELS Oral Reading Fluency probes to monitor Ken's progress. Ms. Smith agreed to locate some reading passages with 50 words that Ken could read to her. They decided to meet again 3 days later before school to review the intervention steps and materials so that intervention could begin later that day.

Dr. Delaney, knowing that she needed to assess whether the intervention was being implemented, decided to create both a monitoring chart and a treatment integrity rating scale for Ms. Smith to complete on a daily basis. Dr. Delaney created a simple chart for Ms. Smith and Ken to monitor progress. Next, she began working on the rating scale and defined the repeated readings intervention:

> Ms. Smith will ask Ken, during independent reading time, to come to her desk before beginning his work. There she will provide Ken with a reading passage of 50 words that is at his instructional level. Ms. Smith will give one passage to Ken and ask him to "Read the passage aloud doing your best reading." While Ken is reading, Ms. Smith will (1) time the reading, (2) count the number of errors, and (3) provide assistance with the unknown words after 3 seconds. After Ken finishes reading, Ms. Smith and Ken will record his reading time as well as the number of words read correctly on a progress chart. They will use different symbols or colors to differentiate between the time and the number of words read correctly on the chart. Ms. Smith will then direct Ken to "Look over the passage, practice words that were hard for you, and then read the passage aloud to me again when you are ready." Again Ms. Smith will monitor Ken's time and errors during reading and provide assistance with difficult words. After Ken finishes reading, they will again chart his progress. Ken will then repeat the process of practicing the difficult words, rereading, and charting his progress one more time. When Ken reaches a grade-level rate of fluency on a particular passage, Ms. Smith will provide him with a new reading passage the next day.

Second, Dr. Delaney determined that (1) Ms. Smith will be responsible for implementing the intervention; (2) the intervention will occur daily, at Ms. Smith's desk, during independent reading time; (3) the duration of intervention sessions will be variable, determined by the amount of practice Ken needs; (4) Ken will be the only recipient of the intervention; and (5) the materials for the intervention will be housed in a special folder at Ms. Smith's desk.

Third, Dr. Delaney broke down the intervention she had defined into smaller components and began creating the treatment integrity rating scale. To do this, she (1) listed the intervention by component, (2) considered the response formats she wanted to use, and (3) determined how deviations would be assessed (see Figure 15.3).

Date: __ / __ / __   Class: <u>2nd Grade Homeroom</u>

Teacher's Name: <u>Ms. Smith</u>   Student's Name: <u>Ken</u>

Directions: The individual implementing the reading intervention with Ken (Ms. Smith or designee when absent) is to complete this form daily regarding how he or she implemented the intervention during *that* day.

The intervention was implemented by	☑ Ms. Smith
	☐ Other: _____
The intervention took place in	☑ Ms. Smith's room at her desk
(check all that apply)	☐ Ms. Smith's room at another location
	☐ Other: _____
The intervention occurred	☑ During independent reading time
(check all that apply)	☐ Other: _____

	Occurred	Did not occur	Deviated
1. Ken was given a reading passage of 50 words.	☑	☐	☐
2. The passage was at Ken's instructional level.	☑	☐	☐
3. Ken was instructed to read the passage aloud the best he could.	☑	☐	☐
4. Ken read the passage aloud.	☑	☐	☐
5. The reading was timed by Ms. Smith (or designee).	☑	☐	☐
6. Ms. Smith (or designee) recorded Ken's errors while he read.	☑	☐	☐
7. Ms. Smith (or designee) provided assistance with unknown words after 3 seconds.	☑	☐	☐
8. When he finished, Ken's time and performance were recorded on the progress chart.	☑	☐	☐
9. Different symbols or colors were used to record time and words read correctly on the progress chart.	☑	☐	☐
10. Ms. Smith (or designee) directed Ken to look over the passage and practice difficult words.	☑	☐	☐
11. Ms. Smith (or designee) asked Ken to read the passage aloud again dong the best he could.	☑	☐	☐
12. Ken read the passage aloud.	☑	☐	☐
13. The reading was timed by Ms. Smith (or designee).	☑	☐	☐
14. Ms. Smith (or designee) recorded Ken's errors while he read.	☑	☐	☐
15. Ms. Smith (or designee) provided assistance with unknown words after 3 seconds.	☑	☐	☐
16. When he finished, Ken's time and performance were recorded on the progress chart.	☑	☐	☐
17. Different symbols or colors were used to record time and words read correctly on the progress chart.	☑	☐	☐
18. Ms. Smith (or designee) directed Ken to look over the passage and practice difficult words again.	☑	☐	☐
19. Ms. Smith (or designee) asked Ken to read the passage aloud again doing the best he could a third time.	☑	☐	☐
20. Ken read the passage aloud.	☑	☐	☐
21. The reading was timed by Ms. Smith (or designee).	☑	☐	☐
22. Ms. Smith (or designee) recorded Ken's errors while he read.	☑	☐	☐
23. Ms. Smith (or designee) provided assistance with unknown words after 3 seconds.	☑	☐	☐
24. When he finished, Ken's time and performance were recorded on the progress chart.	☑	☐	☐
25. Different symbols or colors were used to record time and words read correctly on the progress chart.	☑	☐	☐

FIGURE 15.3. Treatment Integrity Rating Scale completed daily by Ms. Smith.

Dr. Delaney and Ms. Smith met as planned to review the intervention plan as well as the reading materials. Ms. Smith was pleased with the plan and was excited to start later that morning. She agreed to complete the treatment integrity rating scale and the progress chart daily and leave them in Dr. Delaney's mailbox each Friday afternoon. Dr. Delaney agreed to graph these data as well as the DIBELS data for Ms. Smith and leave the graphs in her mailbox each Monday.

Two important pieces of information about the intervention integrity can be seen in Figure 15.4, which illustrates the data from the first week of intervention. First, Ms. Smith rated herself as having a high level of integrity, and the progress chart supports her ratings, as there is data for each time she reported implementing the intervention. Second, Ken's reading fluency increased with the repeated readings intervention according to both the progress chart and the DIBELS probes. Together, these data support the continuation of both the repeated readings intervention and the multifaceted monitoring of both Ken's progress and Ms. Smith's intervention implementation.

SUMMARY

Public schools, including the teachers, school psychologists, and other school personnel who work in them, have a legal and ethical obligation to provide students with an appropriate education in the least restrictive environment. To fulfill this obligation, problem-solving teams often work to create intervention plans to intervene with students who are struggling in

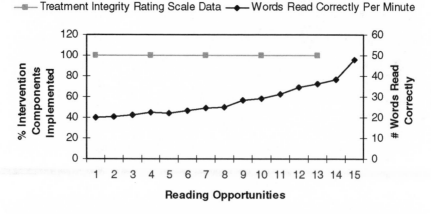

FIGURE 15.4. Treatment integrity data and student progress monitoring data for Ken and Ms. Smith during week 1.

the general education environment. It is often assumed that these interventions are implemented as intended for the duration of the intervention. Several research studies indicate that this assumption is false; intervention implementation cannot be taken for granted and needs to be assessed. Yet, reviews of the intervention outcomes literature tell us that, even under ideal conditions in an intervention study, few researchers assess treatment integrity. It has been hypothesized that the lack of treatment integrity assessment is due to the dearth of treatment integrity measures and the specificity of the treatment integrity measures that have been developed (Schoenwald, Henggeler, Brondino, & Rowland, 2000).

As well as providing background information about the relationship between treatment integrity, treatment outcomes, and current conceptualizations of treatment integrity, this chapter has provided information needed to move toward assessing treatment integrity. When completed step by step, the process for creating a treatment integrity assessment need not be an intimidating task but rather an opportunity to clarify the intervention plan. Utilizing the resulting treatment integrity assessment will allow valid decision making about intervention effectiveness. In addition, when treatment integrity assessment data are coupled with student progress data, the school team will know whether to (1) intervene with the teacher regarding his or her implementation of the intervention, (2) consider another intervention, or (3) continue the current intervention plan. Without question, assessing treatment integrity data is requisite to making data-based decisions about the effectiveness of an intervention within a problem-solving model.

ACKNOWLEDGMENTS

Preparation of this chapter was supported by a grant from the U.S. Department of Education, Office of Special Education and Rehabilitative Services, Student Initiated Research Projects Program (CDFA No. 84.324B). This chapter does not necessarily represent the position or policies of the U.S. Department of Education, and no official endorsement should be inferred. We express sincere appreciation to Katie Streit for her work on this document.

REFERENCES

Eysenck, H. J. (1952). The effects of psychotherapy: An evaluation. *Journal of Consulting Psychology, 16*, 319–324.

Fireman, G. D. (2002). Approaching accountability in psychotherapy. *Journal of Constructivist Psychology, 15*, 219–231.

Foster, S. L., & Cone, J. D. (1986). Design and use of direct observation systems. In A. Ciminero, K. S. Calhoun, & H. E. Adams (Eds.), *Handbook of behavioral assessment* (2nd ed., pp. 253–324). New York: Wiley.

Good, R. H., & Kaminski, R. A. (Eds.). (2002). *Dynamic Indicators of Basic Early Lit-

eracy Skills (6th ed.). Eugene, OR: Institute for the Development of Educational Achievement. Retrieved April 2004 from *dibels.uoregon.edu/*

Gresham, F. M. (1989). Assessment of treatment integrity in school consultation and prereferral intervention. *School Psychology Review, 18,* 37–50.

Gresham, F. M. (1997). Treatment integrity in single-subject research. In R. D. Franklin, D. B. Allison, & B. S. Gorman (Eds.), *Design and analysis of single-case research* (pp. 93–117). Mahwah, NJ: Erlbaum.

Gresham, F. M., Gansle, K. A., & Noell, G. H. (1993). Treatment integrity in applied behavior analysis with children. *Journal of Applied Behavior Analysis, 26,* 257–263.

Gresham, F. M., Gansle, K. A., Noell, G. H., Cohen, S., & Rosenblum, S. (1993). Treatment integrity of school-based behavioral intervention studies: 1980–1990. *School Psychology Review, 22,* 254–272.

Gresham, F. M., MacMillan, D. L., Beebe-Frankenberger, M. E., & Bocian, K. M. (2000). Treatment integrity in learning disabilities intervention research: Do we really know how treatments are implemented? *Learning Disabilities Research and Practice, 15,* 198–205.

Happe, D. (1982). Behavioral intervention: It doesn't do any good in your briefcase. In J. Grimes (Ed.), *Psychological approaches to problems of children and adolescents* (pp. 15–41). Des Moines: Iowa Department of Public Instruction.

Mace, F. C., Page, T., Ivancic, M., & O'Brien, S. (1986). Effectiveness of brief time-out with and without contingent delay: A comparative study. *Journal of Applied Behavior Analysis, 19,* 79–86.

Moncher, F. J., & Prinz, R. J. (1991). Treatment fidelity in outcome studies. *Clinical Psychology Review, 11,* 247–266.

Moretenson, B. P., & Witt, J. C. (1998). The use of weekly performance feedback to increase teacher implementation of a prereferral academic intervention. *School Psychology Review, 27,* 613–627.

Noell, G. H., Witt, J. C., Gilbertson, D. N., Ranier, D. D., & Freeland, J. T. (1997). Increasing teacher intervention implementation in general education settings through consultation and performance feedback. *School Psychology Quarterly, 12,* 77–88.

Noell, G. H., Witt, J. C., LaFleur, L. H., Moretenson, B. P., Ranier, D. D., & LeVelle, J. (2000). Increasing intervention implementation in general education following consultation: A comparison of two follow-up strategies. *Journal of Applied Behavior Analysis, 33,* 271–284.

Peterson, L., Homer, A., & Wonderlich, S. (1982). The integrity of independent variables in behavior analysis. *Journal of Applied Behavior Analysis, 15,* 477–492.

Sanetti, L. H., & Kratochwill, T. R. (2004). *The effects of the Treatment Integrity Planning Protocol (TIPP) on treatment integrity and treatment outcomes in school-based consultation.* Manuscript in progress.

Schoenwald, S. K., Henggeler, S. W., Brondino, M. J., & Rowland, M. D. (2000). Multisystemic therapy: Monitoring treatment fidelity. *Family Process, 39,* 83–103.

Sterling-Turner, H. E., Watson, T. S., Moore, J. W. (2002). The effects of direct training on treatment outcomes in school consultation. *School Psychology Quarterly, 17,* 47–77.

Sterling-Turner, H. E., Watson, T. S., Wildmon, M., Watkins, C., & Little, E. (2001). Investigating the relationship between training type and treatment integrity. *School Psychology Quarterly, 16,* 56–67.

VandenBos, G. R., & Pino, C. D. (1980). Research on the outcome of psychotherapy. In G. R. VandenBos (Ed.), *Psychotherapy: Practice, research, policy* (pp. 23–69). Beverly Hills: Sage.

VonBrock, M. B., & Elliott, S. N. (1987). Influence of treatment effectiveness information on the acceptability of classroom interventions. *Journal of School Psychology,* *25*, 131–144.

Webster-Stratton, C., & Reid, M. J. (2003). The incredible years parents, teachers, and children training series: A multifaceted treatment approach for young children with conduct problems. In A. E. Kazdin & J. R. Weisz (Eds.), *Evidence-based psychotherapies for children and adolescents* (pp. 224–262). New York: Guilford Press.

Wickstrom, K. F., Jones, K. M., LaFleur, L. H., & Witt, J. C. (1998). An analysis of treatment integrity in school-based behavioral consultation. *School Psychology Quarterly, 13,* 141–154.

Witt, J. C., Noell, G. H., LaFleur, L. H., & Moretenson, B. P. (1997). Teacher use of interventions in general education settings: Measurement and analysis of the independent variable. *Journal of Applied Behavior Analysis, 30,* 693–696.

Yeaton, W. H., & Sechrest, L. (1981). Critical dimensions in the choice and maintenance of successful treatments: Strength, integrity, and effectiveness. *Journal of Consulting and Clinical Psychology, 49,* 156–167.

SUGGESTED READINGS

Gresham, F. M. (1989). Assessment of treatment integrity in school consultation and prereferral intervention. *School Psychology Review, 18,* 37–50.

Provides an advanced conceptualization of treatment integrity that builds on that set forth by Yeaton and Sechrest (1981). Specifically, the article discusses additional factors, technical issues, and practical guidelines related to the assessment of treatment integrity. Additional examples of treatment integrity assessments are included.

Yeaton, W. H., & Sechrest, L. (1981). Critical dimensions in the choice and maintenance of successful treatments: Strength, integrity, and effectiveness. *Journal of Consulting and Clinical Psychology, 49,* 156–167.

A seminal work in the area of treatment integrity, this article discusses in more detail the relationship between a treatment's strength, the integrity with which it is implemented, and its effectiveness. The authors discuss assessment and inherent problems within each of these areas.

PART V

♦ ♦ ♦

Implementing and Monitoring Solutions

♦

CHAPTER 16

◆ ◆ ◆

Evaluating Intervention Outcomes

◆

CRAIG A. ALBERS
STEPHEN N. ELLIOTT
RYAN J. KETTLER
ANDREW T. ROACH

The ongoing paradigm shift in education over the past decade has focused on accountability and resulted in demands for *scientifically based research* to justify the use of educational practices, leading to increased interest regarding the use of evidence-based interventions (EBIs) within schools (e.g., Kratochwill & Stoiber, 2002). The EBI movement is predicated on outcome evaluation to identify effective practices. For example, the No Child Left Behind Act of 2001 states that scientifically based research "relies on measurements or observational methods that provide reliable and valid data across evaluators and observers, across multiple measurements and observations, and across studies by the same or different investigators" (§1208(6)(B)(iii)). Additionally, the mere implementation of an intervention that has been supported by scientifically based research is insufficient unless high-quality intervention evaluation occurs throughout the problem-solving process to identify the impact of the intervention. Consequently, the astute practitioner or educator not only will evaluate intervention *outcomes* to document whether the intervention produced the desired effects but also will utilize an evaluative process throughout *all* stages of the Deno (1989) problem-solving model to monitor the effects of the intervention and make changes when indicated.

At the most basic level, a discrepancy between actual and desired behavior indicates the presence of a problem, whether it be within the academic, behavioral, or social–emotional realm. Since interventions can be designed to change the level of the child's functioning by *increasing* positive behavior or by *decreasing* inappropriate behaviors, intervention outcomes can be monitored and evaluated in a significant number of areas. For example, Meyer and Janney (1989) describe nine general categories in which meaningful outcomes can be observed when implementing behavioral interventions, including (1) an improvement in the identified behavior, (2) an increase in more appropriate replacement behaviors, (3) acquisition of strategies that enhance change, (4) an increase in indirect positive behaviors with an absence of negative side effects, (5) a reduced need for related services, (6) a more inclusive placement within the regular education setting, (7) an increase in the student's quality of life, (8) perceived improvement by others, and (9) improved social networks. Similarly, outcome categories to consider when evaluating an academic intervention include (1) changes in the proficiency of an academic skill and frequency of occurrence; (2) changes in work products produced by the student, including quality and quantity; (3) increased academic engaged time; (4) improved achievement test scores; and (5) improved functioning with peers (DiPerna & Elliott, 2000).

Although academic and behavioral difficulties are frequently addressed as being independent of one another, there is ample evidence indicating a reciprocal relationship between academic, behavioral, and social–emotional difficulties (e.g., DiPerna & Elliott, 1999; Malecki & Elliott, 2002; McEvoy & Welker, 2000). For example, academic deficits frequently coexist with behavior difficulties as well as with deficits in prosocial skills. Although exact pathways between academic, behavioral, and social–emotional variables for individual cases have not been delineated, an outcome evaluation should examine whether positive and lasting changes were obtained in areas other than those initially identified.

The recent advances in the field regarding the use of EBIs, as well as the implementation of multitiered levels of intervention, stress the importance of data collection through the use of progress monitoring and outcomes evaluation. Multitiered intervention models are designed to provide levels of service along a continuum, which are frequently referred to as *primary, secondary,* and *tertiary* services (Goldston, 1977) or the corresponding *universal, selective,* and *indicated* (Munoz, Mrazek, & Haggerty, 1996) levels of service. Within these models, the level of service provided is determined by the actual risk factors present, the degree of difficulty experienced, and the student's response to prior implemented interventions. However, to make decisions about a student's need for another level of service, data must be collected throughout the process. Furthermore, there is ample evidence that high-quality progress monitoring and outcomes evaluation can improve the effectiveness of interventions (e.g., Fuchs & Fuchs, 1986; Fuchs, Fuchs, & Hamlett, 1989; Shinn & Hubbard, 1992). With these factors as our foundation, the remainder of this chapter reviews steps involved in the evaluation of intervention outcomes and the connections to the problem-solving model. Following a discussion of the role of theory and assessment in the intervention process, specific procedures are described to assist practitioners in incorporating outcome evaluation methods throughout all stages of the problem-solving model.

INTERVENTION DECISION MAKING: THE ROLE OF THEORY AND ASSESSMENT

There Is Nothing More Practical Than a Good Theory

Common theories of human behavior are often characterized as the medical, psychodynamic, cognitive, social learning, and behavioral models. These models not only impact the interpretation of problem behaviors but also guide practitioners in the selection of interventions. For example, while the medical model posits that problem behaviors are the consequence of an underlying condition, behavioral models are based on the concept that all behavior is learned and, as a consequence, can be influenced by environmental factors. Intervention approaches within the behavioral model tend to focus on the manipulation of environmental variables (e.g., rates and types of reinforcement) to produce the desired behavior change. A specific example of a behavioral model that guides intervention selection is the S-O-R-C model (Kanfer & Goldstein, 1986). The elements of this model include the Stimuli (i.e., variables, such as people or events preceding an action), Organism (i.e., the student), Response (i.e., reactions of the student to the stimulus), and Consequence (i.e., reactions to the response). Based on this model, variables at the four levels can be manipulated as part of the intervention process (Elliott, Witt, Kratochwill, & Stoiber, 2002). The predominant theory of the problem-solving team will provide guidance regarding what measures to evaluate, influence how the data are interpreted, lead to hypotheses regarding the behavior, and suggest types of interventions that should be considered for implementation.

When examining the role of assessment within the problem-solving model, a distinction is necessary between conducting assessment *for* intervention, versus conducting assessment *of* intervention. A high-quality outcomes assessment is a process that begins prior to the implementation of an intervention (i.e., assessment *for* intervention) and continues throughout the duration of, as well as following the completion of, the intervention (i.e., assessment *of* intervention). Given this distinction between assessment *for* and assessment *of* intervention approaches, evaluation components should lend themselves to frequent data-based measurement and should be sensitive to small changes in academic or behavioral performance. While the operational definition and topography of the problem behavior (e.g., academic, behavioral, social–emotional) will provide guidance in determining the appropriate procedures for evaluating the intervention's effectiveness, deficits are frequently not limited to one area and tend to cut across various domains. As a result, the outcome assessment process should utilize a variety of methods (e.g., direct and indirect) from a variety of sources (e.g., teacher, parent, self-report). Although it is preferable to collect data as frequently as possible throughout the problem-solving process, it is essential that data collection occur, at a minimum, during four different times:

1. At the beginning of the process, to serve as baseline data and to aid in problem identification and analysis.
2. During the intervention, to determine whether progress is evident.
3. At the termination of the intervention.
4. During a time period following the termination of the intervention, to determine whether the improvement in performance was maintained.

Assessment *for* Intervention: Problem Identification, Problem Analysis, and Exploring Solutions Stages

Within the five-stage problem-solving model, assessment *for* intervention occurs within the *problem identification, problem analysis,* and *exploring solutions* stages and is designed to guide the selection of an intervention. The data collected throughout the assessment process within these stages serve as the foundation for outcome evaluation at the intervention's termination. Within the problem identification stage, the collection of data is directed toward determining whether discrepancies exist between the student's actual performances as compared to the expected performance. Considering that the collection of data during this stage not only verifies whether a discrepancy between actual and desired behavior exists but also serves as the baseline for evaluating the impact of the implemented intervention, it is essential that clear, concise, and objective definitions of the problem behavior and desired behavior are delineated. If the data collected validate the existence of a meaningful discrepancy, a more in-depth assessment of the deficit is explored within the problem analysis stage. During the problem analysis stage, assessment activities are directed toward specifically identifying what the problem is, how significant the problem is, and whether the discrepancy between actual and desired performance warrants the exploration of intervention possibilities. Ideally, the data collected guide the problem-solving team toward behavior change methods and appropriate goals for the intervention process. This leads to the exploring solutions stage, where a variety of evidence-based interventions should be considered.

During the exploring solutions stage, the intervention approach selected will likely be guided by the theoretical principles endorsed by those involved in the problem-solving process, by the data collected in the first two stages of the problem-solving process, and, ideally, existing research on the effectiveness of the intervention. To aid in intervention selection, Elliott and colleagues developed six "Think Rules" to guide this process (Elliott, DiPirna, & Shapiro, 2001). These include:

1. *Think Behavior*, consisting of focusing on behaviors or permanent products.
2. *Think Positive*, relating to the identification of behaviors for improvement that are incompatible with the defined problem behavior.
3. *Think Solution*, in which focus is on the intervention goal and the change strategy to achieve the goal.
4. *Think Small Steps*, consisting of clearly defining the necessary steps to implement the intervention.
5. *Think Flexible*, in which a variety of intervention possibilities are considered.
6. *Think Future*, which is focused on planning for maintenance and generalizability of the intervention.

These "Think Rules" can guide the intervention team throughout the intervention process.

Assessment *of* Intervention: Intervention Implementation and Treatment Evaluation Stages

The initial three stages of the problem-solving model utilize assessment data for identifying, verifying, and aiding in the selection of an appropriate intervention. During the *intervention implementation* and *treatment evaluation* stages, however, the focus shifts to assessment *of* intervention. During the intervention implementation stage, data collected should assist the problem-solving team in determining whether the intervention is having sufficient impact so that the student can reach defined goals. Essentially, there are three main outcomes possible. If data suggest that the intervention is failing to produce the desired effects, modifications to, or even termination of, the intervention is indicated. If the intervention appears to be insufficient, the problem-solving team reverts to an earlier stage of the process to identify additional intervention possibilities. If a satisfactory level of progress is evident, the intervention and data collection processes continue. The degree to which the intervention is being implemented as intended also is important information to collect during this stage. For example, the data may show that the student's performance has not changed, but this outcome may reflect a lack of correct treatment implementation. In such cases, another trial of the intervention using accurate methods is needed. Documentation that one's intervention goal has been obtained is part of the treatment evaluation stage. However, it is recommended that a broader evaluation of intervention effects be undertaken to understand the collateral impact of the intervention on related behaviors or attitudes.

Understanding and Assessing the Acceptability–Integrity–Outcomes Connections

Using assessment data to understand students' difficulties and identify potential intervention strategies is only the beginning of the journey to improved student outcomes; facilitating the implementation of intervention techniques is often a greater challenge for the school psychologist and school-based consultant or educator. Although the scientist-practitioner model of training has provided most school psychologists with a healthy respect for the value of research-based approaches, predominant methods of intervention utilized by school psychologists and other educational practitioners remain indirect and teacher-mediated (Sladeczek, Kratochwill, Steinbach, Kumke, & Hagermoser, 2003). Unfortunately, it is not uncommon to discover that intervention collaborators are unable or unwilling to implement interventions as originally conceptualized. This lack of treatment acceptability and integrity frequently has deleterious consequences on intervention utility (Gresham, 1989) and thus needs to be monitored and measured as part of the outcome evaluation.

Treatment Acceptability

Acceptability refers to consultees' and clients' perceptions of the utility, fairness, and feasibility of an intervention strategy for addressing students' behavioral or academic concerns (Kazdin, 1981; Zins & Erchul, 2002). Research suggests that interventions viewed as positive (rather than punitive), time-efficient, and minimally intrusive to classroom routines are more likely to be perceived as acceptable by teachers and other educators (Elliott, 1988; Finn, 2000). Because teachers and parents may be resistant to implementing less acceptable interventions, school psychologists and other school-based consultants need to be cognizant of the level of intervention acceptability and potential methods for assessing acceptability to enhance the likelihood of the intervention being implemented as intended.

Treatment Integrity

Treatment integrity refers to the degree to which an intervention is implemented as intended (Gresham, 1989). Some of the more salient factors affecting treatment integrity include (1) the complexity and time required to implement an intervention; (2) resources required; (3) number of people involved in implementing the intervention; (4) degree of motivation of the intervention agents; and (5) perceived, as well as actual, effectiveness of the intervention (Elliott et al., 2002; Gresham, 1989). These factors are also closely related to the acceptability of the intervention. The EBI framework being advocated within school psychology encourages the use of standardized interventions and stresses the need for information regarding treatment utility when implementing and evaluating the effects of an intervention (e.g., Kratochwill & Stoiber, 2002). A manualized treatment is desirable. Simply selecting a high-quality intervention is in itself insufficient unless the intervention is implemented with a high degree of integrity. Examining obtained data and making decisions regarding the effectiveness of the intervention as indicated by the outcomes evaluation is limited without information regarding treatment integrity. If it is unknown to what degree the intervention was implemented, practitioners will be unable to determine whether limited intervention effectiveness was due to (1) a poor match between the presenting concern and the intervention, (2) an intervention that was poorly designed or simply ineffective, or (3) a low degree of treatment integrity.

GENERAL EVALUATION METHODS

Assessing Intervention Process and Integrity

Treatment Acceptability

Intervention acceptability is frequently measured through the use of questionnaire-type instruments. Since acceptability can vary along a continuum from "not being acceptable under any circumstance" to being "completely acceptable," questionnaires generally utilize a Likert-type rating format so that the *degree* of acceptability can be measured. The Academic Intervention Monitoring System (AIMS; Elliott et al., 2001) represents a more recent approach to assessing intervention acceptability. The AIMS, which outlines intervention procedures for over 40 teacher-implemented instructional strategies for improving student's academic skills and enabling behaviors, can be completed by teachers. There are parallel but briefer AIMS forms for parents and students. Raters are asked to identify their perceptions of "how helpful" and "how feasible" implementation of each strategy would be for addressing the student's academic or behavior difficulties. Intervention planning can then focus on the AIMS items that were rated very helpful and feasible to implement. Examples of additional instruments that have been utilized to evaluate treatment acceptability include the Treatment Evaluation Inventory (Kazdin, 1980), the Treatment Evaluation Inventory—Short Form (Kelley, Heffer, Gresham, & Elliott, 1989), the Behavior Intervention Rating Scales (Elliott & Treuting, 1991), the Treatment Acceptability Rating Form—Revised (Reimers, Wacker, Cooper, & DeRaad, 1992), and the Children's Intervention Rating Profile (Witt & Elliott, 1985).

Treatment Integrity

A variety of methods exist for evaluating the degree of treatment integrity, including direct and indirect methods. The most direct method of evaluating treatment integrity is via observation, while indirect methods consist of intervention agent self-reports, completion of checklists, rating scales, and interviews (Gresham, 1989). Treatment integrity is frequently reported as a percentage of intervention components implemented as designed. Innovation Configurations are one of three diagnostic frameworks used in the Concerns-Based Adoption Model (CBAM; Hall & Hord, 1987) and are particularly useful in assessing treatment integrity. The underlying assumption of Innovation Configurations is that individual users' patterns of implementation for an intervention are not identical. Hall and Hord (2001) suggest the primary purpose of Innovation Configurations is the recognition that "(a) in most change efforts, (intervention) adaptation will occur; (b) there is a way to chart these adaptations; and (c) these adaptations have direct and indirect implications for facilitating and assessing change processes" (p. 39). In some cases, implementation of an intervention may be optimal; in others, the actual practice may be diluted or distorted to the point of ineffectiveness. An Innovation Configuration Map is a checklist or rubric that describes the essential "building blocks," or components, of an intervention. Variations of each component or element are described in behavioral terms. Three questions (Hall & Hord, 2001, p. 49) can be used to guide the development of Innovation Configuration Maps for interventions:

1. What does the intervention look like when it is in use?
2. What would I see in classrooms where it is used well (and not used as well)?
3. What will teachers and students be doing when the intervention is in use?

Innovation Configuration Maps can be used as self-report measures, interview protocols, or observation records (Anderson, 1997). Hall and Hord

(1987), however, suggest that components reflecting teacher behaviors are most appropriately assessed through direct classroom observation.

Assessing Intervention Outcomes

Direct Observation Methods and Designs

OBSERVATIONS

Observations are one method of obtaining direct and reliable measures of performance and behavior, and are preferable for a variety of reasons. First, since observations result in data that are collected directly within the environment, inferences are unnecessary. Second, observations allow for the examination of a variety of variables, such as those relating to the classroom environment, a student's academic performance, or a student's behavior. Third, observations can be conducted on a frequent basis and by a variety of individuals. Fourth, observations allow for an examination of setting events, antecedents, and consequences (Hintze, Volpe, & Shapiro, 2002). Finally, conducting an observation can allow one to easily collect data for a comparison student, serving as a reference point for the impact of the intervention on the target student.

When conducting an observation, three different categories of behavior generally are of interest: (1) the amount of time in which the student is actively engaged and experiencing instructional success, which is frequently referred to as academic learning time (Gettinger, 1995); (2) behaviors that interfere with appropriate performance (e.g., off-task behaviors); and (3) interactions with the classroom teacher or classmates (Elliott et al., 2001). While a variety of observation approaches are available, the most appropriate observation format depends upon the topography, frequency, intensity, and duration of the behavior. Regardless of the observation format selected, a clear and unambiguous definition of the behavior is needed to increase the reliability and validity of the observation. Once data are collected, one of the most beneficial methods for evaluating observation data is through the use of graphic analysis, which will be examined later in this chapter.

General Observation Methods. Event/frequency recording is most appropriate for behaviors that have a discrete beginning and end, with data being reported as frequency (e.g., student raised hand five times during a 30-minute observation) or rate (e.g., student raised hand an average of once every 6 minutes). *Duration recording* examines the amount of time that elapses from the beginning to the end of the behavior. Data can be reported as the amount of time the student participated in the behavior during the observation period (e.g., student was out-of-seat for 13 minutes during a 30-minute observation). *Latency recording* is designed to measure the amount of time that elapses before a behavior is initiated, which is then reported as the average amount of time required for a student to comply with the request. Finally, *interval recording* consists of breaking the observation down into intervals of equal length (e.g., the use of 15-second intervals during a 20-minute observation, resulting in 80 intervals) and allows for a sampling of behavior during an observation period. There are three variations in the format of interval recordings:

1. In *whole-interval recording*, the observer notes whether the behavior was present or absent for the entire interval.
2. In *partial-interval recording*, the observer documents whether the behavior occurred during any portion of the interval.
3. In *momentary time sampling*, the observer notes whether the behavior was occurring at the moment the interval began.

In all three interval recording formats, data can be reported as a percentage of intervals during which the behavior was observed.

Standardized Observation Forms. Due to the wide variety of standardized observation forms that have been developed, an extensive review of standardized observation forms is beyond the scope of this chapter (see Chapter 9, this volume). One example of an observation form that is frequently utilized is the Behavior Observation of Students in Schools (BOSS; Shapiro, 1996), which is designed to facilitate the collection of information regarding academic performance within the classroom setting. At the beginning of the 15-second interval, the observer records whether the student was actively or passively engaged in academic behaviors. Throughout the duration of the interval, the observer records whether any additional off-task behaviors (verbal, motor, or passive) occur. Once an off-task behavior occurs and is noted, no additional occurrences of off-task behaviors are recorded until the subsequent interval. The BOSS is also designed to collect observational data from peers during every fifth interval to serve as a classroom norm for behavior. Additional examples of standardized observation forms are the Behavior Assessment Scale for Children—Student Observation System (BASC-SOS; Reynolds & Kamphaus, 1998), Code for Instructional Structure and Student Academic Response (CISSAR; Stanley & Greenwood, 1981), Ecobehavioral Assessment Systems Software (EBASS; Greenwood, Carta, Kamps, & Delquadri, 1995), and State-Event Classroom Observation System (SECOS; Saudargas, 1992).

CURRICULUM-BASED MEASUREMENT

A significant amount of research exists regarding the use of curriculum-based measurement (CBM) as a form of progress monitoring and outcomes evaluation within a problem-solving model (e.g., Deno, 1995; Shinn, 2002; see Chapter 8, this volume). As part of the assessment *for* intervention process, CBM can be utilized to (1) identify a discrepancy between actual and desired performance levels, (2) provide baseline data that can be used throughout the problem-solving model, (3) provide data to aid in goal setting, and (4) provide a direct link between assessment and intervention (Shinn, 2002). Within the assessment *of* intervention stages, CBM provides a method of continual progress monitoring to help in determining whether the intervention is effective or whether the focus and intensity of the instructional level should be modified. Finally, intervention outcomes can be evaluated based on data collected and whether the individual attained the goals that were set regarding performance.

PERMANENT PRODUCTS

When observation data are combined with information obtained from reviewing the student's actual work products completed during the observation period, a more complete understanding of a student's performance is obtained. The examination of permanent products also can be utilized as a method of assessing intervention outcomes. Ways of utilizing these data include examining assignment completion rates, assignment accuracy, and quiz/test scores. This information can be obtained prior to, during, and following the implementation of the intervention as a method of monitoring and assessing its impact. Additionally, naturalistic products such as work samples frequently result in increased intervention acceptability by classroom teachers (Rathvon, 1999).

Indirect Observation Methods and Designs

RATING SCALES

Rating scales provide indirect information regarding the impact of an intervention and can provide additional information when used as part of a multisource, multimethod process. Particularly, the use of rating scales allows for information to be readily obtained from a variety of informants (e.g., teachers, parents) and settings (e.g., school, home) (see Chapter 10, this volume). However, there are various limitations to the use of rating scales to assess intervention progress and outcomes. Specifically, rating scales frequently are not sensitive enough to detect small changes in behavior or performance, especially over a limited time period (Elliott, Busse, & Gresham, 1993). Consequently, their use to monitor progress can be questionable. Further, numerous studies have indicated that rating scale measures have not detected changes in behavior that were documented through observations, which reaffirms the importance of a multisource, multimethod approach (e.g., Harris, Wilkinson, Trovato, & Prior, 1992; Grossman et al., 1997). Finally, the use of rating scales provides indirect measures of behavior and performance, which can be influenced by factors other than actual change.

Recent advances in outcome assessment have resulted in alternative measures for determining the impact of an intervention. For example, the AIMS (Elliott et al., 2001) incorporates the use of goal attainment scales (GAS; discussed in greater detail below) to monitor and evaluate academic interventions and corresponding outcomes. Likewise, Stoiber and Kratochwill (2001) designed Outcomes: Planning, Monitoring, Evaluating (Outcomes: PME) as a method of assisting in the design, implementation, monitoring, and evaluation of academic and behavioral interventions, with GAS being one component of the framework.

GOAL ATTAINMENT SCALING

Kiresuk and Sherman (1968) originally developed GAS for use in evaluating the effectiveness of mental health services. GAS was intended to serve as an alternative to the variety of rating scales, projective techniques, and clinical interviews used by clinicians to document client change. Kratochwill and Elliott (1993) used a modified version of GAS for ongoing monitoring of the effectiveness of teacher- and parent-mediated interventions with preschoolers. Reaching beyond its utility as a follow-up measure of clinician or program effectiveness, Kratochwill and Elliott conceptualized GAS as a formative assessment that could be repeated periodically to monitor students' academic or behavior progress (Robertson-Mjannes, 1999).

As conceptualized by Kratochwill and Elliott (1993), the basic methodology of GAS for assessing students' school performance involves the following steps: (1) selecting a target behavior, (2) describing the desired behavior or academic outcome in objective terms, and (3) developing three to five descriptions of the probable outcomes, from "least favorable" to "most favorable" (Elliott, Sladeczek, & Kratochwill, 1995). By using numerical ratings for each of the five descriptive levels of functioning, the rater can provide a daily or weekly report of student progress. These criterion-referenced reports can accompany direct indicators of progress (e.g., direct observations, CBM) and other indicators such as work samples, student self-reports, or reports from parents or other individuals.

Using GAS as a repeated measure of students' progress required changes in the original scaled descriptions developed by Kiresuk and Sherman (1968). Although Kratochwill and Elliott (1993) maintained the five-point scale used in the original GAS, their modified approach included initial assessments to establish a baseline, which was subsequently assigned a score of zero ("0"). Thus, the new scale levels ranged from the best possible outcome (+2) to the worst possible outcome (-2). This change allowed ratings on the modified GAS to reflect both over- and underattainment of behavioral or academic objectives (Kratochwill, Elliott, & Rotto, 1995).

Although there has been substantial investigation and implementation of GAS in a variety of mental health and medical fields, there has been less extensive research and application of GAS by school psychologists and special educators. Because of its emphasis on operationalizing target behaviors and ongoing (i.e., time-series) evaluation of academic or behavioral progress, GAS is a particularly useful tool for monitoring students' progress and for verifying the need for additional support or intervention (Elliott et al., 2001).

HELPFUL DATA ANALYTIC AND DATA DISPLAY METHODS

Although single-case and small-group data analysis are poor fits for powerful methods of evaluating intervention effectiveness (e.g., regression analysis), a number of methods exist for analyzing or displaying data that are more easily interpretable for practical understanding and organization. Some of those methods, such as calculation of a reliability change index (RCI; Nunnally & Kotsche, 1983) or effect sizes, capitalize on similar logic to that used in larger, more powerful analyses. Other methods, such as convergent evidence scaling (CES) and visual analysis, are more useful for comparing data from different sources or from different points in time. In this section of the chapter, we briefly review four data analytic and display methods that work with individuals or small groups.

Reliability Change Index

Nunnally and Kotsche (1983) proposed RCI as a method for determining whether the impact of an intervention is significant. RCI is calculated like a standard score, by determining the difference between the outcome score and the predicted score with respect to variation, and can be interpreted based on a z-score distribution. Any z-score higher than +1.96 would indicate a difference that would exceed 95% of all differences that are likely occur by chance. Such an RCI would be significant in the sense that there is only a 5% chance that such an extreme positive change would be witnessed if the intervention were not effective. Conversely, any z-score lower than –1.96 would indicate significant change in the negative direction. RCI can be calculated whenever an individual takes the same test, or equivalent forms of a test, both before and after an intervention.

On an individual level, RCI can be calculated by subtracting the pretest score from the posttest score, and dividing by the standard error of measurement—that is, RCI = (posttest score – pretest score) / standard error of measurement. The posttest score is taken after the intervention, and the pretest score is taken during the baseline. The standard error of measurement (SEM) indicates the amount that a score on a test is expected to vary. It is technically the standard deviation (SD) of the error term, and can be found in many test manuals. The formula for calculating the standard error of measurement is $SEM_Y = (SD_Y)\sqrt{1 - r_{XY}}$, where r_{XY} is the expected correlation between the pretest and the posttest. When a test manual provides neither the SEM nor the necessary information to calculate the SEM, an appropriate conservative estimate is 5 (Elliott & Busse, 2004).

The RCI has a couple of advantages that make it attractive for analyzing individual and small-group data. While it is quantifiable on the individual level, it can just as easily be calculated for groups by substituting individual posttest and pretest scores with their respective group means. Another advantage of RCI is that confidence intervals can easily be built to indicate the likely range within which each individual's true score would fall. Although RCI has many advantages, it also has some limitations. Because calculation of the RCI is dependent on collecting pretest and posttest information on an individual, the user must be careful about repeat or practice effects of the selected measure. It is also important to note that for instruments with low reliability, SEMs are likely to be high and statistical significance will be difficult to obtain. This limitation may, however, be more reflective of the danger inherent in using measures with low reliability.

Effect Size

Individual effect size is a more typical measure of magnitude than RCI, although the two are statistically very similar. Like RCI, effect size is calculated by determining the difference between the posttest score and the pretest score within the context of the variation of scores. Consequently, effect size can also be interpreted based on the z-distribution. As with RCI, effect size can be calculated for groups as easily as for individuals, simply by inserting the group means for pretest and posttest scores. The main difference between effect size and RCI is that the former is typically used to quantify magnitude of change (i.e., how large a change is), while the latter is typically used to quantify significance (the likelihood that a change did not occur by chance). Effect size can also be thought of as a more conservative version of RCI.

The individual effect size is calculated by subtracting the pretest score from the posttest score and dividing by the standard deviation: ES = (posttest – pretest) / standard deviation. In cases where pretest and posttest scores can be assumed to have equivalent variances, the variances should be pooled to determine the standard deviation. Otherwise, the standard deviation of the pretest scores should be used, because it is typically a more conservative estimate of variance. Effect sizes that are less than .4 are considered small, while effect sizes between .4 and .8 are considered moderate, and effect sizes that exceed .8 are considered large (Cohen, 1988).

Because *SEM* is calculated by multiplying the standard deviation by some constant less than or equal to 1 (refer to the foregoing formula), standard deviations are always greater than *SEMs*. Because the numerator is always equal between RCIs and effect sizes, and the denominator of RCIs is always smaller, RCIs are always less conservative (larger absolute value) indicators of change. It is also worth noting that because RCIs and effect sizes provide equivalent information on different scales, the correlation between the two measures will always be perfect. Because the two measures are so similar, RCI and effect size share many of the same advantages and disadvantages.

Convergent Evidence Scaling

The "best-practices" push to use multiple and diverse methods for any complete assessment often results in outcome measures on several different metrics. Convergent Evidence Scaling (CES; Stoiber & Kratochwill, 2001) was proposed as a way of combining multiple sources of information on a common metric. CES is reported on a five-point scale (+2 = treatment goal fully met, +1 = treatment goal partially met, 0 = no progress toward goal, –1 = behavior somewhat worse, and –2 = behavior significantly worse). While information from a GAS is already reported on this metric, other information (e.g., RCI, individual effect sizes from observations; Busk & Serlin, 1992) must be converted. For example, an RCI greater than 1.6 or less than –1.6 would correspond to a +2 or –2, respectively. RCIs between .6 and 1.5 SEMs away from the 0 would correspond to +1 or –1, in the appropriate direction, and RCIs within .5 SEMs of 0 would correspond to 0 on the CES. Once data from all sources have been converted to the same scale, the scores can be averaged together to yield a composite score indicating the effectiveness of the intervention.

The advantage of CES is that it converts information from measures on different metrics into a comparable format. Putting multiple measures into a common metric is also advantageous from a research standpoint, as multiple studies can be more easily compared or combined for meta-analysis. The main drawback to CES is that the mean can be a deceptive measure of convergence. While composite CES scores of greater than +1.5 or less than –1.5 would certainly indicate some convergence, CES scores closer to the baseline are more difficult to interpret. For example, consider a case in which a student has a CES score of .8. That score could come from a GAS mean of .7, an RCI of 1, and an individual effect size from an observation of .7. The same score, however, could come from a GAS mean of −.5, an RCI of 2, and an individual effect size from an observation of .9. Clearly the first set of scores is much more convergent than the second set of scores, even though they have the same CES composite.

Graphic Analysis

Perhaps the simplest of descriptive analytic processes, graphic interpretation is a method of organizing data that makes trends more visually apparent. Graphic analyses are relatively easy to calculate, as well as to interpret, because they involve minimal transformation of data. They can be useful for generating hypotheses as well as for drawing conclusions about an individual or sample group. One limitation to graphical analysis is that it is less likely to reveal trends that are relatively subtle.

When selecting the appropriate graphical analytic method, one must consider both the number of different outcomes measured and the likely number of data points. When depicting change in a single outcome variable with a relatively large number of data points, a line graph can be a useful tool. Line graphs are often used in conjunction with GAS. The anchors for different levels of the target behavior provide the scale for the horizontal axis, and intervals of time for the evaluation of intervention provide the scale for the vertical axis. The GAS user adds a data point at the appropriate cross section for the time period and the current behavior level and subsequently draws a line connecting the new point to the point representing the previous rating. The end result is a line graph that effectively communicates the progress a client is making with regard to the target behavior.

It is sometimes useful for a school psychologist or educator to evaluate change on a number of outcome variables at only a few different data points. A bar graph, coded with colors assigned to each point in time, can indicate change in numerous outcome variables measured at multiple points. Using the same conversion system necessary for CES, all variables for a single point in time can be placed adjacent to one another so that the user can see which outcomes are the most troubling at a single point in time. Multiple points in time can again be plotted on the vertical axis, but variables measured at separate points in time should not be adjacent. By focusing on one color/outcome variable, the bar graph user can interpret change over time. (See Steege, Chidsey, and Mace, 2002, for a more in-depth discussion of graphic analysis.)

CASE SCENARIO

Christopher is an 8-year-old boy. Toward the end of the first 9-week grading period, Christopher's third-grade teacher began the *problem identifica-*

tion stage when she noticed that Christopher appeared to have lost motivation and became frustrated when reading. She added Christopher's name to the agenda for the upcoming instructional support team (IST) meeting. As part of the *problem analysis* stage, the school psychologist requested that Christopher's teacher complete the ACES—Teacher Form, which would indicate Christopher's specific strengths and weaknesses. The psychologist observed Christopher during classroom reading instruction, noting that in 6 out of 30 half-minute intervals Christopher exhibited signs of inattention (i.e., daydreaming), and that in 4 intervals Christopher was rocking in his seat.

Christopher's teacher's ratings on the ACES indicated that his academic skills were *below* grade-level expectations, particularly in the area of reading/language arts, but that Christopher exhibited some important academic enablers (e.g., interpersonal skills). Additionally, CBM for reading showed that Christopher was reading at a second-grade instructional level. The IST recommended a prereferral intervention. Christopher's teacher completed a copy of the AIMS Teacher Intervention Form to identify possible intervention strategies, helping the IST move on to the *exploring options* stage.

The IST planned an intervention for Christopher. His reading difficulties were their most serious concern, and they sought a strategy to improve that skill within the instructional environment. Christopher's teacher believed the intervention should focus on Christopher's word-attack skills and reading fluency. The IST team members defined the target behavior: "Christopher will accurately and with an even pace read aloud a page of text from his reading book." Christopher's teacher indicated via the AIMS Teacher Intervention Form that she was considering reinforcement for Christopher to increase his persistence with instructional tasks.

The IST decided that Christopher should work toward the goal of reading materials written at a third-grade instructional level. The IST suggested that he read for an extra 10–12 minutes per day, which Christopher's teacher indicated could be done aloud with a cross-age tutor from sixth grade. Christopher could perform a simple technique known as repeated reading, consisting of reading and rereading short passages aloud, while his tutor provides support and records the reading time and accuracy. The team defined the intervention goal: "Increasing word accuracy and fluent reading with classroom materials written at the second-grade level."

With an intervention goal established and the strategy of "repeated reading to a cross-age tutor" identified, the IST's remaining task was to create a GAS to monitor Christopher's reading progress. Christopher's teacher described his current level of performance: "Christopher accurately reads 30–40% of words in texts written at the third-grade level and has a slow, uneven pace when reading aloud," which was recorded as a "0" on the

GAS worksheet. Christopher's teacher then followed with a description of her goal for Christopher's reading skills: "Christopher accurately reads 85–95% of words in texts written at the third-grade level, with an even pace and some expression when reading aloud," which was recorded as a "+2" on the GAS. The team agreed to the following description of reading for the "–2" on the GAS: "Christopher accurately reads 10%–20% of words in texts written at the third-grade level and cannot finish entire sentences from a page of text when reading aloud." The team also completed descriptions for "+1" (word reading accuracy of 40–85%) and "–1" (word reading accuracy of 20–30%). The team concurred that baseline data should be gathered for 1 week, followed by 8–10 weeks of *intervention implementation*. During this time period, the classroom teacher would monitor the intervention by administering weekly GAS and CBM probes, after which the IST would evaluate the effectiveness of the intervention.

Christopher's teacher closely monitored his reading accuracy and fluency with class material. After training a sixth-grade volunteer to use the repeated-reading technique, Christopher's teacher did not immediately notice gains in Christopher's reading skills, although his motivation to read appeared to increase. During the third week of the intervention, an improvement in Christopher's reading was noted. At the end of the eighth week of intervention, the IST met to review the data collected, which indicated that Christopher was reading third-grade level texts more accurately and fluently during the last 3 weeks of the intervention. During the last week of the intervention, Christopher's teacher completed a second ACES rating of Christopher's academic skills and enablers. As

TABLE 16.1. Summary of Christopher's ACES Scores and RCI

Scale	Scores		Reliability change (RCI)
	Time 1	Time 2	
Academic Skills			
Total Scale	72	87	5.30
Reading/Language Arts	16	25	6.29
Mathematics	17	21	3.88
Critical Thinking	39	41	1.20
Academic Enablers			
Total Scale	154	162	1.69
Interpersonal Skills	44	45	0.69
Engagement	30	31	0.60
Motivation	39	42	1.54
Study Skills	41	44	1.55

indicated in Table 16.1, there were noticeable differences in pre- and postintervention scores (quantified by RCI) on the Reading/Language Arts subscale and on the total Academic Skills and Academic Enablers scales.

The IST met for *treatment evaluation* and to discuss next steps. All members agreed that the intervention appeared to improve Christopher's reading skills; however, since he had not consistently reached his target goal, the team decided that the intervention would continue. Christopher's teacher agreed that the intervention should remain in place and that she would continue to collect weekly GAS and CBM data and report back to the IST. (The case of Christopher is an abbreviated version of a case that appears in Elliott et al., 2001).

SUMMARY: "THINK RULES" TO GUIDE THE EVALUATION OF INTERVENTIONS

Similar to the "Think Rules" developed by Elliott et al. (2001) relating to intervention development and implementation, the following set of "Think Rules" summarize pertinent issues to consider when evaluating the intervention process and corresponding outcomes:

- *Think distinction.* Assessment *for* intervention focuses on the collection of data to (1) verify the existence of a meaningful discrepancy between desired and actual performance, (2) clearly define the problem, and (3) guide the intervention selection process. Assessment *of* intervention focuses on monitoring student progress toward the desired goal as well as evaluating the impact at the end of the intervention process.
- *Think sensitive.* Measures selected to evaluate the intervention process and corresponding outcomes need to be sufficiently sensitive to detect minor changes in performance so that the intervention can be modified when indicated.
- *Think frequent.* To monitor progress, measures need to be frequently collected. Evaluation processes that are time-consuming are unlikely to be used with sufficient frequency to detect progress.
- *Think comprehensive.* The reciprocal relationship between academic, behavior, and social–emotional difficulties suggests that outcome measures should focus on a variety of variables. Changes in one area may correspond to changes in other areas.
- *Think multiple.* A multisource, multimethod evaluation approach is more likely to identify changes in performance as a result of the intervention.

REFERENCES

Anderson, S. E. (1997). Understanding teacher change: Revisiting the concerns based adoption model. *Curriculum Inquiry, 27*, 331–367.

Busk, P. L., & Serlin, R. S. (1992). Meta-analysis for single-case research. In T. R. Kratochwill & J. R. Levin (Eds.), *Single-case research design and analysis: New directions for psychology and education* (pp.187–212). Hillsdale, NJ: Erlbaum.

Cohen, J. (1988). *Statistical power analysis for the behavioral sciences* (2nd ed.). Hillsdale, NJ: Erlbaum.

Deno, S. (1989). Curriculum-based measurement and special education services: A fundamental and direct relationship. In M. R. Shinn (Ed.), *Curriculum-based measurement: Assessing special children* (pp. 1–17). New York: Guilford Press.

Deno, S. (1995). School psychologist as problem solver. In A. Thomas and J. Grimes (Eds.), *Best practices in school psychology III* (pp. 471–484). Washington, DC: National Association of School Psychologists.

DiPerna, J. C., & Elliott, S. N. (1999). The development and validation of the Academic Competence Evaluation Scales. *Journal of Psychoeducational Assessment, 17*, 207–225.

DiPerna, J. C., & Elliott, S. N. (2000). *Academic Competence Evaluation Scales*. San Antonio: Psychological Corporation.

Elliott, S. N. (1988). Acceptability of behavioral treatments: Review of variables that influence treatment selection. *Professional Psychology: Research and Practice, 19*, 68–80.

Elliott, S. N., & Busse, R. T. (2004). Assessment and evaluation of students' behavior and intervention outcomes: The utility of rating scale methods. In R. B. Rutherford, M. M. Quinn, & S. R. Mathur (Eds.), *Handbook of research in emotional and behavioral disorders* (pp. 123–142). New York: Guilford Press.

Elliott, S. N., Busse, R. T., & Gresham, F. M. (1993). Behavior rating scales: Issues of use and development. *School Psychology Review, 22*, 313–321.

Elliott, S. N., DiPerna, J. C., & Shapiro, E. S. (2001). *Academic Intervention Monitoring System*. San Antonio: Psychological Corporation.

Elliott, S. N., Slasdeczek, I., & Kratochwill, T. R. (1995, August). *Goal attainment scaling: Its use as a progress monitoring and outcome effectiveness measure in behavioral consultation*. Paper presented at the annual convention of the American Psychological Association, New York.

Elliott, S. N., & Treuting, M. V. (1991). The Behavior Intervention Rating Scale: Development and validation of a pretreatment acceptability and effectiveness measure. *Journal of School Psychology, 29*, 43–51.

Elliott, S. N., Witt, J. C., Kratochwill, T. R., & Stoiber, K. C. (2002). Selecting and evaluating classroom interventions. In M. R. Shinn, H. M. Walker, & G. Stoner (Eds.), *Interventions for academic and behavior problems II: Preventative and remedial approaches* (pp. 243–294). Bethesda, MD: National Association of School Psychologists.

Finn, C. A. (2000). *Remediating behavior problems of young children: The impact of parent treatment and the efficacy of conjoint behavioral consultation and videotape therapy*. Unpublished doctoral dissertation, McGill University, Montreal.

Fuchs, L. S., & Fuchs, D. (1986). Effects of systematic formative evaluation on student achievement: A meta-analysis. *Exceptional Children, 53*, 199–208.

Fuchs, L. S., Fuchs, D., & Hamlett, C. L. (1989). Effects of instrumental use of Curriculum-Based Measurement to enhance instructional programs. *Remedial and Special Education, 10*(2), 43–52.

Gettinger, M. (1995). Best practices for increasing academic learning time. In A. Thomas and J. Grimes (Eds.), *Best practices in school psychology III* (pp. 943–954). Washington, DC: National Association of School Psychologists.

Goldston, S. (1977). Defining primary prevention. In G. Albee & J. Joffe (Eds.), *Primary prevention of psychopathology* (pp. 18–23). Hanover, NH: University Press of New England.

Greenwood, C. R., Carta, J. J., Kamps, D., & Delquadri, J. (1995). *Ecobehavioral Assessment Systems Software* (EBASS) (Version 3.0): *Manual*. Kansas City: Juniper Gardens Children's Project, University of Kansas.

Gresham, F. M. (1989). Assessment of intervention integrity in school consultation and prereferral interventions. *School Psychology Review, 18,* 37–50.

Grossman, D. C., Neckerman, H. J., Koepsell, T. D., Liu, P. Y., Asher, K. N., Beland, K., Frey, K., & Rivara, F. P. (1997). Effectiveness of a violence prevention curriculum among children in elementary school: A randomized controlled trial. *Journal of the American Medical Association, 277,* 1605–1611.

Hall, G. E., & Hord, S. M. (1987). *Change in schools: Facilitating the process.* Albany, NY: State University of New York Press.

Hall, G. E., & Hord, S. M. (2001). *Implementing change: Patterns, principles, and potholes.* Needham Heights, MA: Allyn & Bacon.

Harris, A. J., Wilkinson, S. C., Trovato, J., & Pryor, C. W. (1992). Teacher completed Child Behavior Checklist ratings as a function of classroom-based interventions: A pilot study. *Psychology in the Schools, 29,* 42–52.

Hintze, J. M., Volpe, R. J., & Shapiro, E. S. (2002). Best practices in the systematic direct observation of student behavior. In A. Thomas & J. Grimes (Eds.), *Best practices in school psychology IV* (pp. 993–1006). Washington, DC: National Association of School Psychologists.

Kanfer, F., & Goldstein, A. P. (Eds.). (1986). *Helping people change: A textbook of methods.* New York: Pergamon.

Kazdin, A. (1980). Acceptability of alternative treatments for deviant child behavior. *Journal of Applied Behavior Analysis, 13,* 259–273.

Kazdin, A. (1981). Acceptability of child treatment techniques: The influence of treatment efficacy and adverse side effects. *Behavior Therapy, 12,* 493–506.

Kelley, M. L., Heffer, R. W., Gresham, F. M., & Elliott, S. N. (1989). Development of a modified Treatment Evaluation Inventory. *Journal of Psychopathology and Behavioral Assessment, 11,* 235–247.

Kiresuk, T. J., & Sherman, R. E. (1968). Goal attainment scaling: A general method for evaluating community mental health programs. *Community Mental Health Journal, 4,* 443–453.

Kratochwill, T. R., & Elliott, S. N. (1993). *An experimental analysis of teacher/parent mediated interventions for preschoolers with behavioral problems.* Unpublished manuscript, Office of Special Educational and Rehabilitation Services, U.S. Department of Education, Wisconsin Center for Education Research, University of Wisconsin–Madison, Madison, WI.

Kratochwill, T. R., Elliott, S. N., & Rotto, P. C. (1995). Best practices in school-based behavioral consultation. In A. Thomas, & J. Grimes (Eds.), *Best practices in school psychology III* (pp. 519–538). Washington, DC: National Association of School Psychologists.

Kratochwill, T. R., & Stoiber, K. C. (2002). Evidence-based interventions in school psychology: Conceptual foundations of the *Procedural and Coding Manual* of Division 16 and the Society for the Study of School Psychology Task Force. *School Psychology Quarterly, 17,* 341–389.

Malecki, C. K., & Elliott, S. N. (2002). Children's social behaviors as predictors of academic achievement: A longitudinal analysis. *School Psychology Quarterly, 17,* 1–23.

McEvoy, A., & Welker, R. (2000). Antisocial behavior, academic failure, and school climate. *Journal of Emotional and Behavioral Disorders, 8,* 130–140.

Meyer, L. H., & Janney, R. E. (1989). User-friendly measures of meaningful outcomes:

Evaluating behavioral interventions. *Journal of the Association for Persons with Severe Handicaps, 14*, 263–270.

Munoz, R. F., Mrazek, P. J., & Haggerty, R. J. (1996). Institute of Medicine report on prevention of mental disorders: Summary and commentary. *American Psychologist, 51*, 1116–1122.

No Child Left Behind Act, Pub. L. No. 107–110 (2001).

Nunally, J., & Kotsche, W. (1983). Studies of individual subjects: Logic and methods of analysis. *British Journal of Clinical Psychology, 22*, 83–93.

Rathvon, N. (1999). *Effective school interventions: Strategies for enhancing academic achievement and social competence.* New York: Guilford Press.

Reimers, T. M., Wacker, D. P., Cooper, L. J., & DeRaad, A. O. (1992). Acceptability of behavioral treatments for children: Analog and naturalistic evaluations by parents. *School Psychology Review, 21*, 628–643.

Reynolds, C. R., & Kamphaus, R. W. (1998). *Behavior Assessment System for Children: Student Observation System (BASC-SOS).* Circle Pines, MN: American Guidance Services.

Robertson-Mjaanes, S. L. (1999). *An evaluation of goal attainment scaling as an intervention monitoring and outcome evaluation technique.* Unpublished doctoral dissertation, University of Wisconsin–Madison.

Saudargas, R. A. (1992). *State–Event Classroom Observation System (SECOS).* Knoxville, TN: Department of Psychology, University of Tennessee.

Shapiro, E. S. (1996). *Academic skills problems workbook.* New York: Guilford Press.

Shinn, M. R. (2002). Best practices in using curriculum-based measurement in a problem-solving model. In A. Thomas & J. Grimes (Eds.), *Best practices in school psychology IV* (pp. 671–697). Bethesda, MD: National Association of School Psychologists.

Shinn, M. R., & Hubbard, D. D. (1992). Curriculum-Based Measurement and problem-solving assessment: Basic procedures and outcomes. *Focus on Exceptional Children, 24*(5), 1–20.

Sladeczek, I. E., Kratochwill, T. R., Steinbach, C. L., Kumke, P., & Hagermoser, L. (2003). Problem-solving consultation in the new millennium. In E. Cole & J. A. Siegel (Eds.), *Effective consultation in school psychology* (2nd ed., pp. 60–86). Ashland, OH: Hogrefe & Huber.

Stanley, S. O., & Greenwood, C. R. (1981). *Code for instructional structure and student academic response; CISSAR.* Kansas City: Juniper Gardens Children's Project, Bureau of Child Research, University of Kansas.

Steege, M., Chidsey, R. B., & Mace, F. C. (2002). Best practices in evaluating interventions. In A. Thomas & J. Grimes (Eds.), *Best practices in school psychology IV* (pp. 517–534). Washington, DC: National Association of School Psychologists.

Stoiber, K. C., & Kratochwill, T. R. (2001). *Outcomes: Planning, monitoring, evaluating.* San Antonio: Psychological Corporation.

Witt, J. C., & Elliott, S. N. (1985). Acceptability of classroom intervention strategies. In T. R. Kratochwill (Ed.), *Advances in school psychology* (Vol. 4, pp. 251–288). Mahwah, NJ: Erlbaum.

Zins, J. E., & Erchul, W. P. (2002). Best practices in school consultation. In A. Thomas & J. Grimes (Eds.), *Best practices in school psychology IV* (pp. 625–643). Washington, DC: National Association of School Psychologists.

SUGGESTED READINGS

Cone, J. D. (2001). *Evaluating outcomes: Empirical tools for effective practice.* Washington, DC: American Psychological Association.

This book provides a comprehensive review of the outcomes evaluation process. Chapters include discussions regarding the need and justification for outcomes evaluation, methods of data collection, tools for evaluating outcomes, analysis methods, case examples, and ethical issues concerning outcomes evaluation.

Elliott, S. N., Witt, J. C., Kratochwill, T. R., & Stoiber, K. C. (2002). Selecting and evaluating classroom interventions. In M. R. Shinn, H. M. Walker, & G. Stoner (Eds.), *Interventions for academic and behavior problems II: Preventative and remedial approaches* (pp. 243–294). Bethesda, MD: National Association of School Psychologists.

Information regarding the process of selecting and evaluating interventions within the educational setting is provided. Topics addressed include the problem-solving process, factors influencing intervention selection and implementation, strategies to consider when selecting interventions, intervention acceptability and integrity, and methods of evaluating outcomes. Examples of self-report and behavior rating scales for treatment integrity are provided.

Steege, M., Chidsey, R. B., & Mace, F. C. (2002). Best practices in evaluating interventions. In A. Thomas & J. Grimes (Eds.), *Best practices in school psychology IV* (pp. 517–534). Washington, DC: National Association of School Psychologists.

This chapter provides an overview of the evaluation process and illustrates various data collection methods and designs. A specific emphasis is placed on single-case experimental designs.

CHAPTER 17

◆ ◆ ◆

Student Success Stories

◆

MARY JEAN O'REILLY
KEVIN TOBIN

A problem-solving assessment model can be implemented effectively in a school district on the district, building, classroom, and/or individual level. The process starts with paying attention to the concerns of parents, students, and teachers and proceeds by gathering objective information about the concerns presented. The problems may take many forms, from a lack of reading fluency to bullying behavior in a hallway. Sometimes the problem is not only with an individual student but may also reflect a problem of instruction, in which directions are not clear or examples are not sufficient to induce student learning. Sometimes the problem is a lack of positive reinforcement for desirable behavior. Creating student success involves concerted efforts at many levels. Concerns are investigated and defined so that the nature of the problem is revealed. Possible solutions are considered along with relative costs and benefits. Then a plan must be written, and the school staff needs to try to implement it with integrity while collecting data to evaluate the efficacy of this effort. Student success comes from solving student problems.

In one school system, the problem-solving process begins with the building assistance meetings. The goal of these meetings is to promote a general, and daily, use of problem-solving methods to promote student success. Parents, teachers, and others who may have an interest in a student's welfare are present and able to consider what strategies might increase the students' skills and motivation. This type of meeting is an essential component of a problem-solving model in schools.

PRACTICING THE PROBLEM-SOLVING MODEL IN THE SCHOOLS

The systematic practice of problem solving in the school setting requires a structure that supports the process. If the school system's process of addressing problems moves directly from noticing a problem to eligibility determination and, from there, to placement in special education if eligibility criteria are met, there is little room for consideration of all possible solutions to the problem. Problem solving can be structured formally, for example, as a district-sanctioned process complete with forms used to document each step, or informally as a way of structuring discussions about student academic and behavioral problems. According to Deno (1989), success in problem solving requires the ability to formulate a variety of strategies to address a problem. Unfortunately, it is not uncommon to see teams attempt to fit a particular strategy to a particular problem over and over again, regardless of the results of the strategy. Evaluating solutions is a step that is often skipped in schools.

There is often confusion about the difference between what Deno (1989) describes as *measurement*, description of the problem, and *evaluation*, the decisions made about the problem. When the process is intervention-focused rather than eligibility-focused, it is easier for team members to understand the importance of collecting data to inform a clear description of the problem before deciding on possible interventions. When the process is eligibility-focused, the problem is often described in terms of IQ/achievement discrepancy or given a standard label such as reading disability. However, a problem-solving team, when faced with a child whose reading skills fall far below those of his same-age peers, might prepare to describe the problem by examining factors such as phonological skills, rapid-naming skills, fluency, accuracy, and instructional factors. A clear description of these factors, rather than the use of a generic label, is far more likely to contribute to the development of a successful intervention.

APPLIED PROBLEM-SOLVING METHODS

Use of the problem-solving model in schools is a matter of applying a structure to the process of planning, implementing, and evaluating interventions based on a clear understanding of the presenting problem. The process is

not applied episodically to immediate or selected individual student problems, but is a general approach to intervention planning and implementation (Deno, 1995), with a primary goal of reducing the gap between the
behavior or skills the student currently has and the level he or she
is expected to reach. Problem-solving approaches provide a systematic
method of directly assessing problems (Tilly, Reschly, & Grimes, 1998)
rather than relying on inferential statements based on assessment data.

The problem-solving process can be applied in both regular and special
education settings. According to Deno (1989), special education itself is
designed to involve problem-solving activities for students who are not
achieving success in regular education programs. A critical first step is to
describe the nature of the problem faced by the student (Deno, 1989). This
includes discriminating between problems involving a student's disability
and a handicapping situation existing within the environment that affects
his or her performance (Deno, 1989). Howell and Hazelton (1998) describe
a survey-level assessment that can be used within the curriculum-based
evaluation model to determine the existence of a problem. The survey
assessment may include parent and teacher interviews, reviews of classwork, standardized achievement scores, and the child's progress toward the
outcome measures used by the district.

Once it is determined through observations, record reviews, and interviews that a problem exists, the next step is to determine the magnitude of
the discrepancy between the child's current level of performance and the
expected level of performance. In this step, it is also essential to determine
whether the discrepancy is significant enough to warrant allocating resources to close the gap (Deno, 1989). Howell and Hazelton (1998) recommend prioritizing "the most important missing prerequisites" (p. 194), as
students will often demonstrate skill deficiencies in a number of areas.
Solution planning, implementation, and evaluation follow, and, ideally, the
process moves in a cyclical manner until the problem is resolved.

In reality, many obstacles hinder the problem-solving process. The
integrity of intervention implementation is often spotty, while solution
planning frequently goes no further than considering a predetermined set of
options commonly used in the current school setting. Program evaluation
processes are often not formalized and, thus, may not occur. Sometimes,
the whole process disintegrates, as steps are skipped or done in an incomplete manner. District-level support, encouragement by building administrators, and active participation in the system by teachers are all critical and
necessary factors in the success of a problem-solving team. Howell and
Hazelton (1998) suggest defining expectations clearly through the use of
checklists that guide the process and by providing feedback to team members on the quality of their adherence to the guidelines. Individual buy-in
on the part of the staff is an important factor in the successful implementation of the problem-solving model in a school setting.

MEASURING SUCCESS:
PROBLEM-SOLVING RESEARCH IN THE SCHOOLS

Traditionally school psychologists have worked to solve student problems on an individual basis. This method can still be employed effectively in a problem-solving model. For example, in a typical situation, a teacher or a parent expresses concern over a student's academic or behavioral performance. As a result, a meeting about the student is held, and data are collected to understand and resolve the problem. However, some problems are systemic in nature and require large-scale data collection and intervention planning.

Educational difficulties at this level defy one-by-one problem solving or case-by-case traditional assessment. Snapp, Hickman, and Conoley (1990) describe system interventions that go beyond the usual gatekeeper role of school psychologists. In one case an individual's routine suspension for drug use led to a review of disciplinary policies and collaboration with students to reduce drug use, which was, apparently, successful. In another case, the problem was a high percentage of students who could not read well in third grade. Rather than advocate for more special education classes, the school psychologist decided to request that the district undertake a pilot study in first grade to determine whether a reading program with explicit phonics instruction could improve student performance and prevent the high rate of failure in third grade.

In this district-based research study, students in four first-grade classes were matched based on scores from assessments that measured phonological awareness and understanding of the conventions of print. Two classes were taught with a direct instruction program and two used a basal reading program. Students were progress-monitored every two weeks using the DIBELS (Kaminski & Good, 1996). Results on measures of phonological skills, reading fluency, and overall reading skills indicated that students who received direct instruction significantly outperformed those who were taught in the basal curriculum (Tobin, 2003).

These results were disseminated to the administration. This resulted in a systemwide dialogue about how to prevent reading difficulties among the most vulnerable students and schools in the district. Several schools soon purchased the direct instruction curriculum used in the study and began to organize teacher training in order to improve instructional practices. Principals started to examine how teachers grouped students for instruction and began making changes in the pacing of instruction to different clusters of students. The following year, state achievement test scores improved among students in those schools that had provided direct instruction in reading. Follow-up research indicated that these gains held steady for students who had received direct instruction, which led to more training and a serious examination of the curriculum by the district.

EXAMPLES OF DISTRICTWIDE DATA COLLECTION
AND ITS USE IN THE PROBLEM-SOLVING MODEL

Data collection that is supported on a districtwide basis can provide an ongoing source of information that can contribute to decision making on all levels. Data collection that focuses on both academic and behavioral factors can provide a relatively integrated system of information that allows educators to gather a more complete picture of an individual child, a classroom system, a particular building, or the district as a whole. A dynamic and systematic data collection plan can make problem solving easier for all involved.

One district is building a data system focused on the reading development of all children in kindergarten through third grade. All elementary schools now administer DIBELS assessments to all kindergarten through third-grade students three times a year for benchmarking purposes. Local norms provide a method for comparing the achievement of peers within the district to that of any individual child; in addition, national benchmarks are used as a comparison to measure student progress. This districtwide process provides information for problem definition. The information, along with other data, is used by the building assistance meeting team when determining the extent of an individual student's discrepancy from the norm. This method of using DIBELS data to contribute to eligibility determination is fairly standard across the district. All elementary schools in the district collect benchmark DIBELS three times a year, and routinely use DIBELS data to inform the problem-solving process.

When it comes to exploring and implementing solutions, however, each school-based team and grade-level teaching team approaches the data differently. The information is used by teaching teams in several schools to develop skill-based flexible groupings, to monitor the make-up of the groups, and to determine which students will shift groups as their skills increase throughout the year. Results are shared with other teams within the school and with personnel from other schools in order to inform districtwide efforts to improve student skills. In each school the principal, as instructional leader, makes the decision as to whether to require skill-based grouping or to allow teachers to decide on how, and whether, to group for reading instruction. In all schools, however, data are collected and provided to staff members and administrators. The superintendent is provided with districtwide data and shares it with the school committee, principals, and other interested parties.

Over the past several years, the DIBELS have become an integral part of the normal data collection cycle that takes place in the school district. Parent meetings are held to describe the assessments, the benchmark goals, and the strategies for reaching those goals. At some schools, small groups of parents of students scoring in the at-risk and at-some-risk ranges gather to learn about the school's plan to help their children reach their goals and the help they can provide at home. Instructional strategies are adjusted as the rate of progress decreases or increases. The graphs available through the DIBELS system provide visual images of the progress of the district, individual schools, classrooms, and individual students. The size of the discrepancy between a particular child's performance and that of his or her peers is mapped out on paper, as is the progress of the child and teachers in closing that gap.

In one middle school, all sixth-grade students were grouped for reading classes based on their scores on a curriculum-based measurement of reading comprehension assessment along with another group-administered comprehension test chosen by the teachers. The next year, one of the four teaching teams opted out of the flexible grouping plan. The principal saw the teachers' request to keep their students for reading as a natural experiment. Data gathering continued, and the progress of the flexibly grouped students was compared to that of the students who had remained in their classrooms. Within-school experiments such as this can provide evidence of successful practice for those who need to see it firsthand, while allowing teachers to examine the data collected and use this information when making instructional decisions under the guidance of the principal and department chair. This type of local ownership of information and decision making based on empirical data is an important piece of the problem-solving process on a schoolwide level.

Districtwide support for problem solving that is focused on positive behavior support is also important. Special education eligibility determination for emotional and behavioral problems typically results in placement decisions, rather than intervention planning. Many school systems are coping with student behavior problems that do not meet criteria for specialized instruction or placement, but nevertheless require significant resources. March, Hawken, and Green (2003) use a triangle to demonstrate the concept of primary, secondary, and tertiary prevention. The majority of the student body is represented in the bottom of the triangle, and general issues are addressed through a primary prevention curriculum. About 15% of the remaining students may be considered to have some at-risk behaviors and need a specialized secondary prevention approach, which may include a mentoring program, more frequent meetings between parents and school, and closer tracking and monitoring of behaviors. The top of the triangle represents the 1–7% of students who demonstrate high-risk behaviors and who need individualized behavior support plans. The focus of the behavior support team meeting is on examining data and making decisions based on current information and past patterns, using a problem-solving approach (Sugai, Kame'enui, Horner, & Simmons, 1998).

Each school-based team began developing a primary prevention behavior plan by clarifying schoolwide behavior expectations and designing procedures for teaching and reinforcing the expectations in nonclassroom settings (Lewis & Sugai, 1999). The use of a data collection system, such as Schoolwide Information Systems (*www.swis.org*) or another graphing program, to collect and graph data is critical in implementing the model. A routine cycle of data collection, reporting, and review allows staff to look at the overall level of referrals as well as trends and patterns (Horner, Sugai, & Todd, 2001).

Through the use of data collection systems, information on referrals according to problem behavior, location, and time of day is available to school personnel working on buildingwide support planning. Smaller teams addressing the issues of individual students or small groups of at-risk students can access information about the most likely time and setting for problem behavior and the types of difficult behavior being displayed, and use that information to develop targeted behavior plans. Graphs of individual student behavior by location, type, and time of day have also been used to involve students and parents in the functional behavior assessment process and to develop behavior plans based on data collected over time. Reliable, useful data can be used throughout the problem-solving process. Visual graphing of the data allows everyone involved to see and understand the trend or pattern shown.

Behavioral problem solving on a primary prevention level typically focuses on issues or conflicts that affect a majority of students and staff. When staff or students complain of a problem such as misbehavior in the cafeteria, data can be used to certify the existence of a problem. For example, the number of cafeteria referrals can be compared to referral rates from other nonclassroom settings. Specific times of day can be identified as more likely to produce referrals. Observations can help to confirm office referral data or provide information on low-level problem behavior that may not rise to the level of a discipline referral. When enough data have been collected to allow the problem to be described according to its frequency or severity, the behavior support team can present the data and lead a solution-focused discussion at a staff meeting to begin generating ideas for solving the problem. Implementing solutions is typically a task shared by all staff involved with the problem, and data collection continues to provide evaluative information, which is reviewed by the team and presented to all staff.

A focus on creating a data-driven system has a positive impact on the ability of school-based teams to use the problem-solving model. Easy access to reliable data means that team decisions, whether for an individual student, a classroom, or a schoolwide system, can be monitored and objectively evaluated. Success is measurable and failure can be caught early and addressed. Successful use of the problem-solving model on a schoolwide basis can provide a structure for the use of the model in many different decision-making settings within the school.

THE BUILDING ASSISTANCE TEAM:
A SCHOOLWIDE PROBLEM-SOLVING TEAM

The building assistance team model is a general problem-solving structure that is applied in a unique way in each school building. The team generally consists of an administrator, such as the principal or vice principal, a school adjustment counselor and school psychologist, other related services personnel as needed (speech and language pathologist, physical therapist, occupational therapist, teacher of the hearing impaired, etc.), and special education and classroom teachers. Typically, parents and older students are invited to the meeting. Problems are initially identified by the teacher or parent as concerns about academic or behavior problems. Teachers are encouraged to complete a building assistance meeting form, which is the first step in the data collection process. The teacher provides information about the child's strengths, a description of the problem behavior or current performance, and a description of what the child is expected to do. This form is submitted to the individual scheduling the meetings in the building, which are held on a designated day each week. Typically the principal or school adjustment counselor manages the scheduling, while paperwork duties are shared by team members. Information gathering by members of the team may begin at any time once the form is submitted.

Staff members bring evidence to demonstrate the severity of the problem being discussed. This evidence may include behavior logs and office referral reports, classroom work products, results of regular education interventions already attempted, DIBELS or CBM scores, or other data relevant to the problem at hand. The focus of the discussion is on the second and third steps in the problem-solving model: determining the severity of the problem, proposing interventions, and deciding upon the resources and personnel needed and available to implement interventions. At the conclusion of the meeting, a method of tracking progress is agreed upon and a follow-up meeting date is set.

Formative evaluation of the proposed interventions as each one is implemented allows the building assistance meeting team to decide on next steps and increases the success of the interventions attempted (Deno, 1995). In addition, ongoing intervention evaluation adds integrity to the implementation process, as one or more staff members are tracking its success (see Chapter 16, this volume). This prereferral process allows a building to apply the problem-solving model on several levels, including individual student issues, classwide problems, and building-level problems, such as attendance rates and truancy.

Particularly on the secondary level, members of a building assistance team may have frequent contact with outside agencies such as the Department of Social Services, Department of Youth Services, services for the mentally retarded and mentally ill, court and juvenile justice employees such as probation officers, staff members from area residential programs, and other community and state agencies involved in children's lives. Introducing a problem-solving model in place of, or in conjunction with, the diagnostic model often used by these agencies can help to improve communication between the school and agencies around intervention planning for students by creating a clear description of the problem. For example, a truancy prevention initiative begun in conjunction with the sheriff's office in one district encouraged communication between the school and outside agencies. The school department truancy officer formed a team with a social worker and a police officer in order to address chronic truancy. The team worked with school building employees to identify issues affecting attendance, such as peer problems on the bus. School refusal problems of children with anxiety disorders were addressed with the help of a school adjustment counselor. In this situation, the severity of the truancy problem was initially measured by attendance records.

The building assistance team developed a list of students to refer to the truancy prevention officer, and relevant information about the specific students was provided in meetings between the school adjustment counselor and the truancy prevention team. Attendance data were used to measure the success of the intervention. In other situations, working closely with agencies may not be as feasible, and funding may not be available for comprehensive services. However, introducing and using the problem-solving model in meetings with outside agencies can often help everyone involved to be more intervention-focused.

PROBLEM SOLVING AT THE CLASSROOM LEVEL

At the classroom level, the problem-solving model supports data-based interventions and changes in instructional practices, curricular choices, and environmental arrangements. The process of asking and answering specific data-based questions provides teachers with a method of gathering relevant information that will help the team make decisions about individual student needs. The model also provides teachers with a way to bring their professional skills to the process rather than handing the problem over to special educators to measure and solve. This level of problem solving can be used by all teachers of a certain grade level to identify grade-level-specific problems and solutions.

An example of problem solving at a specific grade level took place in a small elementary school. The second-grade teachers met with the building-level team to discuss reading instruction and student grouping for the following year. The school-wide implementation of the DIBELS literacy skill assessments had given the teachers hard evidence to back up their own experience—about half of their incoming students were not reading well enough to access the standard reading and language arts instructional program they used. Meetings were held with the remedial reading teacher, the special education teacher, the school psychologist, and the principal to go over the data and investigate potential solutions.

A decision was made to regroup the students based on oral reading fluency scores. Those students below the benchmark of 44 words per minute were placed in a direct instruction program, which was team-taught by the remedial reading teacher and a classroom teacher. The students who had met or exceeded benchmark levels remained in the standard instructional program with the other second-grade teacher. Every student in the direct instruction group was progress-monitored every other week using DIBELS progress-monitoring materials, thus evaluating the solution that was put in place. Flexible grouping allowed students to move out of the direct instruction group as they demonstrated progress. This pilot program spread, as the following year the third-grade teachers who were receiving these students decided to implement flexible grouping for reading instruction across classrooms based on current DIBELS scores, along with weekly progress monitoring for the struggling readers. An additional instructional component to teach students to complete their own progress-monitoring graphs was developed, and the process was described to parents at parent–teacher conferences. The intervention was then expanded to first grade. Through peer modeling and consultation, a pilot program begun by one team of teachers spread within the school building and became a model for other schools within the district.

PROBLEM SOLVING AT THE INDIVIDUAL STUDENT LEVEL

The initial task of the problem-solving team is to define clearly the problem at hand (Deno, 1995). Using measurable terms and descriptions such as frequency, intensity, and severity contributes to a clear problem definition. Without this first step, the problem-solving process is unable to move forward effectively. Team members may use interviews, rating scales, and observations to help delineate the problem and its measurements. In addition, determining who "owns" the problem, or to whom it matters most, is helpful in deciding how to go about defining the problem (Deno, 1995). If the sixth grader being discussed at building assistance meeting is not concerned about her steeply declining math scores, she may not be as helpful in defining the problem as her concerned math teacher might be.

On the elementary level, the problem-solving team often addresses issues of basic skills deficits. At the secondary school level, the problem-solving team is often focused on intransigent problems such as truancy, substance abuse, and school violence, along with more typical interventions for learning problems. Outside service agencies such as juvenile probation, residential programs, crisis teams, and the departments of mental health or social services are sometimes part of the team, depending on student status and need.

ACADEMIC PROBLEM-SOLVING: A CASE EXAMPLE

A first-grader named Denise received reading instruction in an accelerated reading curriculum being piloted by her school. Results of fall DIBELS testing indicated that she was having trouble associating letter sounds with the letters that represented them. A parent interview revealed that Denise had spent considerable time working with her mother at home to improve her reading. As the autumn went by, Denise mastered fluent letter-naming and phonemic segmentation but did not make expected progress in developing oral reading fluency skills. At a building assistance meeting in late November, her teacher expressed concern about her lack of sufficient progress. The team decided to schedule an observation of Denise, as well as a consultation with the teacher and the educational consultant who was responsible for assisting in the implementation of the reading curriculum. It was also decided to conduct another assessment using oral reading fluency probes and first-grade subtests from the DIBELS.

The observation and teacher interview revealed that Denise appeared to learn new letter-sound associations and to have them firmly in mind one day but not remember them the next. The consultant proposed that Denise and three other students be taught each lesson twice each day. The classroom routine was for students to enter and put their things away and then to sit down and do about 15 minutes of seatwork from the board. In order to provide Denise and others with additional instruction during the 15-minute period at the beginning of the day, Denise and three of her peers went to a table in the back of the classroom and learned the key elements of the day's reading lesson before the rest of the class. Once everyone arrived and reading time began, shortly after 9 A.M., Denise was again taught this same material.

Following the implementation of the preview lessons, Denise's progress was monitored weekly. Several weeks later her chart was reviewed, and it was found she was able to read nonsense words fluently, but that her oral reading was not yet at the expected rate of fluency. It was decided to examine the pace of the curriculum as a factor. As noted, Denise was in a pilot accelerated reading program. It was designed for students of average to above-average ability with good prerequisite phonological skills. Despite double lessons, Denise was not making sufficient progress.

Rather than undertake a special education eligibility determination process at that time, instruction was begun in a different reading program using direct instruction methods. Denise's progress continued to be monitored using oral reading fluency probes. By the end of the year, she had achieved reading fluency benchmarks, and her nonsense-word reading fluency and phonological segmentation fluency were solidly in the average range based on local norms.

Denise's case shows how application and reapplication of the problem-solving model resulted in successful outcomes for the student. Schoolwide screening data on early literacy skills initially provided information indicating her insufficient progress. Data were collected to determine the severity of the problem, intervention planning was based on the hypothesized problem, and data were gathered on her progress during each intervention phase. The collection of ongoing formative data allowed the consultant and teacher to monitor the success of their efforts. When more frequent instruction did not result in improved outcomes, the pace of the curriculum was considered. This second intervention proved successful. In this situation, effort was expended in intervention planning and implementation rather than in eligibility assessment for special education, resulting in improved student outcomes.

A CASE OF INATTENTION

Mike, a 9-year-old fourth-grader, had normal development in early childhood. In second grade he began to receive speech therapy as well as remedial reading services. The school psychologist initially assessed Mike because his fourth-grade teacher reported that he appeared inattentive. On a behavior rating scale completed by his teacher, Mike had significant weaknesses in attention and social skills, but all other scores were average. Further assessment outside of the school setting indicated that Mike had a deficit in written expression and significant problems with inattention. The building assistance team decided to begin the problem-solving process by examining the environmental and instructional factors that may have contributed to his poor achievement.

First, an observation of Mike in his classroom was conducted, because this was the environment in which his inattention was most problematic. Mike attended a general education fourth-grade class. His classroom was well-lit, spacious, and cheerful-looking. There were 24 students in his class, seated in clusters of four. His classroom was adjacent to the playground, and at recess his class could exit directly to the playground. The clear and easy view of the playground seemed to be distracting to Mike. His teacher tended to give long verbal explanations when teaching and seldom used visual aids or prompts. Instruction involved lecture interspersed with questions to the students. Mike would often stare out the window during the teacher's lectures.

When he was on task, Mike responded to teacher instructions and completed worksheets. Mike seldom raised his hand to volunteer answers, and the teacher seldom called on him. When he was attentively completing his worksheet in the morning, he was not reinforced or given verbal feedback, with the exception of occasional verbal correction from his teacher as she circulated throughout the room.

In addition to difficulties with attention to task, Mike appeared to struggle with writing. He did not appear to approach the writing process with a plan or a strategy. When he was writing, he would stop and not persist in the task. Assessment using curriculum-based measures of written language indicated that his writing skills were below the expected level for a fourth-grade student. His sentences were simple and his vocabulary was immature. He used no linking words or expressions, nor did he attempt to elaborate on his initial ideas, and the overall quality of his written expression was poor.

Written expression has many task demands, including graphomotor skills, working memory, word choice, syntax, spelling, and the ability to plan and initiate the written assignment. A breakdown or weakness in any area can make effective written expression quite difficult to achieve. Individuals with attention deficits often have weaknesses in working memory, executive functioning, response inhibition, and task vigilance, which may contribute to written language problems (Cherkes-Julkowski, Sharp, & Stolzenberg, 1997). Barkley (1990) estimated that 25% of students with ADHD may also have a specific learning disability in written language. Students typically demonstrate their academic knowledge through the written word. Consequently, interventions designed to improve written expression can be quite useful for students with attention problems who have academic achievement weaknesses.

An intervention was developed for Mike by the building assistance team. He was given a brief overview before the lesson in order to focus his attention and had his understanding of the purpose of the lesson briefly checked afterward by his teacher. He received more frequent feedback and reinforcement once his teacher was instructed to notice Mike's attentive behavior and provide verbal praise for attentive behavior. Because it appeared that Mike had difficulty learning from intermittent reinforcement, it was suggested that he be reinforced frequently and immediately following productive and task-oriented behavior.

Given the hypothesis that Mike's inattention and his poor writing skills were related, it was recommended that he receive specialized instruction in writing. Two other students in his class were also having writing difficulties, and together with Mike, they participated in a direct instruction writing curriculum. These were inclusion services provided by special education staff. Two goals were written by the psychologist and the resource room teacher: (1) after 20 weeks of instruction, when presented with a story starter, Mike will write 30 correct word sequences in three minutes, and (2) after 20 weeks of instruction, Mike will display on-task and productive behavior for four out of five 5-minute periods during two randomly selected time sampling intervals in one day.

Throughout the intervention phase, Mike's writing fluency was monitored weekly using CBM probes. At the end of 12 weeks, Mike had made significant progress. More frequent verbal praise and the opportunity to earn incentives for productive work significantly improved his attention and level of accomplishment as well. Long-term follow-up in middle school indicated that he was doing well and appeared to be a productive writer.

In Mike's case, the problem-solving process was used to address two related concerns: written expression and inattention in class. His inattention to the lesson was addressed through a brief interaction with his teacher meant to help him focus his attention on the topic along with a postlesson check of his understanding of that lesson. His teacher was supported in developing a more effective reinforcement plan for Mike's attentive and on-task behavior. In addition, specialized instruction in written language was provided and his progress was monitored over time. In this case, an integrated plan of behavioral and academic support helped Mike to achieve academic success.

It is not unusual for students to exhibit more than one skill deficit or behavior of concern; often, behavioral difficulties are linked to academic problems. When one problem is addressed at a time, other issues may continue to develop or worsen. As shown through Mike's example, integrated academic and behavioral support plans can support students who are receiving special education as well as regular education. The components of the problem-solving process remain the same for all students.

Another feature of the problem-solving process that can be used to describe and plan interventions is the inclusion consultation agreement (ICA). The ICA is a good way to clarify staff responsibilities and roles in serving special education students in the general education classroom. An ICA specifies the amount and type of support for instruction special education students will receive in general education. Ideally, an ICA deals with the factors that affect low-performing students. These include:

- Classroom management techniques.
- Curriculum modifications and accommodations (one should take advantage of existing material for modifications included with the standard curriculum).
- Learning strategies.
- Study skills.

These plans should specify the roles and responsibilities of regular and special education teachers, the student, parent, and other school staff who may be involved with the student (see Table 17.1).

SUMMARY

Adopting a problem-solving process to address individual, classroom, building, and school-district concerns can be an effective and efficient way to improve instructional practices and student achievement. This process requires a focus on how the instructional, curricular, and environmental factors in the situation can be harnessed to accomplish the goal of improving student academic or behavioral skills. A collaborative approach among school staff in regular and special education is an essential piece of the process. It is important to define the questions that need to be answered and to use data-based decision making to answer the questions.

Adopting a problem-solving process involves every member of the team. Shapiro (2000) has argued that working to solve problems child-by-child, although admirable, is inefficient because while we focus on small

TABLE 17.1. Example of an Inclusion Consultation Agreement for Mike

Statement of problem: Mike has trouble following directions, does not ask for help when he does not understand an assignment, and fails to complete written classwork.

Student responsibilities	Parent responsibilities	General education responsibilities	Special education responsibilities
Look up at the teacher frequently. Put homework in correct places. Get back to his seat and have homework pad out and start to copy the assignment from the board. Come to writing group without prompting.	Have a quiet homework place set up. Mike's mother will prompt him to get him started. He will be monitored after 5 minutes to see if he is making progress. He can use a tape recorder to dictate stories and an electronic spell checker.	A tape recorder will be used to help Mike create essays. His teacher will try to notice and reinforce any effort Mike makes to be more productive. Mike can earn points for remembering to go to the writing group without verbal prompting.	Mike will have special instruction designed to improve his written expression in his classroom with a small group of students. The resource room teacher will administer writing probes on a weekly basis and graph the results.

problems, big problems only increase. Many districts have begun to address the issues of solving "big rather than little problems" (Shapiro, 2000). Use of early literacy screening tools such as the DIBELS (Kaminski & Good, 1996) allows schools to be proactive in addressing student skill needs and allocating resources as needed. The use of progress-monitoring tools allows schools to evaluate the long-term progress of students taught with different programs and instructional methods. A structured prereferral process allows for collaborative problem solving and discussion. However, there are obstacles to establishing a problem-solving model in public schools. If the problem behavior of an individual student is given priority without considering the context in which the behavior occurs, then problem solving is less effective. It is essential to focus continuously on the instructional, environmental, and curricular variables that can be changed and to emphasize data-based decision making.

By using curriculum-based measurement (CBM) as Fuchs and Fuchs (1986) advocate, it is possible to assess student response to instruction and to track the dynamic process of skill acquisition in reading, writing, and arithmetic. Although the use of CBM has not replaced the use of commercial standardized tests for eligibility determination in most districts, it has made progress monitoring possible once specialized instruction has begun. In addition, changes in instructional groups can be made at the classroom level as a result of systemic screening for skill development, and students can be flexibly grouped based on their response to instruction. These instructional changes can be assessed through regular progress monitoring, and program evaluation can occur through collaboration among general education teachers, remedial reading teachers, school psychologists, and special education teachers.

Solving individual problems is still a concern. A child's problem may not be big to a school system, but it can be very big for an individual child and his or her family. A systematic problem-solving approach with ongoing monitoring of progress allows school-based teams to do more than just determine eligibility for special education. Periodic meetings among involved teachers, parents, school psychologists, and administrators in which progress-monitoring data are shared and instructional strategies are refined are a productive and effective use of valuable staff time.

REFERENCES

Barkley, R. A. (1990). *Attention-deficit/hyperactivity disorder: A handbook for diagnosis and treatment.* New York: Guilford Press.

Cherkes-Julkowski, M,, Sharp, S., & Stolzenberg, J. (1997). *Rethinking attention deficit disorders.* Cambridge, MA: Brookline Books.

Deno, S. L. (1989). Curriculum-based measurement and special education services:

A fundamental and direct relationship. In M. R. Shinn (Ed.), *Curriculum-based measurement: Assessing special children* (pp. 1–17). New York: Guilford Press.

Deno, S. L. (1995). School psychologist as problem solver. In A. Thomas & J. Grimes (Eds.), *Best practices in school psychology* (pp. 471–484). Washington, DC: National Association of School Psychologists.

Fuchs, L. S., & Fuchs, D. (1986). Linking assessment to instructional interventions: An overview. *School Psychology Review, 15*, 318–323.

Horner, R. H., Sugai, G., & Todd, A. W. (2001). "Data" need not be a four-letter word: Using data to improve schoolwide discipline. *Beyond Behavior: A Magazine for Exploring Behavior in Our Schools 11*, 20–26.

Howell, K. W., & Hazelton, S. C. (1998). Curriculum-based evaluation: Finding solutions to educational problems. In D. J. Reschly, W. D. Tilly, III, & J. P. Grimes (Eds.), *Functional and noncategorical identification and intervention in special education* (pp. 181–200). Des Moines: Iowa State Department of Education.

Kaminski, R. A., & Good, R. H. (1996). Toward a technology for assessing basic early literacy. *School Psychology Review, 25*, 215–227.

Lewis, T. J., & Sugai, G. (1999). Effective behavior support: A systems approach to proactive schoolwide management. *Focus on Exceptional Children, 31*(6), 1–24.

March, R., Hawken, L., & Green, J. (2003). Schoolwide behavior support: Creating urban schools that accommodate diverse learners. *Journal of Special Education Leadership, 16*, 15–22.

Shapiro E. S. (2000). School psychology from an instructional perspective: Solving big, not little problems. *School Psychology Review, 29*, 560–573.

Snapp, M., Hickman, J. A., & Conoley, J. C. (1990). Systems interventions in school settings: Case studies. In T .B. Gutkin & C. R. Reynolds (Eds.), *The handbook of school psychology* (pp. 920–934). New York: Wiley.

Sugai, G. M., Kame'enui, E. J., Horner, R. H., & Simmons, D. C. (1998). *Effective instructional and behavioral support systems: A school-wide approach to discipline and early literacy.* Washington, DC: U.S. Office of Special Education Programs.

Tilly, W. D., Reschly, D. J., & Grimes, J. (1998). Disability determination in problem-solving systems: Conceptual foundations and critical components. In D. J. Reschly, W. D. Tilly, & J. Grimes (Eds.), *Functional and noncategorical identification and intervention in special education* (pp. 221–254). Des Moines: Iowa State Department of Education.

Tobin, K. G. (2003). The effects of the Horizons reading program and prior phonological awareness training on the reading skills of first graders. *Journal of Direct Instruction. 3*, 1–17.

SUGGESTED READINGS

Reschley, D., Tilly, W., & Grimes, J. (1999). *Special education in transition: Functional assessment and noncategorical programming.* Longmont, CO: Sopris West.

This edited book focuses on functional and noncategorical approaches to the delivery of special education services.

Sugai, G., Horner, R., & Gresham, F. M. (2002). Behaviorally effective school environments. In M. R. Shinn, H. M. Walker, & G. Stoner (Eds.), *Interventions for academic and behavior problems II: Preventive and remedial approaches* (pp. 315–350). Bethesda, MD: National Association of School Psychologists.

This volume provides a clear and concise discussion of how to establish and sustain a safe and socially competent environment in schools.

Sugai, G., Kame'enui, E., Horner, R., & Simmons, D. (1998). *Effective instructional and behavioral support systems: A schoolwide approach to discipline and early literacy.* Washington, DC: U.S. Office of Special Education Programs.

The authors present a model and guide to developing an integrated program of academic and behavioral support.

Index

♦